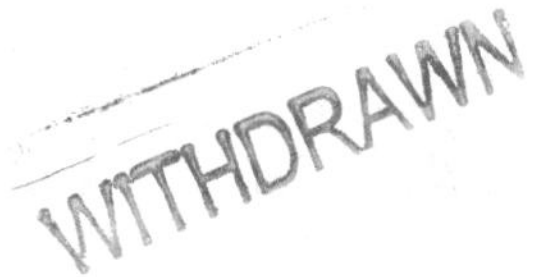

DEATH AND DYING

END-OF-LIFE CONTROVERSIES

ISSN 1532-2726

DEATH AND DYING

END-OF-LIFE CONTROVERSIES

Mark Lane

INFORMATION PLUS® REFERENCE SERIES
Formerly Published by Information Plus, Wylie, Texas

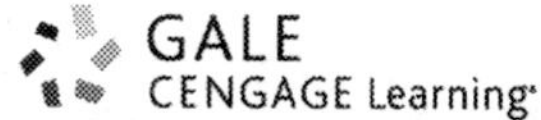

Farmington Hills, Mich • San Francisco • New York • Waterville, Maine
Meriden, Conn • Mason, Ohio • Chicago

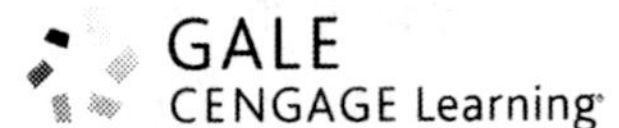

Death and Dying: End-of-Life Controversies

Mark Lane
Kepos Media, Inc.: Steven Long and Janice Jorgensen, Series Editors

Project Editors: Tracie Moy, Laura Avery

Rights Acquisition and Management: Lynn Vagg

Composition: Evi Abou-El-Seoud, Mary Beth Trimper

Manufacturing: Rita Wimberley

Gale
27500 Drake Rd.
Farmington Hills, MI 48331-3535

ISBN-13: 978-0-7876-5103-9 (set)
ISBN-13: 978-1-57302-695-6

ISSN 1532-2726

This title is also available as an e-book.
ISBN-13: 978-1-57302-674-1 (set)
Contact your Gale sales representative for ordering information.

Printed in the United States of America
1 2 3 4 5 6 7 18 17 16 15 14

TABLE OF CONTENTS

through the Patient Protection and Affordable Care Act are considered, as is the continued viability of Medicare, which is imperiled by the dual pressures of an aging population and rising medical costs.

PREFACE

Death and Dying: End-of-Life Controversies is part of the *Information Plus Reference Series*. The purpose of each volume of the series is to present the latest facts on a topic of pressing concern in modern American life. These topics include the most controversial and studied social issues of the 21st century: abortion, capital punishment, care for the elderly, crime, the environment, health care, immigration, race and ethnicity, social welfare, women, youth, and many more. Although this series is written especially for high school and undergraduate students, it is an excellent resource for anyone in need of factual information on current affairs.

By presenting the facts, it is the intention of Gale, Cengage Learning to provide its readers with everything they need to reach an informed opinion on current issues. To that end, there is a particular emphasis in this series on the presentation of scientific studies, surveys, and statistics. These data are generally presented in the form of tables, charts, and other graphics placed within the text of each book. Every graphic is directly referred to and carefully explained in the text. The source of each graphic is presented within the graphic itself. The data used in these graphics are drawn from the most reputable and reliable sources, such as from the various branches of the U.S. government and from private organizations and associations. Every effort has been made to secure the most recent information available. Readers should bear in mind that many major studies take years to conduct and that additional years often pass before the data from these studies are made available to the public. Therefore, in many cases the most recent information available in 2014 is dated from 2011 or 2012. Older statistics are sometimes presented as well, if they are landmark studies or of particular interest and no more-recent information exists.

Although statistics are a major focus of the *Information Plus Reference Series*, they are by no means its only content. Each book also presents the widely held positions and important ideas that shape how the book's subject is discussed in the United States. These positions are explained in detail and, where possible, in the words of their proponents. Some of the other material to be found in these books includes historical background, descriptions of major events related to the subject, relevant laws and court cases, and examples of how these issues play out in American life. Some books also feature primary documents or have pro and con debate sections that provide the words and opinions of prominent Americans on both sides of a controversial topic. All material is presented in an evenhanded and unbiased manner; readers will never be encouraged to accept one view of an issue over another.

HOW TO USE THIS BOOK

Death is one of the universal human experiences. This and its ultimately unknowable nature combine to make it a topic of great interest to most Americans. How we die and how we deal with the deaths of others evokes profound religious or ethical issues, or both, about which many people hold strong beliefs. When these beliefs are in conflict with those of others, this can result in some of the most serious and divisive controversies in the United States. This book examines how Americans deal with death, with a particular focus on the highly charged political and moral issues of living wills, life-sustaining treatments, funding for end-of-life care, and physician-assisted suicide.

Death and Dying: End-of-Life Controversies consists of 10 chapters and three appendixes. Each chapter is devoted to a particular aspect of death and dying in the United States. For a summary of the information that is covered in each chapter, please see the synopses that are provided in the Table of Contents. Chapters generally begin with an overview of the basic facts and background information on the chapter's topic, then proceed to examine subtopics of particular interest. For example, Chapter 5: Older Adults first addresses the rapid expansion of the 65-and-over population during the late 20th and early 21st centuries. The chapter then examines the demographic characteristics of the older population and describes the health issues and morbidity trends that inform broader cultural discussion of end-of-life issues. Finally, the chapter discusses the urgent need, given the rapid aging of the U.S. population, for geriatricians (physicians who specialize in the health needs of the elderly). Readers can find their way through a chapter by looking for the section and subsection headings, which are clearly set off from the text. They can also refer to the book's extensive Index if they already know what they are looking for.

Statistical Information

The tables and figures featured throughout *Death and Dying: End-of-Life Controversies* will be of particular use to readers in learning about this issue. These tables and figures represent an extensive collection of the most recent and important statistics on death, as well as related issues—for example, graphics cover the death rates for the 15 leading causes of death, the percentage of high school students who attempt suicide, the growth in Medicare expenditures, and public opinion on the moral acceptability of physician-assisted suicide. Gale, Cengage Learning believes that making this information available to readers is the most important way to fulfill the goal of this book: to help readers understand the issues and controversies surrounding death and dying in the United States and reach their own conclusions.

Each table or figure has a unique identifier appearing above it, for ease of identification and reference. Titles for the tables and figures explain their purpose. At the end of each table or figure, the original source of the data is provided.

To help readers understand these often complicated statistics, all tables and figures are explained in the text. References in the text direct readers to the relevant statistics. Furthermore, the contents of all tables and figures are fully indexed. Please see the opening section of the Index at the back of this volume for a description of how to find tables and figures within it.

Appendixes

Besides the main body text and images, *Death and Dying: End-of-Life Controversies* has three appendixes. The first is the Important Names and Addresses directory. Here, readers will find contact information for a number of government and private organizations that can provide further information on aspects of death and dying. The second appendix is the Resources section, which can also assist readers in conducting their own research. In this section, the author and editors of *Death and Dying: End-of-Life Controversies* describe some of the sources that were most useful during the compilation of this book. The final appendix is the detailed Index. It has been greatly expanded from previous editions and should make it even easier to find specific topics in this book.

COMMENTS AND SUGGESTIONS

The editors of the *Information Plus Reference Series* welcome your feedback on *Death and Dying: End-of-Life Controversies*. Please direct all correspondence to:

Editors
Information Plus Reference Series
27500 Drake Rd.
Farmington Hills, MI 48331-3535

CHAPTER 1

DEATH THROUGH THE AGES: A BRIEF OVERVIEW

Strange, is it not? That of the myriads who
Before us pass'd the door of Darkness through,
Not one returns to tell us of the Road,
Which to discover we must travel too.

—Omar Khayyám, *Rubáiyát of Omar Khayyám*

Death is the inevitable conclusion of life, a universal destiny that all living creatures share. Although all societies throughout history have realized that death is the certain fate of human beings, different cultures have responded to it in different ways. Death is central to all major world religions, all of which address the fate of the individual after the body ceases to function. Individual religions answer the challenges posed by death in different ways, however. Many promise an afterlife in which the soul survives bodily death, but there is little agreement among religions about the nature of that afterlife, and this diversity of views has centrally shaped the customs and attitudes of cultures, nations, and individuals. Philosophical inquiry into the nature of death has likewise varied from culture to culture over time, ensuring an ongoing diversity of beliefs and customs. Increased scientific understanding in the 19th and 20th centuries has not made earlier religious and philosophical approaches to death obsolete, but in some cases it has diminished the universality of these traditional modes of understanding, and it has complicated the overall approach to death at the societal level. The medical advances of the 20th and 21st centuries, by prolonging life dramatically, have further reshaped some of humanity's most basic assumptions about the relation between life and death, raising a host of ethical issues that would have been unimaginable to past generations.

ANCIENT TIMES

Archaeologists have found that as early as the Paleolithic period, around 2.5 million to 3 million years ago, humans held metaphysical beliefs about death and dying—those beyond what humans can know with their senses. Tools and ornaments excavated at burial sites suggest that the earliest human ancestors believed that some element of a person survived the dying experience.

The earliest civilizations likewise typically believed in the existence of an eternal soul or something like it. For example, the ancient Egyptians (c. 3100–332 BC) believed that a person had a dual soul: the *ka* and the *ba*. The *ka* was the spirit that dwelled near the body, whereas the *ba* was the vitalizing soul that lived on in the netherworld (the world of the dead) but that could not survive without the body. Accordingly, early ancient Egyptians left their deceased loved ones in the open air of the desert, the aridity of which allowed bodies to be preserved long after they would have decomposed in wetter environments. Later Egyptians relied on a more active form of bodily preservation, mummification, to allow their loved ones access to a happy afterlife.

The mummification process, which may have taken more than two months to complete, included the ritual washing of the corpse and the removal of the brain and organs, with the exception of the heart, which was believed to be vital for the deceased person's continued existence. The body was then dried, padded for the retention of its lifelike shape, and preserved through the use of embalming chemicals. After being blessed by a priest, the mummified body was wrapped in bandages, decorated, and entombed. Mummification remained a common practice in Egypt for approximately 3,000 years.

The ancient Mesopotamians (c. 3100–539 BC), whose civilization flowered near present-day Iraq at roughly the same time as the ancient Egyptian civilization, also believed in an afterlife, but in their cosmology the afterlife was uniformly dismal. After the death of the body, the immortal element of the spirit was believed to exist in a dark underworld, where it ate dust and clay and had no access to water. The dead could find relief from this onerous existence only when their living relatives ritually contributed food and other offerings to them. Thus, the living had a significant responsibility toward their dead loved ones and ancestors, and one of the worst fates that could befall a person who had died was for his or her remains to be removed from the care of the living family. It was believed, however, that the dead would haunt the living if they were not given a proper burial. As a result, even the bodies of fallen enemies were typically buried so as to prevent the spirit's vengeful return.

The ancient Chinese (c. 2100–256 BC) believed in an afterlife that in most respects represented a continuation of the individual's worldly life. The dead were thus buried with possessions they would need in the afterlife, and living relatives were expected to continue making offerings and attending to the needs of their deceased loved ones. Royal and noble people were buried with particular extravagance, in some cases in houses complete with stables and grounds rivaling those that they had enjoyed in life. Beginning in the Shang dynasty (1600–1046 BC), some royal or noble people were buried not only with vast amounts of riches and material possessions but also with their servants and concubines. It is believed that in some cases these people may have been buried alive. By the end of the ancient period, this practice had largely been discontinued, and human figures made of pottery were used in their place. The burial of possessions and figures continued well into the second millennium AD.

In ancient Greece (1200 BC–AD 600), it was believed that the souls of the dead passed into an underworld ruled by Hades and his wife, Persephone. Depending on the life that the individual had lived, the soul might be remanded to the Fields of Asphodel or to Tartarus. The Fields of Asphodel were the abode of those whose lives had been neither excessively good nor excessively evil. Tartarus was a pit where those who had been wicked suffered in torment. Some accounts of the Greek afterlife also refer to Elysium, an idyllic part of the underworld reserved for heroes and others who had lived exceptional lives. The ancient Romans (c. 800 BC–AD 476) derived many of their religious and cultural traditions from their Greek predecessors, including those parts of their cosmology relating to the afterlife.

Greek and Roman attitudes toward death were strongly influenced by the mythological epic poems of Homer (c. seventh century BC), the *Iliad* and the *Odyssey*. Greek mythology was freely interpreted by writers after Homer, and belief in eternal judgment and retribution evolved throughout the ancient period. Certain Greek philosophers also influenced conceptions of death. For example, Pythagoras of Samos (c. 570–c. 490 BC) opposed euthanasia ("good death" or mercy killing) because it might disturb the soul's journey toward final purification as planned by the gods. On the contrary, Socrates (469–399 BC) and Plato (428–347 BC) believed that people could choose to end their life if they were no longer useful to themselves or the state.

Like Socrates and Plato, the classical Romans (c. 509–264 BC) believed that a person suffering from intolerable pain or an incurable illness should have the right to choose a "good death." They considered euthanasia a "mode of dying" that allowed a person to take control of an intolerable situation. The Romans distinguished euthanasia from suicide, an act considered to be a shirking of responsibilities to one's family and to humankind.

The historical sense and attitudes of the ancient Hebrews (c. 1800 BC–AD 363) toward death are described in the Tanakh, or Hebrew Bible (which also constitutes the Old Testament of the Christian Bible). The ancient Jewish people, whose destinies overlapped with those of the ancient Egyptians, Mesopotamians, Greeks, and Romans, did not generally live in the expectation of an immediate individual afterlife. They lived according to the commandments of their god, to whom they entrusted their eternal destiny. The Tanakh describes the end of days, a time when the world will end. At that time, according to ancient prophets, God will return the Jewish people to the Land of Israel, resurrect the dead, and create a new heaven and a new earth. The Tanakh also includes references to the coming of the Messiah, a human leader who will unite the people of Israel and bring about an age of peace and well-being for the living and the dead.

THE MIDDLE AGES AND THE RENAISSANCE

During the European Middle Ages (500–1485) the tenets of Christianity, as adjudicated by the medieval Roman Catholic Church, established many of the cultural and social conventions relating to death and dying. Although the Christian Bible references an afterlife in which believers will be united with God, concrete descriptions of heaven and hell have been more the creation of various interpreters of the Bible than of the text itself. In the medieval view, to ascend to heaven after death, one had to be not only a believer but an observer of proper Christian behavior. Those who were impious or guilty of sin risked eternal damnation if they did not confess their sins prior to death.

Because life expectancy during this period commonly extended to little more than 30 years, death and the necessity of being prepared for it were a constant and looming presence in the lives of many. Because medical practices during this era were crude and imprecise, the ill or dying person often endured prolonged suffering. This long period of suffering gave the dying individual an opportunity to feel forewarned about impending death, to put his or her affairs in order, and to confess his or her sins.

By the late Middle Ages, the fear of death had intensified because of the Black Death—the great plague of 1347 to 1351. The Black Death killed more than 25 million people in Europe alone. Commoners watched not only their neighbors but also church officials and royalty struck down: King Alfonso XI (1311–1350) of Castile met with an untimely death, as did many at the papal court in Avignon, France. With their perceived "proper order" of existence shaken, the common people became increasingly preoccupied with their own death and with the Last Judgment—God's final and certain determination of the character of each individual.

From the 14th through the 16th centuries Europe experienced a cultural rebirth, the Renaissance, in which Christian doctrine and art forms were supplemented by notions of earthly beauty and the good life derived from the cultures of ancient Greece and Rome. New directions emerged in economics, the arts, and social, scientific, and political thought. This flowering occurred especially in the city-states of what is now Italy but also in the rest of Continental Europe and the British Isles. Despite a renewed focus on the things of this world, medicine remained rudimentary, and life expectancy was low by modern standards. Outbreaks of plague continued to erupt periodically, especially in the urban centers of art, intellectual life, and commerce.

Furthermore, the new self-awareness and emphasis on humans as the center of the universe may have fueled the fear of dying. In *The Hour of Our Death*, an influential study of Western attitudes toward death first published in France in 1977, the French historian Philippe Ariès (1914–1984) suggests that whereas the ancient and medieval attitude toward death involved casual acceptance, the increasing rationalism and individualism characteristic of the Renaissance brought an increased focus on death as a moment of fear and crisis.

The Catholic Church remained a dominant influence on perceptions of death and dying during the Renaissance. The generally accepted Christian attitude was that believers should continually meditate on death as a means of staying mindful of their soul's destiny and their duty to God. By the 16th century, however, the Protestant Reformation had begun, representing a diminution of the church's power, including its authority to dictate what Christians believed about death and dying. In general, the doubt cast on the Roman Catholic Church's cosmology translated into increased uncertainty about death and dying.

THE 17TH AND 18TH CENTURIES

Although Christianity remained the dominant arbiter of Western attitudes toward death throughout the 17th and 18th centuries, science progressed, bringing about an increasing reliance on reason. As such, death became an object for medical and scientific study as well as religious meditation. However, increasing rationalism did not result in an immediate break with historical beliefs in an afterlife. René Descartes (1596–1650), the philosopher most responsible for inaugurating the period of modern philosophy (from the 17th century to the early 20th century), was both a committed rationalist and a believer in the immortality of the soul. His *Meditations on First Philosophy* (1641), one of the most influential works of philosophy in history, is famous for formulating the idea of mind–body dualism, as encapsulated in the phrase *Cogito ergo sum* (I think, therefore I am), which Descartes had first used several years earlier. This suggestion that the mind, as distinct from all aspects of the body, is the starting point for all identity and existence has been one of the central preoccupations of Western thought in the centuries since Descartes advanced the idea. Less commonly discussed is the fact that Descartes's stated reason for establishing the mind as the seat of existence in this way was to prove that it "is immortal by its very nature."

Also during the 17th and 18th centuries, people began questioning the medical definition of death. Reports of unconscious patients mistakenly believed to be dead and hurriedly prepared for burial by the clergy, only to "come back to life" during transport to the cemetery or burial, led to an increased focus on understanding the physiological processes of death. Some physicians believed that the body retained some kind of "sensibility" after death. Thus, many people preserved cadavers so that the bodies could "live on." Alternatively, some physicians applied the teachings of the Catholic Church to their medical practice and believed that once the body was dead, the soul proceeded to its eternal fate and the body could no longer survive. These physicians did not preserve cadavers and pronounced them permanently dead.

The fear of "apparent death," a condition in which people appeared to be dead but were not, increased in intensity during the 18th century. Coffins were built with contraptions that enabled any prematurely buried person to survive and communicate from the grave. Figure 1.1, which dates from the 19th century, shows such a device. In some cases Christianity was blamed for the hasty burial of those who were only apparently dead because religious authorities had actively deemphasized such pagan burial traditions as protracted mourning rituals. In the wake of apparent death incidents, some older burial traditions were revived.

THE 19TH CENTURY

Throughout most of the 19th century, as in previous eras, death typically took place in the home following a long deathbed watch. Family members then prepared the

FIGURE 1.1

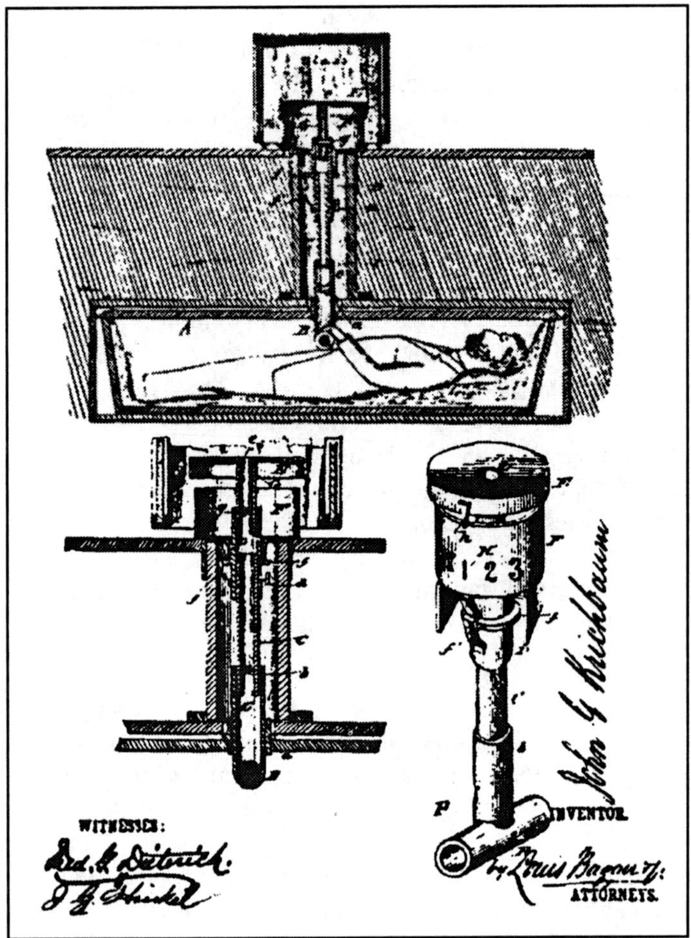

Device for indicating life in buried persons, 1882. *Source: U.S. Government Printing Office.*

corpses of their loved ones for viewing in the home. During the late 19th century, however, a new class of professional undertakers emerged, and they began taking over the job of preparing and burying the dead. Undertakers provided services such as readying the corpse for viewing and burial, building the coffin, digging the grave, and directing the funeral procession. Professional embalming and cosmetic restoration of bodies became widely available, all carried out in a funeral parlor, where bodies were then viewed.

Cemeteries changed as well. Before the early 19th century U.S. cemeteries were unsanitary, overcrowded, and weed-filled places that bore an odor of decay. The graveyard environment began to change in 1831, when the Massachusetts Horticultural Society purchased 72 acres (29 ha) of fields, ponds, trees, and gardens in Cambridge and built Mount Auburn Cemetery. This cemetery became a model for the landscaped garden cemetery in the United States. Such cemeteries were tranquil places where mourners could visit the graves of loved ones and find comfort in the beautiful surroundings.

Literature of the time often focused on and romanticized death. Death poetry, consoling essays, and mourning manuals became available after 1830. These works comforted the grieving with the concept that the deceased were in heaven—released from worldly cares and reunited with other deceased loved ones. During the 19th century the deadly lung disease tuberculosis was pervasive in Europe and the United States. The disease caused sufferers to develop a certain appearance—an extreme pallor and thinness, with a look often described as haunted—that actually became a kind of fashion statement. The fixation on the subject by writers such as Edgar Allan Poe (1809–1849) and the English romantic poets helped fuel the public's fascination with death and dying.

Spiritualism

In the mid-19th century one of the most notable trends in attitudes about the end of life was the rise of spiritualism. This belief system centered on the idea that certain "mediums" could communicate with the dead. In 1848 in the United States, the sisters Margaret Fox (1833–1893) and Kate Fox (1839–1892) of Hydesville, New York, became celebrated for their supposed ability to receive messages from the dead. The sisters claimed to have communicated with the spirit of a man who had been murdered by a former tenant in their house. The practice of conducting "sittings" to contact the dead gained instant popularity. Mediums such as the Fox sisters were supposedly sensitive to "vibrations" from the disembodied souls who temporarily lived in that part of the spirit world just outside Earth's limits.

Efforts to communicate with the dead have been practiced for millennia in cultures all over the world. For example, many Native Americans believe that shamans (priests or medicine men) have the power to communicate with the spirits of the dead. In the Judeo-Christian tradition, the first book of Samuel in the Old Testament of the Christian Bible recounts the visit of King Saul to a medium at Endor. The medium summoned the spirit of the prophet Samuel, who predicted the death of Saul and his sons. The outbreak of spiritualism in the United States is noteworthy, however, because the country was among the most rapidly modernizing in the world and because increased scientific understanding had begun to extinguish many of humanity's lingering beliefs in the supernatural.

During the 1860s and 1870s the mood in the United States was ripe for spiritualist séances. Most people had lost a son, a husband, or another loved one during the U.S. Civil War (1861–1865). Some survivors wanted assurances that their loved ones were all right; others were simply curious about life after death. Those who had drifted away from traditional Christianity embraced this new spiritualism, which claimed scientific evidence of survival after physical death. This so-called evidence included table rapping, levitation, and materialization that occurred during the séances. In May 1875 a 12-member commission organized by the Russian chemist and inventor Dmitry Ivanovich Mendeleyev (1834–1907) concluded that spiritualism had no scientific basis and that the séance phenomena resulted from fraud—from mediums consciously deceiving those in attendance by using tricks to create illusions.

Nineteenth-century spiritualism was not a purely American philosophy. In 1882 the British poet and classicist Frederic William Henry Myers (1843–1901), who coined the word *telepathy* to describe the supposed phenomenon of two minds communicating without words or any sensory interactions, established the Society for Psychical Research. The organization, which was devoted to the "scientific" investigation of paranormal phenomena—especially those providing evidence for the continued existence of deceased individuals—attracted some of the most prominent intellectuals of the late 19th and early 20th centuries. Among them were the American philosopher and psychologist William James (1842–1910), the French philosopher Henri Bergson (1859–1941), the Nobel Prize–winning French physiologist Charles Robert Richet (1850–1935), the British writers John Ruskin (1819–1900) and Alfred, Lord Tennyson (1809–1892), and leading British politicians, including William Gladstone (1809–1898) and Arthur James Balfour (1848–1930). *The Immortalization Commission* (2011), by the British political philosopher John Gray (1948–), describes the outbreak of such belief in the supernatural at a time otherwise characterized by the dominance of science-based views of death. Gray argues that the burgeoning of spiritualism was not merely a continuation of a previous era's superstitions but a desperate response to scientific rationalism, which had "disclosed a world in which humans were no different from other animals in facing final oblivion when they died and eventual extinction as a species."

THE 20TH AND 21ST CENTURIES

In the 20th century advances in medicine and public health revolutionized humans' relationship with death, at least in the developed world. People continued to wrestle with the idea of death and to look to religion and philosophy for ways of understanding and coping with it. By the end of the 20th century, however, vaccines and other public health initiatives had eradicated or brought under control many previously fatal diseases, and few developed countries were regularly ravaged by war in the decades after World War II (1939–1945). In this environment it became the norm, for the first time in human history, for most people to expect to live into old age. No longer an imminent threat to most young and middle-aged people, death became less interwoven into the fabric of daily life than it had been in other periods of history.

Moreover, whereas death throughout history most commonly resulted from unexpected diseases for which there was no treatment, in the late 20th and early 21st centuries most people became able to stave off disease through preventive care or to manage illness through treatment. Thus, people were more likely to die of a chronic illness, treated by medical professionals, over a protracted period. As a consequence, most deaths began occurring in hospitals or other institutionalized settings, rather than in the home. This fact, as well as the fact that burial and funerary rituals were still largely managed by professional undertakers, resulted in what many observers characterize as a depersonalization of death.

The removal of death from daily life, from the home, and from community life posed challenges for individuals. Death remained as inevitable as ever, of course, but in the absence of the cultural and community structures that once helped people cope with loss and with the eventuality of their own death, many people were left alone to grieve and to prepare for their own death. New societal institutions have, to some extent, arisen to compensate for these absences and to address the challenges death poses for the modern individual. For example, death has become the subject of intense sociological and psychological study, much of which has resulted in new forms of understanding the ways humans cope with the deaths of loved ones and with the prospect of their own death. Many of the insights from such research are used by grief counselors (mental health professionals who specialize in helping bereaved people navigate the challenges of mourning).

One of the most influential theoreticians of death in the modern world was Elisabeth Kübler-Ross (1926–2004), an American psychologist. Her pioneering first book, *On Death and Dying* (1969), established the widely accepted notion that individuals confront death (either their own death or the death of a loved one) in five distinct stages, commonly called the five stages of grief: denial, anger, bargaining, depression, and acceptance. In the denial stage, the individual refuses to admit the reality of the situation, believing, for example, that a loved one's death is not final or that one's own terminal illness can be cured. As the reality of the situation becomes evident, the individual feels pain and responds with anger. Often, this anger is directed inappropriately, such as at the loved one who has died or at other grieving family members or friends. The bargaining stage may involve attempts to make a deal with God, or it may include a reassessment of past choices ("If I had not done X, my mother would still be alive"), both of which represent attempts to regain control. These attempts at control typically give way to depression, as the individual faces the inconsolable nature of the loss and regrets practical mistakes made in relationships with those from whom he or she is being permanently separated. The last phase, acceptance, is not reached by all who are facing their own death or who are mourning a loved one. Acceptance does not suggest happiness or forgetting but an integration of memories into the process of going about daily life.

The "five stages" model is not meant to imply that all individuals respond to death in exactly these ways or that all people move through the stages in order. Rather, the theory suggests that people move back and forth through the first four stages prior to reaching the stage of acceptance and a renewed commitment to life. Still, many researchers and analysts have contested Kübler-Ross's model, noting that it has never been substantiated in scientific studies, that it may suggest a normative model for grief that can be counterproductive for those who experience loss differently, and that the very concept of dividing grief into discrete "stages" bears little relation to reality.

Alternative models of the grief process include Margaret Stroebe and Henk Schut's "dual process" model, which is presented in "The Dual Process Model of Coping with Bereavement: Rationale and Description" (*Death Studies*, vol. 23, no. 3, April–May 1999). Stroebe and Schut suggest that, rather than moving through distinct stages, grief is a process characterized by alternating confrontation and avoidance of the loss and the feelings associated with it. The periods of avoidance provide needed respite from the difficult periods of confrontation and allow the individual to progress toward integration of the loss in a piecemeal fashion.

Another influential theory of the grief process is the "four tasks of mourning" model pioneered by the psychologist J. William Worden (1932–), the author of *Grief Counseling and Grief Therapy* (4th ed., 2009), an influential textbook for grief counselors. Worden maintains that an individual must accomplish four tasks before completing the grieving process: accepting the reality of the loss, working through the pain of grief, adjusting to the environment characterized by the absence of the loved one, and finding a way to relocate the emotions related to the deceased so that the living person can form new relationships.

Common Attitudes toward Death and Dying

RELIGION AND THE AFTERLIFE. In the United States, attitudes toward death and dying are strongly tied to the country's persistent religiosity as compared with other developed countries, most of whose populations are far less likely to claim religious affiliation of any kind. According to the Gallup Organization, in *Religion* (2014, http://www.gallup.com/poll/1690/religion.aspx), in 2013 a majority (56%) of U.S. adults claimed that religion was "very important" in their life, little changed from the percentage (58%) who gave the same answer in 1992. Gallup finds that 41% of respondents were Protestant, 24% were Roman Catholic, 2% were Jewish, 2% were Mormon, and 9% were affiliated with nonspecific forms of Christianity. Another 5% of Americans were believers in other religions, and 15% were affiliated with no religion.

Surveys undertaken by the Pew Research Center largely confirm these findings. In *Trends in American Values: 1987–2012* (June 4, 2012, http://www.people-press.org/files/legacy-pdf/06-04-12%20Values%20Release.pdf), the organization notes that on numerous measures of religiosity, Americans have changed little since the 1980s. For example, in 2012, 80% of respondents agreed with the statement "I never doubt the existence of God," down slightly from 88% in 1987; 76% agreed with the statement "Prayer is an important part of my daily life," unchanged from 1987; and 76% agreed with the statement "We will all be called before God at Judgment Day," down from 81% in 1987.

Polling by Harris Interactive reveals that since 2005 Americans' belief in an afterlife, along with belief in other supernatural events and beings, has declined slightly but remains very high by world standards. The organization reports in *Americans' Belief in God, Miracles and Heaven Declines* (December 16, 2013, http://www.harrisinteractive.com/vault/Harris%20Poll%2097%20-%20Beliefs_12.16.2013.pdf) that in 2013, 64% of Americans claimed to believe that the soul survives death, down from 69% in 2005. A slightly higher percentage of Americans (68%) expressed a belief in heaven, down from 75% in 2005. Additionally, the Harris poll found that as of 2013, 72% of Americans believed in miracles, 58% believed in the devil and hell, 42% believed in ghosts, 26% believed in witches, and 24% believed in reincarnation.

ANXIETIES ABOUT DEATH. Medical researchers in the late 20th and early 21st centuries have often found that young adults are typically more fearful of death than are older adults and that women typically report higher levels of anxiety about death than do men. In "Death Anxiety across the Adult Years: An Examination of Age and Gender Effects" (*Death Studies*, vol. 31, no. 6, July 2007), R. J. Russac et al. confirm these findings, noting that anxiety about death peaks around age 20 and that women report higher levels of concern about death than do men. However, the researchers also show that the decline in death anxiety after age 20 differed between men and women. Concern about death declined after age 20 in both sexes, but in women a secondary peak in anxiety about death occurred during their early 50s.

In attempting to explain these differences in attitudes toward death by age and sex, Russac et al. note that other researchers argue that older Americans come to terms with death as they age. Other hypotheses suggest that death is more appealing to older people (especially those with chronic conditions and illnesses) than to younger people, that older people are more religious and that their beliefs affect their views, and that older people have more experience with death over their lifetime and are thus less anxious about it. Russac et al. suggest that the differences might have to do with the concurrent peak in younger people's reproductive years. People of this age are likely concerned about their children and might wonder what would happen to their children if they died. Likewise, some researchers suggest that women report more anxiety about death than do men because women are the primary caretakers, not only of children but also of the elderly and those who might be dying. One hypothesis for women's secondary peak of anxiety about death in their 50s is that women reach menopause during those years, and this change of life may remind them that they are getting older and closer to death.

Ann Bowling et al. observe in "Fear of Dying in an Ethnically Diverse Society: Cross-Sectional Studies of People Aged 65+ in Britain" (*Postgraduate Medical Journal*, vol. 86, no. 1014, April 2010) that fears about dying differ among social and ethnic groups. The researchers find that in an ethnically diverse sample of study participants aged 65 years and older, Pakistani participants expressed the greatest fear of dying, whereas Chinese participants expressed the least fear. Bowling et al. conclude that when the combined ethnically diverse group of older participants was compared with an ethnically homogeneous group of older British participants, the "older people from ethnic minorities had more anxieties about dying than others, and were more likely to express fears the more extensive their family support."

CHILDREN. Prior to the 20th century, when it was the norm for people to die at home surrounded by their families and for bodies to be prepared for burial by loved ones, children experienced death as part of daily life and were part of the communal grieving that took place. In the 20th and 21st centuries, however, as death was moved into hospitals and bodies were prepared for burial by professional undertakers, children became less likely to spend time in the presence of dying people and to become acquainted with the process of grieving. Thus, children are often left to develop their attitudes toward death on their own, in accordance with their stages of development and their individual experiences (e.g., witnessing the deaths of pets and insects or characters on television). Mental health professionals strongly encourage parents to learn to communicate with their children about death. Parents must be sensitive to their children's readiness to communicate on the subject, allowing them to feel free to discuss their concerns, being attentive to children's feelings, explaining situations honestly within the limits of their understanding, and being careful not to overwhelm children with answers that are too long, elaborate, or sophisticated.

THE SERIOUSLY ILL. Daren K. Heyland et al. explain in "What Matters Most in End-of-Life Care: Perceptions of Seriously Ill Patients and Their Family Members" (*Canadian Medical Association Journal*, vol. 174, no. 5, February 28, 2006) that when patients with advanced chronic illnesses and advanced cancer were asked whether they agreed or strongly agreed about the importance of various end-of-life issues, their concerns were quite different from those of the general population. Although dying at home appears to be a priority for many Americans, dying in the location of choice (home or hospital) was 24th on the chronically ill patients' ranked list of concerns. Their top priorities (very or extremely important) were trusting their physician (ranked first), not being kept on life support when there is little hope (ranked second), having their physician communicate with them honestly (ranked third), and completing tasks and preparing for death (such as resolving conflicts and saying good-bye; ranked fourth). Seriously ill patients also revealed that they did not want to be a physical or emotional burden on their families (ranked fifth), they wanted to have an adequate plan of home care and health services when discharged from the hospital (ranked sixth), and they wanted to have relief from their symptoms (ranked seventh).

REGRETS. In *The Top Five Regrets of the Dying: A Life Transformed by the Dearly Departing* (2012), Bronnie Ware, an Australian palliative-care nurse, reports that the most common regrets of her dying patients were as follows:

1. I wish I'd had the courage to live a life true to myself, not the life others expected of me.
2. I wish I hadn't worked so hard.
3. I wish I'd had the courage to express my feelings.
4. I wish I had stayed in touch with my friends.
5. I wish I had let myself be happier.

Public Health Advances and an Aging Population

Between 1900 and 1999 the average life span of U.S. residents increased more than 30 years. According to the Centers for Disease Control and Prevention, in "Ten Great Public Health Achievements—United States, 1900–1999" (*Morbidity and Mortality Weekly Report*, vol. 48, no. 12, April 2, 1999), the most recent publication on this topic as of April 2014, "25 years of this gain are attributable to advances in public health." The introduction of compulsory vaccination led to the eradication or control of a number of life-threatening diseases, such as smallpox, polio, and measles. Expanded access to clean water and improved sanitation contributed to the prevention of other deaths resulting from infectious diseases. Elevated standards for motor-vehicle and workplace safety led to large reductions in deaths on the road and on the job, and improvements in food safety and nutrition led to decreases in harmful food-borne illnesses as well as the elimination of nutritional deficiencies. Better understanding of heart disease and stroke risks, as well as advances in treatment and early detection, led to dramatic decreases in the death rates for these conditions. Improvements in prenatal and neonatal care transformed the risks associated with pregnancy and birth: infant mortality decreased 90% over the course of the 20th century, and maternal mortality decreased 99%. With the 1964 U.S. surgeon general's report on the dangers of smoking, tobacco use began to decline, and by the early 21st century, smoking-related deaths had declined dramatically.

According to Donna L. Hoyert of the National Center for Health Statistics, in *75 Years of Mortality in the United States, 1935–2010* (March 2012, http://www.cdc.gov/nchs/data/databriefs/db88.pdf), the age-adjusted rate of death (the chance that a person of any age will die in a given year, measured in terms of deaths per 100,000 people) dropped 60% between 1935 and 2010, from 1,860.1 to 746.2. (See Figure 1.2.) Death rates for all age groups except those aged 85 years and older fell more than 50%, and the risk of dying declined most dramatically for the young. (See Figure 1.3.) For individuals under the age of one year, aged one to four years, and aged five to 14 years, death rates fell more than 80%.

The major strides made in protecting the health of children represent one of the signature features of modernity in the developed world. Throughout human history, low life expectancy was intimately linked with high rates of infant and child mortality, and until the mid-20th century, the loss of a child was a commonplace experience within families. By the early 21st century the death of a child had become a rarity for families in the United States and other similarly developed countries.

These public health trends, together with the enormous size of the Baby Boom generation (people born between 1946 and 1964, the first of whom reached retirement age in 2011), have transformed the nature of the U.S. population. Carrie A. Werner of the U.S. Census Bureau notes in *The Older Population: 2010* (November 2011, http://www.census.gov/prod/cen2010/briefs/c2010br-09.pdf) that

FIGURE 1.2

Number of deaths, crude death rate, and age-adjusted death rate, 1935–2010

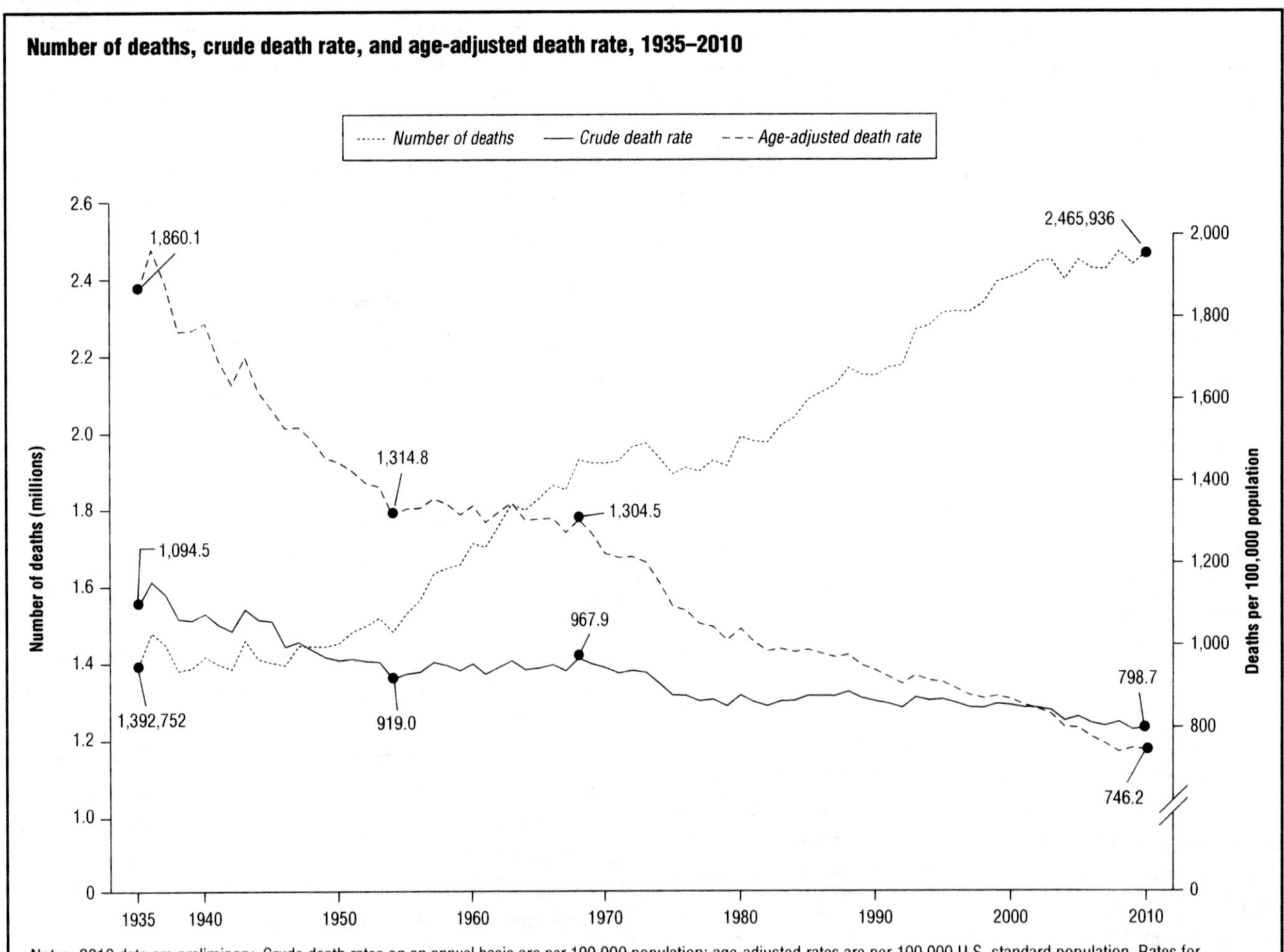

Notes: 2010 data are preliminary. Crude death rates on an annual basis are per 100,000 population; age-adjusted rates are per 100,000 U.S. standard population. Rates for 2001–2009 are revised and may differ from rates previously published.

SOURCE: Donna L. Hoyert, "Figure 1. Number of Deaths, Crude and Age-Adjusted Death Rates: United States, 1935–2010," in "75 Years of Mortality in the United States, 1935–2010," *NCHS Data Brief*, no. 88, Centers for Disease Control and Prevention, National Center for Health Statistics, March 2012, http://www.cdc.gov/nchs/data/databriefs/db88.pdf (accessed December 28, 2013)

FIGURE 1.3

Percentage change in death rates, by age, 1935–2010

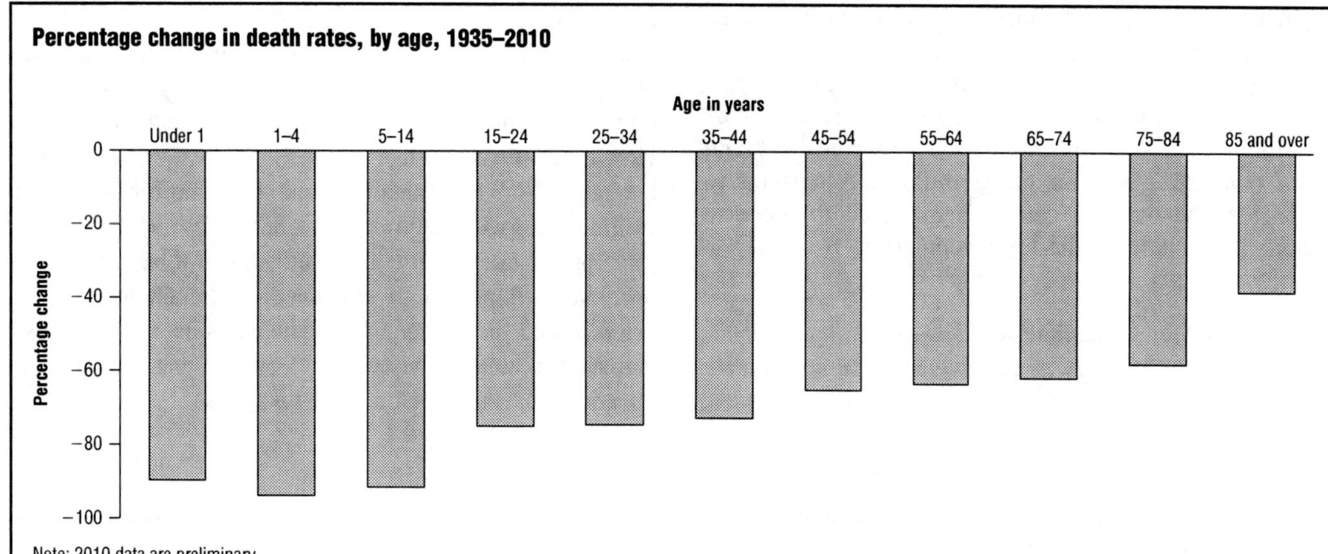

Note: 2010 data are preliminary.

SOURCE: Donna L. Hoyert, "Figure 3. Percentage Change in Death Rates by Age: United States, 1935–2010," in "75 Years of Mortality in the United States, 1935–2010," *NCHS Data Brief*, no. 88, Centers for Disease Control and Prevention, National Center for Health Statistics, March 2012, http://www.cdc.gov/nchs/data/databriefs/db88.pdf (accessed December 28, 2013)

FIGURE 1.4

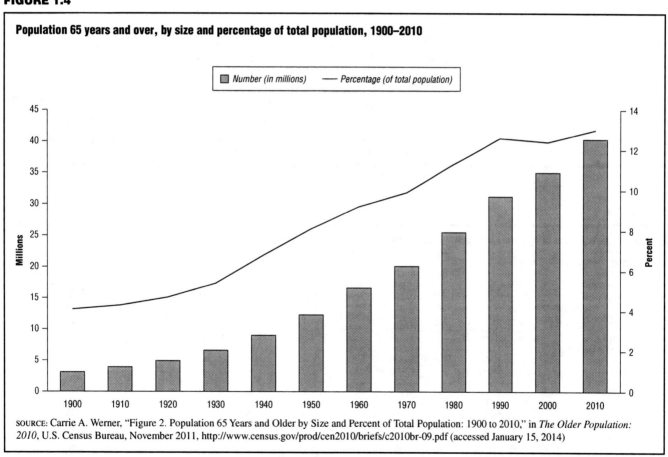

Population 65 years and over, by size and percentage of total population, 1900–2010

Number (in millions) — *Percentage (of total population)*

Millions: 0, 5, 10, 15, 20, 25, 30, 35, 40, 45

Percent: 0, 2, 4, 6, 8, 10, 12, 14

1900 1910 1920 1930 1940 1950 1960 1970 1980 1990 2000 2010

SOURCE: Carrie A. Werner, "Figure 2. Population 65 Years and Older by Size and Percent of Total Population: 1900 to 2010," in *The Older Population: 2010*, U.S. Census Bureau, November 2011, http://www.census.gov/prod/cen2010/briefs/c2010br-09.pdf (accessed January 15, 2014)

there were more people aged 65 years and older in the United States in 2010 than in any previous decennial census and that this sector of the population was growing more rapidly (at a rate of 15.1%) than the population at large (9.7%). As Figure 1.4 shows, in 1900 only around 3 million people in the United States were aged 65 years and older, and they accounted for a little over 4% of the population. By 2010, 40.3 million Americans were aged 65 years and older, and they accounted for 13% of the total population. These trends were expected to continue. As Table 1.1 shows, the Census Bureau projects a near-doubling of the over-65 population between 2015 and 2060, from 47.7 million to 92 million. According to Table 1.2, the over-65 cohort is expected to increase steadily as a share of the total population, from 14.8% in 2015 to 21.9% in 2060.

The growing population of older people and the medical ability to prolong life far beyond historical norms have generated a host of societal changes and pressing issues. These issues are, for the most part, unique to the late 20th and early 21st centuries, and many of them are far from being conclusively settled. Given the ability to keep people's bodies alive through medical technology even when they are in a nonresponsive state, how do we define death? How much medical intervention should be harnessed when extending life? How should people be cared for at the end of life? Who will pay for their care? What role should the government take? Is it ethical, and should it be legal, for a terminally ill person to stop medical treatment or even actively end his or her life? At what point in the illness can such judgments be made? These are just some of the questions that this book seeks to address.

TABLE 1.1

Population projections, 2015–60

[Resident population as of July 1. Numbers in thousands.]

Sex and age	2015	2020	2025	2030	2035	2040	2045	2050	2055	2060
	321,363	**333,896**	**346,407**	**358,471**	**369,662**	**380,016**	**389,934**	**399,803**	**409,873**	**420,268**
Under 18 years	74,518	76,159	78,190	80,348	81,509	82,621	84,084	85,918	87,744	89,288
Under 5 years	21,051	21,808	22,115	22,252	22,516	23,004	23,591	24,115	24,479	24,748
5 to 13 years	36,772	37,769	39,511	40,366	40,790	41,190	41,936	42,951	43,969	44,758
14 to 17 years	16,695	16,582	16,565	17,730	18,203	18,427	18,558	18,852	19,296	19,782
18 to 64 years	199,150	201,768	203,166	205,349	210,838	217,675	224,562	230,147	234,819	238,947
18 to 24 years	30,983	30,028	30,180	30,605	32,125	33,199	33,680	33,967	34,469	35,239
25 to 44 years	84,327	88,501	91,833	93,878	95,013	96,078	98,725	101,609	104,331	106,303
45 to 64 years	83,839	83,238	81,152	80,865	83,700	88,398	92,157	94,570	96,020	97,404
65 years and over	47,695	55,969	65,052	72,774	77,315	79,719	81,288	83,739	87,309	92,033
85 years and over	6,306	6,693	7,389	8,946	11,579	14,115	16,512	17,978	18,201	18,187
100 years and over	78	106	143	168	188	230	310	442	564	690
16 years and over	255,161	266,024	276,558	286,967	297,259	306,634	315,152	323,314	331,770	340,868
18 years and over	246,845	257,737	268,218	278,123	288,153	297,395	305,850	313,885	322,129	330,980
15 to 44 years	127,847	130,958	134,451	137,764	140,793	143,114	146,337	149,714	153,263	156,374

SOURCE: "Table 2. Projections of the Population by Selected Age Groups and Sex for the United States: 2015 to 2060," in *2012 National Population Projections: Summary Tables*, U.S. Census Bureau, May 15, 2013, http://www.census.gov/population/projections/files/summary/NP2012-T2.xls (accessed December 30, 2013)

TABLE 1.2

Percentage distribution of the projected population, 2015–60

[Percent of total resident population as of July 1.]

Sex and age	2015	2020	2025	2030	2035	2040	2045	2050	2055	2060
Both sexes	**100.00**	**100.00**	**100.00**	**100.00**	**100.00**	**100.00**	**100.00**	**100.00**	**100.00**	**100.00**
Under 18 years	23.19	22.81	22.57	22.41	22.05	21.74	21.56	21.49	21.41	21.25
Under 5 years	6.55	6.53	6.38	6.21	6.09	6.05	6.05	6.03	5.97	5.89
5 to 13 years	11.44	11.31	11.41	11.26	11.03	10.84	10.75	10.74	10.73	10.65
14 to 17 years	5.20	4.97	4.78	4.95	4.92	4.85	4.76	4.72	4.71	4.71
18 to 64 years	61.97	60.43	58.65	57.28	57.04	57.28	57.59	57.57	57.29	56.86
18 to 24 years	9.64	8.99	8.71	8.54	8.69	8.74	8.64	8.50	8.41	8.38
25 to 44 years	26.24	26.51	26.51	26.19	25.70	25.28	25.32	25.41	25.45	25.29
45 to 64 years	26.09	24.93	23.43	22.56	22.64	23.26	23.63	23.65	23.43	23.18
65 years and over	14.84	16.76	18.78	20.30	20.92	20.98	20.85	20.95	21.30	21.90
85 years and over	1.96	2.00	2.13	2.50	3.13	3.71	4.23	4.50	4.44	4.33
100 years and over	0.02	0.03	0.04	0.05	0.05	0.06	0.08	0.11	0.14	0.16
16 years and over	79.40	79.67	79.84	80.05	80.41	80.69	80.82	80.87	80.94	81.11
18 years and over	76.81	77.19	77.43	77.59	77.95	78.26	78.44	78.51	78.59	78.75
15 to 44 years	39.78	39.22	38.81	38.43	38.09	37.66	37.53	37.45	37.39	37.21

SOURCE: "Table 3. Percent Distribution of the Projected Population by Selected Age Groups and Sex for the United States: 2015 to 2060," in *2012 National Population Projections: Summary Tables*, U.S. Census Bureau, May 15, 2013, http://www.census.gov/population/projections/files/summary/NP2012-T3.xls (accessed December 30, 2013)

CHAPTER 2
REDEFINING DEATH

THE CHANGING DEFINITION OF DEATH

Prior to the age of modern medicine, determining that a person was dead consisted of determining whether he or she was breathing or had a detectable heartbeat. Respiration and blood circulation provide the body's cells with the oxygen that is needed to perform their life functions. When injury or disease prevents these operations and the supply of oxygen to the body is interrupted, the body's cells deteriorate and life ceases.

Modern life-saving measures such as cardiopulmonary resuscitation or defibrillation (electrical shock) can restart cardiac activity, however, and modern medical technologies such as the mechanical respirator, which was developed in the 1950s, can breathe on behalf of a patient whose respiratory functions would otherwise have ceased. Based on the heart and lung criteria, then, many people who would have been declared dead in prior eras can continue to live and, in some cases, recover from their injuries and diseases.

Further complicating the traditional definition of death was the development of the capacity to transplant the human heart. Experimental organ transplantations were first performed during the early decades of the 20th century, and by the 1960s transplantation of organs such as kidneys became routine practice. Kidneys could be harvested from a patient whose heart had stopped and who therefore could be declared legally dead. By contrast, a successful heart transplant required a beating heart from a "dead" donor.

On December 3, 1967, the South African surgeon Christiaan Barnard (1922–2001) transplanted a heart from a fatally injured accident victim, who was being kept alive by mechanical means, into the South African businessman Louis Washkansky (1913–1967). The transplanted heart functioned in Washkansky's body, but the drugs required to prevent his body from rejecting the organ weakened his immune system, and he died of pneumonia 18 days later. Following Barnard's success, dozens of transplant teams globally tried to improve on the transplantation process. By the end of the decade, approximately 150 patients had received transplanted hearts, but few patients lived longer than one year after the surgery due to the difficulties of suppressing the body's tendency to reject the organ. The 1980s saw improvements in the drugs needed to prevent rejection of the transplanted heart, and the increased ability to keep patients alive after surgery led to increased numbers of heart transplants across the world. In "A Brief History of Heart Transplants" (Time.com, November 16, 2009), Laura Fitzpatrick indicates that by the early 21st century over 2,000 heart transplants were being performed annually, and over 85% of patients survived more than one year after surgery.

Because heart donors must be both fatally injured or otherwise compromised at the same time that their hearts continue to function and respirators breathe on their behalf, a new definition of death was necessary to ensure that a patient was truly dead before his or her heart was removed. Physicians in the late 1960s first proposed a new criterion: irreversible cessation of brain activity, or what many called brain death.

The Harvard Criteria

In 1968 the Ad Hoc Committee of the Harvard Medical School to Examine the Definition of Brain Death was organized. The goal of the Harvard Brain Death Committee, as it was also known, was to redefine death. In August 1968 the committee published the report "A Definition of Irreversible Coma" (*Journal of the American Medical Association*, vol. 205, no. 6). This landmark report, known as the Harvard Criteria, listed the following guidelines for identifying irreversible coma:

- Unreceptivity and unresponsivity—the patient is completely unaware of externally applied stimuli and inner need. He or she does not respond even to intensely painful stimuli.

- No movements or breathing—the patient shows no sign of spontaneous movements and spontaneous respiration and does not respond to pain, touch, sound, or light.
- No reflexes—the pupils of the eyes are fixed and dilated. The patient shows no eye movement even when the ear is flushed with ice water or the head is turned. He or she does not react to harmful stimuli and exhibits no tendon reflexes.
- Flat electroencephalogram (EEG)—this shows lack of electrical activity in the cerebral cortex.

The Harvard Criteria could not be used unless reversible causes of brain dysfunction, such as drug intoxication and hypothermia (abnormally low body temperature—below 90 degrees Fahrenheit [32.2 degrees Celsius] core temperature), had been ruled out. The committee further recommended that the four criteria be repeated 24 hours after the initial test.

The Harvard committee stated, "Our primary purpose is to define irreversible coma as a new criterion for death." Despite this, the committee in effect reinforced brain death (a lack of all neurological activity in the brain and brain stem) as the legal criterion for the death of a patient. A patient who met all four guidelines could be declared dead, and his or her respirator could be withdrawn. The committee added, however, "We are concerned here only with those comatose individuals who have no discernible central nervous system activity." Brain death differs somewhat from irreversible coma; patients in deep coma may show brain activity on an EEG, although they may not be able to breathe on their own. People in a persistent vegetative state are also in an irreversible coma; however, they show more brain activity on an EEG than patients in deep coma and are able to breathe without the help of a respirator. Such patients were not considered dead by the committee's definition because they still had brain activity.

Criticisms of the Harvard Criteria

In 1978 Public Law 95-622 established the ethical advisory body called the President's Commission for the Study of Ethical Problems in Medicine and Biomedical and Behavioral Research. President Ronald Reagan (1911–2004) assigned the commission the task of defining death. In *Defining Death: A Report on the Medical, Legal and Ethical Issues in the Determination of Death* (July 1981, http://bioethicsarchive.georgetown.edu/pcbe/reports/past_commissions/defining_death.pdf), the commission reported that "the 'Harvard criteria' have been found to be quite reliable. Indeed, no case has yet been found that met these criteria and regained any brain functions despite continuation of respirator support."

However, the commission noted the following deficiencies in the Harvard Criteria:

- The phrase "irreversible coma" is misleading. Coma is a condition of a living person. A person lacking in brain function is dead and, therefore, beyond the condition called coma.
- The Harvard Brain Death Committee failed to note that spinal cord reflexes can continue or resume activity even after the brain stops functioning.
- "Unreceptivity" cannot be tested in an unresponsive person who has lost consciousness.
- The committee had not been "sufficiently explicit and precise" in expressing the need for adequate testing of brain stem reflexes, especially apnea (absence of the impulse to breathe, leading to an inability to breathe spontaneously). Adequate testing to eliminate drug and metabolic intoxication as possible causes of the coma had also not been spelled out explicitly. Metabolic intoxication refers to the accumulation of toxins (poisons) in the blood resulting from kidney or liver failure. These toxins can severely impair brain functioning and cause coma, but the condition is potentially reversible.
- Although all people who satisfy the Harvard Criteria are dead (with irreversible cessation of whole-brain functions), many dead individuals cannot maintain circulation long enough for retesting after a 24-hour interval.

THE GOVERNMENT REDEFINES DEATH

The president's commission proposed in *Defining Death* a model statute, the Uniform Determination of Death Act, the guidelines of which would be used to define death:

- [Determination of Death.] An individual who has sustained either (1) irreversible cessation of circulatory and respiratory functions, or (2) irreversible cessation of all functions of the entire brain, including the brain stem, is dead. A determination of death must be made in accordance with accepted medical standards.
- [Uniformity of Construction and Application.] This act shall be applied and construed to effectuate its general purpose to make uniform the law with respect to the subject of this act among states enacting it.

Brain Death

In *Defining Death*, the president's commission incorporated two formulations or concepts of the "whole-brain definition" of death. It stated that these two concepts were "actually mirror images of each other. The Commission has found them to be complementary; together they enrich one's understanding of the 'definition' [of death]."

The first whole-brain formulation states that death occurs when the three major organs (heart, lungs, and brain) suffer an irreversible functional breakdown. These organs are closely interrelated, so that if one stops functioning permanently, the other two will also stop working. Although traditionally the absence of the "vital signs" of respiration and circulation have signified death, this is simply a sign that the brain, the core organ, has permanently ceased to function. Individual cells or organs may continue to live for many hours, but the body as a whole cannot survive for long. Therefore, death can be declared even before the whole system shuts down.

The second whole-brain formulation "identifies the functioning of the whole brain as the hallmark of life because the brain is the regulator of the body's integration." Because the brain is the seat of consciousness and the director of all bodily functions, when the brain dies, the person is considered dead.

Reason for Two Definitions of Death

The president's commission claimed in *Defining Death* that its aim was to "supplement rather than supplant the existing legal concept." The brain-death criteria were not being introduced to define death in a new way. In most cases the cardiopulmonary definition of death would be sufficient. Only comatose patients on respirators would be diagnosed using the brain-death criteria.

Criteria for Determination of Death

The president's commission did not include in the proposed Uniform Determination of Death Act any specific medical criteria for diagnosing brain death. Instead, it had a group of medical consultants develop a summary of currently accepted medical practices. The commission stated in *Defining Death* that "such criteria—particularly as they relate to diagnosing death on neurological grounds—will be continually revised by the biomedical community in light of clinical experience and new scientific knowledge." These Criteria for Determination of Death read as follows (with medical details omitted here):

1. An individual with irreversible cessation of circulatory and respiratory functions is dead. A) Cessation is recognized by an appropriate clinical examination. B) Irreversibility is recognized by persistent cessation of functions during an appropriate period of observation and/or trial of therapy.

2. An individual with irreversible cessation of all functions of the entire brain, including the brainstem, is dead. A) Cessation is recognized when evaluation discloses findings that cerebral functions are absent and brainstem functions are absent. B) Irreversibility is recognized when evaluation discloses findings that the cause of coma is established and is sufficient to account for the loss of brain functions; the possibility of recovery of any brain functions is excluded; and the cessation of all brain functions persists for an appropriate period of observation and/or trial of therapy.

The Criteria for Determination of Death further warn that conditions such as drug intoxication, metabolic intoxication, and hypothermia may be confused with brain death. Physicians should practice caution when dealing with young children and people in shock. Infants and young children, who have more resistance to neurological damage, have been known to recover brain function. Shock victims might not test well due to a reduction in blood circulation to the brain.

Since the development of brain-death criteria in the United States, most countries have adopted the brain-death concept. Nevertheless, determining brain death varies worldwide. One reason has to do with cultural or religious beliefs. For example, in Japan it is believed that the soul lingers in the body for some time after death. Such a belief may influence the length of time the patient is observed before making the determination of death.

There is no federally mandated definition for brain death or method for certifying brain death. Thus, states have adopted the previously described Uniform Determination of Death Act. However, within each hospital, clinical practice is determined by the medical staff and administrative committees. A simplified list of criteria for brain death, which was current as of early 2014, is listed in Table 2.1.

Although the practice parameter has been published, several questions arose regarding the American Academy of Neurology's (AAN) guidelines, which were established in 1995. These questions are based on historical criteria. In

TABLE 2.1

Criteria for brain death

Coma
Absence of motor responses
Absence of pupillary responses to light and pupils at midposition with respect to dilatation (4–6 mm)
Absence of corneal reflexes
Absence of caloric responses
Absence of gag reflex
Absence of coughing in response to tracheal suctioning
Absence of respiratory drive at $PaCO_2$ that is 60 mm Hg or 20 mm Hg above normal baseline values

SOURCE: Eelco F. M. Wijdicks and Ronald E. Cranford, "Table 3. Clinical Criteria for Brain Death," in "Clinical Diagnosis of Prolonged States of Impaired Consciousness in Adults," *Mayo Clinic Proceedings*, vol. 80, no. 8, August 2005, http://download.journals.elsevierhealth.com/pdfs/journals/0025-6196/PIIS0025619611615863.pdf (accessed January 31, 2012). Data from E. F. M. Wijdicks, "The Diagnosis of the Brain," *New England Journal of Medicine*, no. 344, 2001: 1215–21.

"Evidence-Based Guideline Update: Determining Brain Death in Adults" (*Neurology*, vol. 74, no. 23, June 8, 2010), Eelco F. M. Wijdicks et al. articulate the questions and seek to answer them. The questions are:

1. Are there patients who fulfill the clinical criteria of brain death who recover neurologic [nervous system] function?
2. What is an adequate observation period to ensure that cessation of neurologic function is permanent?
3. Are complex motor movements that falsely suggest retained brain function sometimes observed in brain death?
4. What is the comparative safety of techniques for determining apnea?
5. Are there new ancillary [secondary] tests that accurately identify patients with brain death?

The researchers reviewed studies between January 1996 and May 2009, and they limited their focus to adults aged 18 years and older. The answers that Wijdicks et al. report, which are endorsed by the Neurocritical Care Society, the Child Neurology Society, the Radiological Society of North America, and the American College of Radiology, are:

1. The criteria for the determination of brain death given in the 1995 AAN practice parameter have not been invalidated by published reports of neurologic recovery in patients who fulfill these criteria.
2. There is insufficient evidence to determine the minimally acceptable observation period to ensure that neurologic functions have ceased irreversibly.
3. Complex-spontaneous motor movements and false-positive triggering of the ventilator may occur in patients who are brain dead.
4. There is insufficient evidence to determine the comparative safety of techniques used for apnea testing.
5. There is insufficient evidence to determine if newer ancillary tests accurately confirm the cessation of function of the entire brain.

Wijdicks et al.'s results confirm that the parameters described in Table 2.1 remain accurate guidelines for diagnosing brain death. In addition, Wijdicks's editorial "The Clinical Criteria of Brain Death throughout the World: Why Has It Come to This?" (*Canadian Journal of Anesthesia*, vol. 53, no. 6, June 2006) maintains his premise that "what is required is standardization of policy, appropriate education of staff, introduction of checklists in intensive care units, and brain death examination by designated, experienced physicians who have documented proficiency in brain death examination."

The need to improve implementation of the existing guidelines for brain death was underscored by Claire N. Shappell et al. in "Practice Variability in Brain Death Determination" (*Neurology*, vol. 81, no. 23, December 3, 2013). The authors, reporting on a survey of organ donors from 68 hospitals in the midwestern United States, note that in 44.7% of cases AAN guidelines were strictly followed and that in 37.2% of cases AAN guidelines were loosely followed. The authors report wide variation in the standards for documenting determinations of brain death and they surmise that these variations correspond to a similar level of variation in the clinical practice of the physicians making the determinations. As a result of their research, the authors point out the need for "improved documentation, better uniformity of policies, and comprehensive and strategically targeted educational initiatives to ensure consistently contemporary approaches to BD [brain death] determination in every patient."

Diagnosing brain death in children corresponds to the process for making diagnoses in adults, but there are variations in protocol and guidelines specific to newborns, in whom diagnosis differs from older children and adults. The American Academy of Pediatrics first issued guidelines for children in 1987. They were updated in 2011, in keeping with the recommendations of Thomas A. Nakagawa et al. in "Clinical Report—Guidelines for the Determination of Brain Death in Infants and Children: An Update of the 1987 Task Force Recommendations" (*Pediatrics*, vol. 128, no. 3, September 2011).

Brain Death and Persistent Vegetative State

In the past, when someone suffered an injury that caused them to stop breathing—such as a severe head injury—they typically died shortly thereafter. Beginning in the 20th century, however, the development of rapid emergency medical interventions makes it possible to place individuals in these dire situations onto respirators before they die. Sustained by respirators, some of these people go on to recover from their condition to various degrees. However, in other cases lack of oxygen has already caused serious, irreversible brain damage.

The brain stem, traditionally called the lower brain, is usually more resistant to damage from anoxia (oxygen deprivation). Thus, oxygen deprivation may cause irreversible damage to the cerebrum, or higher brain, but may spare the brain stem. (See Figure 2.1.) When the cerebrum is irreversibly damaged yet the brain stem still functions, the patient goes into a persistent vegetative state. Persistent vegetative state patients, lacking in the higher-brain function, are awake but unaware. They swallow, grimace when in pain, yawn, open their eyes, and may even breathe without a respirator.

Table 2.2 lists the criteria for the diagnosis of the persistent vegetative state, which is also called unresponsive wakefulness syndrome. Steven Laureys et al. explain

FIGURE 2.1

Parts of the brain

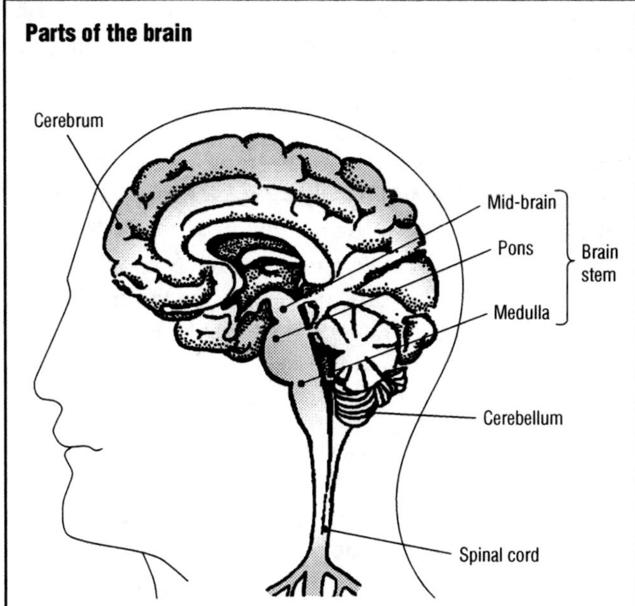

SOURCE: Adapted from "Figure 2. Anatomic Interrelationships of Heart, Lungs, and Brain," in *Defining Death: A Report on the Medical, Legal and Ethical Issues in the Determination of Death*, President's Commission for the Study of Ethical Problems in Medicine and Biomedical and Behavioral Research, July 1981, http://bioethics.georgetown.edu/pcbe/reports/past_commissions/defining_death.pdf (accessed January 31, 2012)

TABLE 2.2

Criteria for persistent vegetative state (PVS)

- Unaware of surroundings or self
- Exhibits eye-opening and eye-closing cycles
- Has enough autonomic nervous system and hypothalamus function to allow long-term survival with medical care
- Unable to interact with others
- Does not respond in a sustained, reproducible, or purposeful way to sights, sounds, touches, or smells
- Does not provide evidence of understanding language nor an ability to communicate with language
- Cannot control bladder and bowel functions
- May exhibit certain cranial nerve reflexes, such as dilation and constriction of pupils and the gag reflex

SOURCE: Created by Sandra Alters for Gale, © 2014

in "Unresponsive Wakefulness Syndrome: A New Name for the Vegetative State or Apallic Syndrome" (*BMC Medicine*, vol. 8, no. 68, November 1, 2010) that the use of the term *unresponsive wakefulness syndrome* is more appropriate, neutral, and descriptive. According to the researchers:

> Our proposal offers the medical community the possibility to adopt a neutral and descriptive name, unresponsive wakefulness syndrome, as an alternative to vegetative state (or apallic syndrome) which we view as outdated. We feel this is a real necessity, given that the term [persistent vegetative state] continues to have strong negative connotations after over 35 years of use, while inadvertently risking comparisons between patients and vegetables and implying persistency from the moment of diagnosis. It should be stressed that [unresponsive wakefulness syndrome] is a clinical syndrome describing patients who fail to show voluntary motor responsiveness in the presence of eyes-open wakefulness which can be either transitory on the way to recovery from (minimal) consciousness or irreversible.

Patients in a persistent vegetative state are not dead, so the brain-death criteria do not apply to them. They can survive for years with artificial feeding and antibiotics for possible infections. In *Defining Death*, the president's commission reported on a patient who remained in a persistent vegetative state for 37 years: Elaine Esposito (1934–1978) lapsed into a coma after surgery in 1941 and died in 1978.

The case of Karen Ann Quinlan (1954–1985) called attention to the ramifications of the persistent vegetative state. In 1975 Quinlan suffered a cardiopulmonary arrest after ingesting a combination of alcohol and drugs. In 1976 Joseph Quinlan was granted court permission to discontinue artificial respiration for his comatose daughter. Even after life support was removed, Karen remained in a persistent vegetative state until she died of multiple infections in 1985.

A more recent case that refocused national attention on the persistent vegetative state was that of Terri Schiavo (1963–2005), who entered a persistent vegetative state in 1990, when her brain was deprived of oxygen during a heart attack that was brought on by an eating disorder. Michael Schiavo, her husband, argued that she would never recover and that she would not want to be kept alive by artificial means. He petitioned a Florida court to remove her feeding tube. In October 2003 a Florida judge ruled that the tube should be removed. However, Schiavo's parents believed their daughter would recover and requested that Jeb Bush (1953–), the governor of Florida, intervene. The Florida legislature subsequently gave Governor Bush the authority to override the courts, and the feeding tube was reinserted six days after its removal. In May 2004 the law that allowed Governor Bush to intervene in the case was ruled unconstitutional by a Florida appeals court. The case was then appealed to the U.S. Supreme Court, which in January 2005 refused to hear the appeal and reinstate the Florida law. In March 2005 doctors removed Terri's feeding tube. She died 13 days later. An autopsy showed extensive damage throughout the cerebrum.

A similar case followed four years later, in 2009, when Eluana Englaro (1970–2009) died in Italy. She had been in a vegetative state for 17 years after a car accident resulted in her irreversible brain damage. Eluana's father, Beppino, tried for a decade to have his daughter's feeding tube removed, because she did not want to be kept alive by artificial means. He finally succeeded in spite of protests by the Catholic Church. Eluana died four days into the process of having her food and water diminished.

That same year the case of Rom Houben (1963–) was publicized worldwide. When Houben was 20, he was injured in an automobile accident, and his doctors eventually determined that he fell into a persistent vegetative state. Twenty-three years later he was suddenly able to communicate. Houben's doctors were convinced that he had been misdiagnosed and that he had not really been in a persistent vegetative state for all those years. However, experts questioned the man's method of communication, which is called facilitated communication. Maria Cheng explains in "Belgian Coma Patient Can't Talk after All" (Associated Press, February 19, 2010) that facilitated communication is a method by which a speech therapist helps the patient type out his or her thoughts by having the patient guide the therapist's hand. In response to questions raised about the technique, one of Houben's doctors performed tests on the method and determined that it did not work. Further tests have revealed that facilitated communication does not work with patients such as Houben. Claims that Houben could communicate were proven to be false.

Martin M. Monti et al. reveal in "Willful Modulation of Brain Activity in Disorders of Consciousness" (*New England Journal of Medicine*, vol. 362, no. 7, February 18, 2010) that they used functional magnetic resonance imaging technology to determine whether patients in a persistent vegetative state or a minimally conscious state (patients with partial preservation of conscious awareness) had brain activity that reflected "some awareness and cognition." The researchers scanned the brains of 54 previously unresponsive patients. Five of the patients showed brain activity (responsiveness) when researchers asked the patients to imagine themselves playing tennis. One of those five patients was also able to respond to questions with brain activity that is consistent with yes or no answers. Monti et al. expect that using such techniques with patients in a persistent vegetative or minimally conscious state may help to better refine the diagnosis of their condition, provide more appropriate treatment to those who show responsiveness, and establish basic communication with patients who otherwise appear to be unresponsive. See Chapter 4 for more information on disorders of consciousness and the minimally conscious state.

THE NEAR-DEATH EXPERIENCE

The term *near-death experience* was first used by Raymond A. Moody Jr. in *Life after Life: The Investigation of a Phenomenon—Survival of Bodily Death* (1976), a compilation of interviews with people who claimed to have come back from the dead. A decade earlier, the American psychiatrist Elisabeth Kübler-Ross (1926–2004) investigated out-of-body episodes that were recounted by her patients.

The near-death experience is not a phenomenon limited to modern times. It has been recounted in various forms of mysticism and by well-known historical figures such as the Greek philosopher Plato (428–347 BC) and the Benedictine historian and theologian St. Bede the Venerable (c. 673–c. 735). It appears, however, that the development and administration of emergency resuscitation has contributed to widespread reports of near-death experiences.

Some people who were revived after having been declared clinically dead have recounted remarkably similar patterns of experiences. They report leaving their body and watching, in a detached manner, while others tried to save their lives. They felt no pain and experienced complete serenity. After traveling through a tunnel, they encountered a radiant light. Some claim to have met friends and relatives who had already died; many attest to seeing their whole lives replayed and of being given a choice or a command to return to their bodies. Many people who have had such an experience believe it to be a spiritual event of great importance. For example, they may believe that they saw, or even entered, the afterlife.

Scientists have investigated whether there are potential physical explanations for near-death experiences. Studies conducted during the 1990s indicated that the near-death experience might be related to one or more physical changes in the brain. These changes include the gradual onset of anoxia in the brain, residual electrical activity in the brain, the release of endorphins in response to stress, or drug-induced hallucinations produced by drug therapies that are used during resuscitation attempts or resulting from previous drug abuse. In "Near-Death Experiences and the Temporal Lobe" (*Psychological Science*, vol. 15, no. 4, April 2004), Willoughby B. Britton and Richard R. Bootzin of the University of Arizona discuss the results of their study of temporal lobe functioning in 43 individuals who had experienced life-threatening events. Of the 43 participants, 23 reported having had near-death experiences during these events. The researchers find that people who reported near-death experiences had more of certain types of temporal lobe activity than those who did not have such experiences. Britton and Bootzin conclude that "altered temporal lobe functioning may be involved in the near-death experience and that individuals who have had such experiences are physiologically distinct from the general population."

In "Heaven Can Wait—or Down to Earth in Real Time: Near-Death Experience Revisited" (*Netherlands Heart Journal*, vol. 16, no. 10, October 2008), C. van Tellingen describes a neurophysiological explanation for near-death experiences. Van Tellingen suggests that as the body's nerve cells and their connections break down, "reminiscences, memories and building stones of the personal identity are 'released' and strengthen a feeling of time travel and life review. Perhaps this situation is more or less comparable with the situation in old age when literally loss of neurons and their connections bring back 'buried' memories and reminiscences." Dean Mobbs and Caroline Watt agree and conclude in "There Is Nothing Paranormal about Near-Death Experiences: How Neuroscience Can Explain Seeing Bright Lights, Meeting the Dead, or Being Convinced You Are One of Them" (*Trends in Cognitive Sciences*, vol. 15, no. 10, August 18, 2011) that "near-death experiences are the manifestation of normal brain function gone awry, during a traumatic, and sometimes harmless, event."

Jimo Borjigin et al. shed further light on what may occur in the brain as the body approaches death in "Surge of Neurophysical Coherence and Connectivity in the Dying Brain" (*Proceedings of the National Academy of Sciences of the United States of America*, vol. 110, no. 28, July 9, 2013). In research conducted on dying rats, the authors found that, contrary to the conventional wisdom maintaining that the brain became inactive at the point of clinical death, brain activity spikes at the point of death, exceeding comparable activity during periods of wakefulness. Furthermore, the researchers found increased levels of gamma oscillations (a form of high-frequency brainwave) near the visual cortex, the part of the brain responsible for the processing of visual sensations, which could be linked to the reports of near-death experiences involving radiant light. Experts noted that these findings were extremely preliminary, however. "This is an interesting and well-conducted piece of research," Chris Chambers of Cardiff University told Rebecca Morrelle in "Near-Death Experiences Are Electrical Surge in Dying Brain" (BBC.co.uk, August 12, 2013). "We know precious little about brain activity during death, let alone conscious brain activity.... [But] we should be extremely cautious before drawing any conclusions about human near-death experiences: it is one thing to measure brain activity in rats during cardiac arrest, and quite another to relate that to human experience."

Pam Reynolds, a singer-songwriter who had a near-death experience while undergoing brain surgery in Arizona in 1991, lived to tell a compelling story of her experience. Barbara Bradley Hagerty reports in "Decoding the Mystery of Near-Death Experiences" (NPR.org, May 22, 2009) that Reynolds was undergoing a rare form of neurosurgery to remove an aneurysm, which involved "chilling her body, draining the blood out of her head like oil from a car engine, snipping the aneurysm and then bringing her back from the edge of death." As part of the procedure, the medical team placed special headphones in her ears and played deafening sounds that they believed would make it impossible for Reynolds to hear anything else. They also taped her eyes shut. Reynolds, who was deeply comatose during the procedure, with a stopped heart and no brain activity, later described a near-death experience in which she "popped out" of the top of her head and watched her body being attended to by 20 physicians, accompanied by her deceased grandmother and uncle. She heard the sound of a drill and observed the saw that her neurosurgeon was using to perform the surgery; she heard a female voice say, "Her arteries are too small" in reference to her groin area; and she heard the classic rock song "Hotel California" by the Eagles.

Reynolds initially took these sensations for a hallucination, but a year after the operation, she discussed the details of her experience with the neurosurgeon who had led the surgery, and her account matched his own memory of the procedure. Years later, Michael Sabom, a cardiologist who was researching near-death experiences, examined the records from Reynolds's surgery and found that her account of what had happened matched the records with startling exactitude. There were 20 doctors in the room, there was a conversation about the veins in her left leg, "Hotel California" was playing on the stereo, and the saw that the neurosurgeon used matched Reynolds's description. "She could not have heard [it]," Sabom told Hagerty, "because of what they did to her ears.... In addition, both of her eyes were taped shut, so she couldn't open her eyes and see what was going on. So her physical sensory perception was off the table." Although some see Reynolds's experience and others like it as evidence that consciousness—and, by extension, an entity such as the soul or spirit—can exist outside of the body, anecdotes such as hers do not rise to the level of scientific evidence. And critics charge that there are other possible explanations for her experience. Anesthesiologist Gerald Woerlee, who studied Reynolds's case, told Hagerty that he believes she experienced "anesthesia awareness," a condition in which a person is conscious but cannot move, and that she heard parts of the operation because her headphones did not work as intended. In any case, scientific proof of what happens in near-death experiences such as Reynolds's may be impossible to achieve given the moral, ethical, and legal issues that would be involved in experimentally inducing death or near-death in human beings.

CHAPTER 3
THE END OF LIFE: ETHICAL CONSIDERATIONS

Difficulties in defining death present but one of the many ethical dilemmas related to end-of-life care and decision making. Decisions concerning the withdrawal of life-support efforts for people who are in persistent vegetative states are often even more controversial. Because of the diversity of religious and other belief systems that influence people's opinions about such matters of life and death, there exist no universal standards for making determinations about when, and for whom, such measures are appropriate. Besides the fact that the intentional discontinuation of life support is itself controversial, in many cases such decisions must be made by the spouses, parents, or adult children of the individuals involved, complicating matters still further. How much weight should be given to the patient's wishes versus the ethical convictions of the decision makers and the physicians and other personnel charged with carrying out the decision? Who should determine when medical care is futile and no longer benefits the dying patient?

RELIGIOUS TEACHINGS

All major religions consider life sacred. When it comes to death and dying, they take seriously the fate of the soul, be it eternal salvation (as in Christian belief) or reincarnation (as in Buddhist philosophy). Much of the debate surrounding end-of-life issues centers on the strongly held beliefs of people and institutions with religious affiliations.

Roman Catholicism

According to Catholic teachings, death is contrary to God's plan for humankind. When God created the first human beings, Adam and Eve, he did not intend for them to die. However, when Adam and Eve disobeyed God in the Garden of Eden, physical death was the consequence of their sin. The New Testament of the Bible explains that Jesus was the son of God who, out of love for humankind, was born into the world and died as a man. God raised Jesus from the dead after his crucifixion to live eternally with him in heaven, and Jesus promised humankind the same opportunity. The Vatican notes in *Catechism of the Catholic Church* (August 23, 2002, http://www.vatican.va/archive/ccc_css/archive/catechism/ccc_toc.htm) that according to Christian doctrine, Jesus "transformed the curse of death into a blessing."

HISTORY. Early Christians believed that God was the giver of life and that he alone could take life away. They viewed euthanasia (hastening the death of a dying, suffering patient who requests death) as usurping that divine right. The Christian philosopher St. Augustine of Hippo (354–430) taught that people must accept suffering because it comes from God. According to Augustine, suffering not only helps Christians grow spiritually but also prepares them for the eternal joy that God has in store for them. Moreover, the healthy were exhorted to minister to the sick not for the purpose of helping to permanently end their suffering, but to ease their pain.

St. Thomas Aquinas (c. 1225–1274), the most influential Catholic thinker after Augustine, taught that ending one's suffering by ending one's life was sinful. To help another take his or her life was just as sinful. Not all Catholic thinkers have always agreed. In 1516 Sir Thomas More (1478–1535), an English statesman, humanist, and loyal defender of the Catholic Church, published *Utopia*, which described an ideal country governed by reason. If a disease is not only incurable but also causes pain that is hard to control, in More's *Utopia* it is permissible to free the sufferer from his or her painful existence. This was a major departure from the medieval acceptance of suffering and death as the earthly price to be paid for eternal life.

RULE OF DOUBLE EFFECT. Aquinas is believed to have first formulated the ethical principle of "double effect," which has been influential among Catholic theologians and other moral philosophers. According to this principle, an action that might be wrong if committed intentionally is acceptable if committed unintentionally. Aquinas introduced the idea in the context of killing an assailant in self-defense, a situation that creates two effects: the saving of one's life and the ending of the life of another. The rule of double effect was not unconditional, however. Even a well-intentioned person who killed in self-defense might err in moral terms if his response was disproportionate, for example by being excessively violent.

The rule of double effect has been applied by Catholics to discussions surrounding end-of-life care. For example, a physician may prescribe an increased dosage of the painkiller morphine to ease a patient's pain, even if the physician reasonably foresees that it might bring about the patient's death. Pain relief, not death, is the intent, although both effects may result from the administration of the drugs. In *Catechism of the Catholic Church*, the Vatican states that "the use of painkillers to alleviate the sufferings of the dying, even at the risk of shortening their days, can be morally in conformity with human dignity if death is not willed as either an end or a means, but only foreseen and tolerated as inevitable."

ON EUTHANASIA. Since the mid-20th century Catholic theologians have debated balancing the preservation of God-given life with the moral issue of continuing medical treatments that are of no apparent value to patients. In "The Prolongation of Life" (1957), Pope Pius XII (1876–1958) states that if a patient is hopelessly ill, physicians may discontinue heroic measures "to permit the patient, already virtually dead, to pass on in peace." He adds that if the patient is unconscious, relatives may request withdrawal of life support under certain conditions.

The Vatican's 1980 *Declaration on Euthanasia* (http://www.vatican.va/roman_curia/congregations/cfaith/documents/rc_con_cfaith_doc_19800505_euthanasia_en.html) outlines the official Catholic Church stance on euthanasia today. It defines the term thus: "By euthanasia is understood an action or an omission which of itself or by intention causes death, in order that all suffering may in this way be eliminated." The declaration notes that a person cannot ask for euthanasia no matter what the situation, because it is a "violation of the divine law" and it is almost always an "anguished plea for help and love." The declaration indicates, however, that a dying patient may be administered painkilling medications at the end of life to help him or her be more comfortable.

The Committee for Pro-Life Activities of the National Conference of Catholic Bishops states in *Nutrition and Hydration: Moral and Pastoral Reflections* (April 1992, http://www.priestsforlife.org/magisterium/bishops/92-04nutritionandhydrationnccbprolifecommittee.htm) that "in the final stage of dying one is not obliged to prolong the life of a patient by every possible means: 'When inevitable death is imminent in spite of the means used, it is permitted in conscience to take the decision to refuse forms of treatment that would only secure a precarious and burdensome prolongation of life, so long as the normal care due to the sick person in similar cases is not interrupted.'" However, the Vatican's Congregation for the Doctrine of the Faith ruled in 2007 that a person in a persistent vegetative state must receive nutrition and hydration. Pope Benedict XVI (1927–) approved the ruling. Moreover, the Vatican explains in *Catechism of the Catholic Church* that "direct euthanasia" is "morally unacceptable" in any situation under the Fifth Commandment.

The Eastern Orthodox Church

The Eastern Orthodox Church, which resulted from the division between eastern and western Christianity during the 11th century, does not have a single worldwide leader such as the Roman Catholic pope. Instead, national jurisdictions called sees are each governed by a bishop. Accordingly, Eastern Orthodoxy relies on the scriptures, traditions, and decrees of the first seven ecumenical councils to regulate its daily conduct. Concerning matters of morality in the 21st century, such as the debates on end-of-life issues, contemporary Orthodox ethicists explore possible courses of action that are in line with the "sense of the church." The sense of the church is deduced from church laws and dissertations of the church fathers, as well as from previous council decisions. Their recommendations are subject to further review.

In "The Stand of the Orthodox Church on Controversial Issues" (2014, http://www.goarch.org/ourfaith/ourfaith7101), the Reverend Stanley S. Harakas of the Greek Orthodox Archdiocese of America (a branch of the larger Eastern Orthodox faith), states, "The Orthodox Church has a very strong pro-life stand which in part expresses itself in opposition to doctrinaire advocacy of euthanasia." However, Harakas notes that "as current Orthodox theology expresses it: 'The Church distinguishes between euthanasia and the withholding of extraordinary means to prolong life. It affirms the sanctity of human life and man's God-given responsibility to preserve life. But it rejects an attitude which disregards the inevitability of physical death.'"

Protestantism

The different denominations of Protestantism have varying positions on end-of-life care. Many hold that euthanasia is morally wrong, but they also believe that prolonging life by extraordinary measures is not necessary. In other words, few leaders of any Protestant church would condone active euthanasia, but many approve of the withdrawal of life support from a dying patient. Among the Protestant denominations that support this latter view are the Jehovah's Witnesses, the Church of

Jesus Christ of Latter-Day Saints (Mormons), the Lutheran Church, the Reformed Presbyterians, the Presbyterian Church in America, the Christian Life Commission of the Southern Baptist Convention, and the General Association of the General Baptists.

Some denominations have no official policy on euthanasia. However, many individual ethicists and representatives within these churches agree with other denominations that euthanasia is morally wrong but that futile life support serves no purpose. Among these churches are the Seventh-Day Adventists, the Episcopal Church, and the United Methodist Church.

Christian Scientists believe that prayer heals all diseases. They claim that illnesses are mental in origin and therefore cannot be cured by outside intervention, such as medical help. Some also believe that seeking medical help while praying diminishes or even cancels the effectiveness of the prayers. Because God can heal even those diseases that others see as incurable, euthanasia has no practical significance among Christian Scientists.

The Unitarian Universalist Association, a union of the Unitarian and Universalist Churches, is perhaps the most liberal when it comes to the right to die. The association states in "The Right to Die with Dignity: 1988 General Resolution" (August 24, 2011, http://www.uua.org/socialjustice/socialjustice/statements/14486.shtml) that "human life has inherent dignity, which may be compromised when life is extended beyond the will or ability of a person to sustain that dignity." Furthermore, "Unitarian Universalists advocate the right to self-determination in dying, and the release from civil or criminal penalties of those who, under proper safeguards, act to honor the right of terminally ill patients to select the time of their own deaths."

Judaism

There are three main branches of Judaism in the United States. The Orthodox tradition adheres strictly to Jewish laws. Conservative Judaism advocates adapting Jewish precepts to a changing world, but all changes must be consistent with Jewish laws and tradition. Reform Judaism, while accepting the ethical laws as coming from God, generally considers the other laws of Judaism as "instructional but not binding."

Like the Roman Catholics, Jews believe that life is precious because it is a gift from God. No one has the right to extinguish life, because one's life is not his or hers in the first place. Generally, rabbis from all branches of Judaism agree that euthanasia is not morally justified. It is tantamount to murder, which is forbidden by the Torah. Moreover, Jewish teaching holds that men and women are stewards entrusted with the preservation of God's gift of life and therefore are obliged to hold on to that life as long as possible.

PROLONGING LIFE VERSUS HASTENING DEATH. Although Jewish tradition maintains that a devout believer must do everything possible to prolong life, this admonition is subject to interpretation even among Orthodox Jews.

The Torah and the Talmud (the definitive rabbinical compilation of Jewish laws, lore, and commentary) provide the principles and laws that guide Jews. The Talmud offers continuity to Jewish culture by interpreting the Torah and adapting it to the constantly changing situations of Jewish people.

On the subject of prolonging life versus hastening death, the Talmud narrates a number of situations that involve people who are considered "goses" (literally, "the death rattle is in the patient's throat" or "one whose death is imminent"). Scholars often refer to the story of Rabbi Hanina ben Teradyon, who, during the second century, was condemned to be burned to death by the Romans. To prolong his agonizing death, the Romans wrapped him in some wet material. At first, the rabbi refused to hasten his own death; however, he later agreed to have the wet material removed, thus bringing about a quicker death.

Some Jews interpret this Talmudic narration to mean that in the final stage of a person's life, it is permissible to remove any hindrance to the dying process. In this modern age of medicine, this may mean implementing a patient's wish, such as a do-not-resuscitate order or the withdrawal of artificial life support.

Islam

Islam was founded by the prophet Muhammad (c. 570–632) during the seventh century. The Koran, which is composed of Allah's (God's) revelations to Muhammad, and the sunna, Muhammad's teachings and deeds, are the sources of Islamic beliefs and practice. Although there are many sects and cultural diversities within the religion, all Muslims (followers of Islam) are bound by a total submission to the will of Allah. The basic doctrines of Allah's revelations were systematized into definitive rules and regulations that now make up the sharia (the religious law that governs the life of Muslims).

Muslims look to the sharia for ethical guidance in all aspects of life, including medicine. Sickness and pain are part of life and must be accepted as Allah's will. They should be viewed as a means to atone for one's sins. By contrast, death is simply a passage to another existence in the afterlife. Those who die after leading a righteous life will merit the true life on Judgment Day. The Koran states, "How do you disbelieve in God seeing you were dead and He gave you life and then He shall cause you to die, then He shall give you life, then unto Him you shall be returned?"

Islam teaches that life is a gift from Allah; therefore, no one can end it except Allah. Muhammad said, "Whosoever takes poison and thus kills himself, his poison will be in his hand; he will be tasting it in Hell, always abiding therein, and being accommodated therein forever" (compiled in *Sahih Bukhari*). Although an ailing person does not have the right to choose death, even if he or she is suffering, Muslims heed the following admonition from the *Islamic Code of Medical Ethics* (1981): "[The] doctor is well advised to realize his limit and not transgress it. If it is scientifically certain that life cannot be restored, then it is futile to diligently [maintain] the vegetative state of the patient by heroic means.... It is the process of life that the doctor aims to maintain and not the process of dying. In any case, the doctor shall not take a positive measure to terminate the patient's life."

Hinduism

The Eastern religious tradition of Hinduism is based on the principle of reincarnation (the cycle of life, death, and physical rebirth). Hindus believe that death and dying are intricately interwoven with life and that the individual soul undergoes a series of physical life cycles before uniting with Brahman (God or the ultimate reality). Karma refers to the ethical consequences of a person's actions during a previous life, which determine the quality of his or her present life. A person can neither change nor escape his or her karma. By conforming to dharma (religious and moral law), an individual is able to fulfill obligations from the past life. Life is sacred because it offers one the chance to perform good acts toward the goal of ending the cycle of rebirths.

Therefore, a believer in Hinduism views pain and suffering as personal karma, and serious illness as a consequence of past misdeeds. Death is simply a passage to another rebirth, which brings one closer to Brahman. Artificial medical treatments to sustain life are not recommended, and medical intervention to end life is discouraged. Euthanasia simply interrupts one's karma and the soul's evolution toward final liberation from reincarnation.

Buddhism

Buddhism, like Hinduism, has a cosmology involving a cycle of reincarnation. To Buddhists, the goals of every life are the emancipation from samsara (the compulsory cycle of rebirths) and the attainment of nirvana (enlightenment or bliss). Like the Hindus, Buddhists believe that sickness, death, and karma are interrelated. The followers of Buddha (563–480 BC), the founder of Buddhism, claim that Buddha advised against taking too strict a position when it comes to issues such as the right to die.

Tenzin Gyatso (1935–), the 14th Dalai Lama, the spiritual leader of Tibetan Buddhism, has commented on the use of mechanical life support when the patient has no chance of recovery. Sogyal Rinpoche explains in *The Tibetan Book of Living and Dying* (1992) that the Dalai Lama advises that each case be considered individually: "If there is no such chance for positive thoughts [Buddhists believe that a dying person's final thoughts determine the circumstances of his or her next life], and in addition a lot of money is being spent by relatives simply to keep someone alive, then there seems to be no point. But each case must be dealt with individually; it is very difficult to generalize."

SECULAR PERSPECTIVES

Atheists and others whose moral beliefs are human-centered, or secular, rather than based on divine law or religious dogma, share no single set of beliefs on end-of-life issues such as the prolongation of life and euthanasia. Nevertheless, secular belief systems are generally more likely to privilege human dignity and the wishes of the individual person, rather than adhering to one-size-fits-all rules regarding the sanctity of life. Secularists are more likely than most religious people to agree with the idea that every case must be considered individually rather than in accordance with belief systems that cannot, in a modern world characterized by a diversity of religions and moral systems, claim universal applicability. Many of the strongest arguments in favor of allowing people to make their own choices regarding the end of life are rooted in secular viewpoints.

There are a number of secular, rights-based arguments in favor of ending life either through the withdrawal of life support or through active euthanasia. One argument is that humans have the right to die at a time and in the manner of their choosing; another, similar argument is that the right to life implies a right to die; still others argue that the rights to privacy and to determine one's own belief system imply a right to die. However, many secular thinkers would place limits on each of these arguments by maintaining that these rights must be balanced with the individual's obligations. For example, a terminally ill person may not have an unconditional right to die when and how he or she chooses when dependent children or other loved ones will be affected by the death. In such cases, the individual's rights should be balanced against the obligations he or she has to those other people.

Other secular thinkers argue that it is immoral to require people to suffer against their will and in situations in which they have no hope for meaningful life. Against religious arguments maintaining that life in all its manifestations is sacred and must be defended, some secularists maintain that forcing people to prolong a life that presents them only with agony represents a degradation of life.

MEDICAL ETHICS AND THE PERSPECTIVES OF HEALTH CARE PROFESSIONALS

Medical practice has always been governed by ethical codes and concerned with ethical issues that arise in matters of life, death, and illness. Physicians since the mid-20th century, however, have been faced with far more—and far more complicated—ethical dilemmas than their counterparts in earlier eras of human history.

The Hippocratic Oath

The earliest written document to deal with medical ethics is generally attributed to Hippocrates (460–377 BC), an ancient Greek physician traditionally considered the father of medicine. For more than 2,000 years the Hippocratic oath has stood as the centerpiece of medical ethics in the Western world, defining the conduct of health care providers in the discharge of their duties. In part, the oath states: "I will follow that method of treatment, which, according to my ability and judgment, I consider for the benefit of my patients, and abstain from whatever is deleterious [harmful] and mischievous. I will give no deadly medicine to anyone if asked, nor suggest any such counsel."

Some scholars claim that the giving of "deadly medicine" does not refer to euthanasia. During the time of Hippocrates, helping a suffering person end his or her life was common practice. Therefore, the oath might have been a commitment to avoid acting as an accomplice to murder, rather than a promise to refrain from the practice of euthanasia.

Most physicians, moreover, believe that a literal interpretation of the oath is not necessary. It simply offers guidelines that allow for adaptation to 21st-century situations. In fact, in 1948 the World Medical Association modified the Hippocratic oath to call attention to the atrocities that were committed by Nazi physicians. Known as the Declaration of Geneva (June 6, 2002, http://www.cirp.org/library/ethics/geneva/), the document reads in part: "I will practice my profession with conscience and dignity; the health of my patient will be my first consideration.... I will not permit considerations of religion, nationality, race, party politics or social standing to intervene between my duty and my patient. I will maintain the utmost respect for human life from the time of conception, even under threat, I will not use my medical knowledge contrary to the laws of humanity."

The Changing Patient–Physician Relationship

In all periods of human history, the practice of medicine has presupposed that physicians are able to determine what is best for their patients, often more effectively than the patients themselves. Prior to the middle of the 20th century, it was common for patients to rely on their doctors' abilities and judgment without question. Doctors were not even required to tell their patients the details of their illnesses or to disclose that an illness was terminal. Beginning in the 1960s, however, patients generally began to assume a more active role in their medical care. An emphasis on preventive medicine encouraged people to take responsibility for their own health, and physicians encouraged patients to be active participants in the health care process. Patients have also generally become more attentive to technologies and procedures that have changed the practice of medicine. As a result of this new patient–physician relationship, health care providers have become responsible for fully informing and educating patients, and they have been found increasingly legally liable for failing to inform patients of the consequences of medical treatments and procedures.

To compound the complexity of the changing patient–physician relationship, modern technology can prolong death as well as life. Historically, physicians had been trained to prevent and combat death, rather than to deal with dying patients, communicate with the patient and the family about a terminal illness, prepare them for an imminent death, or respond to a patient requesting assisted suicide.

Contemporary Ethical Guidelines for Physicians

For most of history, physicians' training has been focused on the saving of lives, not on the process of dying. Ira R. Byock, a well-known palliative care physician (palliative care is focused on relieving pain and stress in seriously ill patients) and a former president of the American Academy of Hospice and Palliative Medicine, admits in one of his early books, *Dying Well: The Prospect for Growth at the End of Life* (1997), that "a strong presumption throughout my medical career was that all seriously ill people required vigorous life-prolonging treatment, including those who were expected to die, even patients with advanced chronic illness such as widespread cancer, end stage congestive heart failure, and kidney or liver failure. It even extended to patients who saw death as a relief from suffering caused by their illness."

More recent medical education, however, has changed the focus from life-prolonging treatment for all patients to one of understanding the futility of prolonging the life, and process of dying, of a terminally ill and actively dying patient. Medical ethics now recognizes the obligation of physicians to shift the intent of care for dying patients from that of futile procedures that may only increase patient distress to that of comfort and closure.

The AMA provides ethical guidelines to help educate and support physicians in such end-of-life care. The AMA's *Code of Medical Ethics: Principles, Opinions, and Reports* (2014, http://www.ama-assn.org/ama/pub/physician-resources/medical-ethics/code-medical-ethics.shtml) provides end-of-life ethical guidelines in the following areas: 2.037 "Medical Futility in End-of-Life Care"; 2.20 "Withholding or Withdrawing Life-Sustaining Medical Treatment"; 2.201 "Sedation to Unconsciousness in End-of-Life Care"; 2.21 "Euthanasia"; 2.211 "Physician-Assisted Suicide"; 2.22 "Do-Not-Resuscitate Orders"; and 2.225 "Optimal Use of Orders-Not-to-Intervene and Advance Directives." For example, the section on "Withholding or Withdrawing Life-Sustaining Medical Treatment" (1994, http://www.ama-assn.org/ama/pub/physician-resources/medical-ethics/code-medical-ethics/opinion220.page?) states in part: "The principle of patient autonomy requires that physicians respect the decision to forgo life-sustaining treatment of a patient who possesses decision making capacity. Life-sustaining treatment is any treatment that serves to prolong life without reversing the underlying medical condition."

The American College of Physicians also provides clinical practice guidelines in end-of-life care. Examples of articles that provide such guidelines include "Evidence-Based Interventions to Improve the Palliative Care of Pain, Dyspnea, and Depression at the End of Life: A Clinical Practice Guideline from the American College of Physicians" (*Annals of Internal Medicine*, vol. 148, no. 2, January 15, 2008) by Amir Qaseem et al. and "Evidence for Improving Palliative Care at the End of Life: A Systematic Review" (*Annals of Internal Medicine*, vol. 148, no. 2, January 15, 2008) by Karl A. Lorenz et al.

MEDICAL EDUCATION IN DEATH AND DYING. Training in end-of-life care, accordingly, increased beginning in the mid- to late 20th century. In "Educating Medical Students about Death and Dying" (*Archives of Disease in Childhood*, vol. 64, no. 5, May 1989), D. Black, D. Hardoff, and J. Nelki note that, in a review of the medical literature between 1960 and 1971, they found no articles about the teaching of death and dying to medical students. This began to change in the 1970s. George E. Dickinson of the College of Charleston (South Carolina) studied medical school offerings on end-of-life issues by mailing brief questionnaires to all accredited U.S. medical schools in 1975, 1980, 1985, 1990, 1995, 2000, and 2005. His findings, published in "Teaching End-of-Life Issues in US Medical Schools: 1975 to 2005" (*American Journal of Hospice and Palliative Medicine*, vol. 23, no. 3, June–July 2006) provide an overview of the growing attention paid to these issues. Only 7% of medical schools offered separate courses in death and dying in 1975, according to Dickinson. By 1990 this figure stood at 18%. The percentage of lectures and short courses that incorporated death and dying information was much higher, ranging between 70% and 87% over the years covered by Dickinson's survey. Likewise, the number of students enrolled in death and dying offerings increased, slowly at first (from 71% in 1975 to 77% in 1995) and then rapidly, with medical schools reporting 96% of their students enrolled in death and dying offerings in both 2000 and 2005.

Training in palliative care also became more common during the late 20th and early 21st centuries. In "Palliative Care in Medical School Curricula: A Survey of United States Medical Schools" (*Journal of Palliative Medicine*, vol. 11, no. 9, November 2008), Emily S. Van Aalst-Cohen, Raine Riggs, and Ira R. Byock report on their survey of 128 medical schools and other information from the Association of American Medical Colleges Curriculum Management and Information Tool database. They determine that palliative care was a required course in 30% of medical schools, was an elective in 15% of medical schools, and was integrated into required courses in 53% of medical schools as of 2007.

PATIENT AUTONOMY

Principles of patient autonomy have increasingly informed the physician–patient relationship and influenced the process of end-of-life care. Competent patients, as defenders of personal autonomy argue, have the right to self-rule—to choose among medically recommended treatments and to refuse any treatment they do not want. To be truly autonomous, patients have to be told about the nature of their illness, the prospects for recovery, the course of the illness, alternative treatments, and treatment consequences. After thoughtful consideration, a patient makes an informed choice and grants "informed consent" to treatment or decides to forgo treatment. Decisions about medical treatment may be influenced by the patient's psychological state, family history, culture, values, and religious beliefs.

Cultural Differences

Although patient autonomy is a fundamental aspect of medical ethics, not all patients want to know about their illnesses or be involved in decisions about their terminal care. In "Cultural Diversity at the End of Life: Issues and Guidelines for Family Physicians" (*American Family Physician*, vol. 71, no. 3, February 1, 2005),

H. Russell Searight and Jennifer Gafford of the Forest Park Hospital Family Medicine Residency Program in St. Louis, Missouri, note that the concept of patient autonomy is not easily applied to members of some racial and ethnic groups. Searight and Gafford explain the three basic dimensions in end-of-life treatment that vary culturally: communication of bad news, locus of decision making, and attitudes toward advance directives and end-of-life care.

Members of some ethnic groups, including a variety of people from African nations and people from Japan, soften bad news with terms that do not overtly state that a person has a potentially terminal condition. For example, the term *growth* or *blood disease* may be used rather than telling a person he or she has a cancerous tumor or leukemia. This concept is taken one step further in many Hispanic, Chinese, and Pakistani communities, in which the terminally ill are generally protected from knowledge of their condition. Many reasons exist for this type of behavior, such as viewing the discussion of serious illness and death as disrespectful or impolite, not wanting to cause anxiety or eliminate hope in the patient, or believing that speaking about a condition makes it real. Many people of Asian and European cultures believe that it is cruel to inform a patient of a terminal diagnosis.

Another excellent study on multiculturalism in death and dying issues is Jessica Doolen and Nancy L. York's "Cultural Differences with End-of-Life Care in the Critical Care Unit" (*Dimensions of Critical Care Nursing*, vol. 26, no. 5, September–October 2007). In this study, the researchers add similar cultural scenarios in communication about death and dying to those outlined by Searight and Gafford. Doolen and York note that South Koreans generally do not talk about the dying process because it fosters sadness and because such discussions may quicken the dying process. According to the authors Filipinos similarly believe that such discussions may hasten death and interfere with God's will.

The phrase "locus of decision making" refers to the network of people who make end-of-life decisions together: the physician, the family, and/or the patient. Searight and Gafford explain that the locus of decision making varies among cultures. For example, in North America the patient typically plays the primary role in the decision-making process. South Koreans and Mexicans often approach end-of-life decision making differently, abiding by a collective process in which relatives make treatment choices for a family member without that person's input. Eastern Europeans and Russians often look to the physician as the expert in end-of-life decision making. In Indian, Pakistani, and other Asian cultures, physicians and family members may share decision making. Doolen and York note that among Afghans, health care decisions are made by the head of the family, possibly in consultation with an educated younger family member.

An advance directive (often called a living will) is a written statement that explains a person's wishes about end-of-life medical care. Completion of advance directives varies among cultures. For example, Searight and Gafford note that approximately 40% of elderly whites have completed advance directives, whereas only 16% of elderly African Americans have done the same. Doolen and York add that Mexican Americans, African Americans, Native Americans, and Asian Americans do not necessarily share the typical American philosophy that end-of-life decisions are the individual's responsibility and are much less likely than the general American population to sign advance directives or do-not-resuscitate orders.

Health Care Proxies and Surrogate Decision Makers

When a patient is not competent to make informed decisions about his or her medical treatment, a proxy or a surrogate must make the decision for that patient. Some patients, in anticipation of being in a position of incompetence, will execute a durable power of attorney for health care by designating a proxy. Most people choose family members or close friends who will make all medical decisions, including the withholding or withdrawal of life-sustaining treatments.

When a proxy has not been named in advance, health care providers usually involve family members in medical decisions. Most states have laws that govern surrogate decision making. Some states designate family members, by order of kinship, to assume the role of surrogates.

THE DESIRE TO DIE: EUTHANASIA AND ASSISTED SUICIDE

The prospect of being allowed to end one's own life by active means, with the help of a physician, has become more relevant in an age when life can often be prolonged past the point when an individual wants to continue living. Euthanasia became a topic of mainstream conversation in the 1990s, thanks in large part to the activities of Jack Kevorkian (1928–2011), a physician who publicized his role in administering lethal injections to more than 130 terminally ill people. Kevorkian, an advocate for the right to die, attempted to further his cause by euthanizing a terminally ill man on videotape in 1998 and providing the footage to the CBS television show *60 Minutes*. After the show broadcast the footage, Kevorkian was arrested and charged with second-degree murder. In 1999 he was convicted and sentenced to

10 to 25 years in prison, in spite of emotional pleas on his behalf from the widow and the brother of the man who had sought out Kevorkian's services. He was paroled in 2007, and he died in 2011.

Although the type of active euthanasia championed by Kevorkian remains illegal everywhere in the United States, some states have legalized physician-assisted suicide in which the patient takes the dominant role in death. Oregon became the first U.S. state to legalize physician-assisted suicide in 1997, when it enacted the Death with Dignity Act. Under the law, terminally ill adults are allowed to obtain prescriptions for lethal doses of medication to be self-administered. In 2009 the state of Washington enacted its own Death with Dignity Act, closely modeled on Oregon's, and Vermont followed suit in 2013. In Montana, the state Supreme Court ruled in 2009 that state law permitted physician-assisted suicide, but as of 2014 no legislation or regulatory framework had been created to implement the practice.

CHAPTER 4

THE END OF LIFE: MEDICAL CONSIDERATIONS

TRENDS IN CAUSES OF DEATH AND IN DEATH RATES

The public-health advances described in Chapter 1 have brought about a change in the primary causes of death in the United States. During the 19th and early 20th centuries infectious (communicable) diseases such as influenza, tuberculosis, and diphtheria (a potentially deadly upper respiratory infection) were leading causes of death. Vaccinations, antibiotics, increased public awareness, improved sanitation, and advances in treatment have eliminated or drastically circumscribed the effects of these conditions. Progress has also been made at reducing the fatality of chronic noninfectious conditions, such as heart disease, cancer (often referred to as "malignant neoplasms"), and chronic lower respiratory diseases, but the impact on their effects has been more modest. Thus, as rates of infectious diseases have fallen, chronic noninfectious diseases, although they are less likely to strike any given person in any given year, have come to account for a majority of deaths in the United States. (See Figure 4.1.)

As Figure 4.1 shows, in every year since the middle of the 20th century heart disease and cancer have accounted for half or more of all deaths in the United States; furthermore, heart disease, cancer, and stroke were among the five leading causes of death every year between 1935 and 2010. Some conditions appeared and then disappeared from the ranks of the five leading causes of death over this time. For example, kidney disease was among the five leading causes of death from 1935 to 1948; influenza and pneumonia were among the five leading causes from 1935 to 1945, in 1963, and between 1965 and 1978; and diseases of early infancy were among the five leading causes from 1949 to 1962 and in 1964. All of these conditions have since fallen out of the top five, due to the effectiveness of prevention and treatment. Meanwhile, chronic lower respiratory diseases appeared as one of the five leading causes in 1979 and has remained there in the decades since.

Table 4.1 shows the top 15 causes of death in 2011 for residents of the United States. Heart disease accounted for 596,339 deaths and cancer (malignant neoplasms) accounted for 575,313 deaths—making both conditions more than four times as deadly as the third-leading cause of death, chronic lower respiratory diseases (143,382). Strokes (cerebrovascular diseases; 128,931) and accidents (122,777) accounted for similar numbers of deaths. Alzheimer's disease, the sixth-leading cause of death in 2011, took the lives of 84,691 people, and diabetes took the lives of 73,282.

Not surprisingly, the leading causes of death vary by age. (See Table 4.2.) For the four youngest age groups (children between one and four years old, children five to 14 years old, young people 15 to 24 years old, and adults 25 to 44 years old) tracked by the U.S. Centers for Disease Control and Prevention, accidents were the leading cause of death in 2011. For each of these groups, however, the second-leading cause of death differed. Among those aged one to four years, birth defects (congenital malformations, deformations, and chromosomal abnormalities) were the second-leading cause of death; among those aged five to 14 years, cancer was the second-leading cause of death; among those aged 15 to 24 years, suicide was the second-leading cause of death (followed closely by homicide and cancer); and among those aged 25 to 44 years, cancer was the second-leading cause of death (followed closely by heart disease and suicide).

Older Americans' causes of death more closely tracked the overall national trends. This is unsurprising, because those aged 45 years and older accounted for approximately 2.3 million (93%) of the total 2.5 million deaths in 2011. (See Table 4.2.) Those over the age of

FIGURE 4.1

Percentage of all deaths due to five leading causes of death, by year, 1935–2010

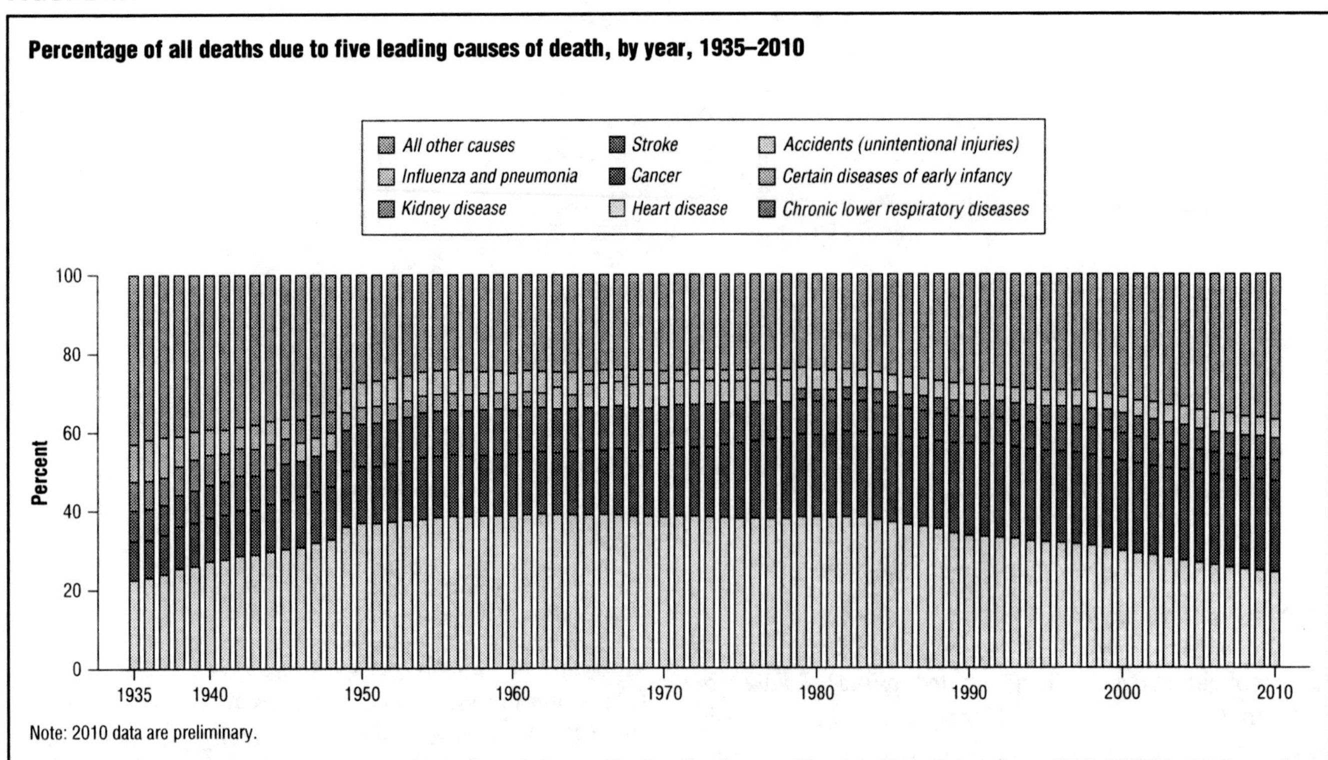

Note: 2010 data are preliminary.

SOURCE: Donna L. Hoyert, "Figure 2. Percentage of All Deaths Due to Five Leading Causes of Death by Year: United States, 1935–2010," in "75 Years of Mortality in the United States, 1935–2010," *NCHS Data Brief*, no. 88, Centers for Disease Control and Prevention, National Center for Health Statistics, March 2012, http://www.cdc.gov/nchs/data/databriefs/db88.pdf (accessed December 28, 2013)

65 years accounted for 1.8 million, or 72.8%, of total 2011 deaths. The two leading causes of death for adults aged 45 to 64 years were cancer and heart disease, in that order. The same causes of death were most common for adults aged 65 years and older, but for this age group heart disease was more common than cancer. Chronic lower respiratory disease, strokes, and Alzheimer's disease were much more common causes of death for the over-65 cohort than for any other age group.

Age-adjusted death rates differed significantly by sex, race, and ethnicity in the early 21st century. As Table 4.3 shows, the 2011 death rate for men was 874.5 deaths per 100,000 people, whereas the rate for women was 631.9. The death rate for African American men (1,067.3), however, far exceeded that of white men (869.3). Meanwhile, the death rate for African American women (740.1) exceeded that for white women (629.7) but was lower than that of white men. The infant mortality rate was much higher for African Americans (11.42 per 1,000 live births) than for whites (5.11).

These disparities translated into differences in life expectancy. Non-Hispanic African American men had the lowest life expectancy of any demographic subgroup between 2006 and 2011, followed by non-Hispanic white men. (See Figure 4.2.) Non-Hispanic African American women had a slightly lower life expectancy during this period than Hispanic men. Non-Hispanic white women had a life expectancy of over 80 years throughout this period, and Hispanic women had a life expectancy of over 83 years in 2011, the highest of any demographic subgroup in the United States.

As of 2011 there were also significant disparities in death rates by geography. As Table 4.4 shows, that year the age-adjusted death rate was highest in Mississippi (956.2 per 100,000 people), followed by West Virginia (953.3), Alabama (933.7), Kentucky (910.3), and Oklahoma (910.1). Of the 50 states, Hawaii (584.8) had the lowest age-adjusted death rate, followed by California (638.8), Minnesota (659.2), Connecticut (660.9), and New York (664.2).

LIFE-SUSTAINING TREATMENTS

As people succumb to the chronic, noninfectious diseases that are the leading causes of death in the United States, life-sustaining treatments, commonly called life support, are often used. Such treatments are not controversial when a patient suffers from a treatable illness, in which cases life support is a temporary measure used until the body can function on its own. Debate arises when life-sustaining treatments are used in cases involving the incurably ill and permanently unconscious.

TABLE 4.1

Death rates for the 15 leading causes of death, 2011, and percentage change, 2010–11

[Date are based on a continuous file of records received from the states. Rates are per 100,000 population age-adjusted rates per 100,000 U.S. standard population based on the year 2000 standard. Figures for 2011 are based on weighted data rounded to the nearest individual, so categories may not add to totals.]

				Age-adjusted death rate		
Rank[a]	Case of death (based on the *International Classification of Diseases, Tenth Revision*, 2008 Edition, 2009)	Number	Death rate	2011	2010	Percent change
—	All causes	2,512,873	806.5	740.6	747.0	−0.9
1	Diseases of heart (I00–I09, I11, I13, I20–I51)	596,339	191.4	173.7	179.1	−3.0
2	Malignant neoplasms (C00–C97)	575,313	184.6	168.6	172.8	−2.4
3	Chronic lower respiratory diseases (J40–J47)	143,382	46.0	42.7	42.2	1.2
4	Cerebrovascular diseases (I60–I69)	128,931	41.4	37.9	39.1	−3.1
5	Accidents (unintentional injuries) (V01–X59, Y85–Y86)[b, c]	122,777	39.4	38.0	38.0	0.0
6	Alzheimer's disease (G30)	84,691	27.2	24.6	25.1	−2.0
7	Diabetes mellitus (E10–E14)	73,282	23.5	21.5	20.8	3.4
8	Influenza and pneumonia (J09–J18)[d]	53,667	17.2	15.7	15.1	4.0
9	Nephritis, nephrotic syndrome and nephrosis (N00–N07, N17–N19, N25–N27)[e]	45,731	14.7	13.4	15.3	−12.4
10	Intentional self-harm (suicide) (U03, X60–X84, Y87.0)[b]	38,285	12.3	12.0	12.1	−0.8
11	Septicemia (A40–A41)	35,539	11.4	10.5	10.6	−0.9
12	Chronic liver disease and cirrhosis (K70, K73–K74)	33,539	10.8	9.7	9.4	3.2
13	Essential hypertension and hypertensive renal disease (I10, I12, I15)	27,477	8.8	8.0	8.0	0.0
14	Parkinson's disease (G20–G21)[f]	23,107	7.4	7.0	6.8	2.9
15	Pneumonitis due to solids and liquids (J69)	18,090	5.8	5.3	5.1	3.9
—	All other causes (residual)	512,723	164.6	—	—	—

—Category not applicable.
[a]Rank based on number of deaths.
[b]For unintentional injuries, suicides, preliminary and final data may differ significantly because of the truncated nature of the preliminary file.
[c]New ICD–10 subcategories were introduced for the existing X34 (Victim of earthquake).
[d]New ICD–10 code J12.3 (Human metapneumovirus pneumonia) was added to the category in 2011.
[e]New subcategories replaced previous ones for N18 (Chronic kidney disease) in 2011. Changes affect comparability with previous year's data.
[f]New ICD–10 code G21.4 (Vascular parkinsonism) was added to the category in 2011.
Notes: Data are subject to sampling and random variation. For information regarding the calculation of standard errors and further discussion of the variability of the data.

SOURCE: Donna L. Hoyert and Jiaquan Xu, "Table B. Deaths and Death Rates for 2011 and Age-Adjusted Death Rates and Percentage Changes in Age-Adjusted Rates from 2010 to 2011 for the 15 Leading Causes of Death in 2011: United States, Final 2010 and Preliminary 2011," in "Deaths: Preliminary Data for 2011," *National Vital Statistics Reports*, vol. 61, no. 6, October 10, 2012, http://www.cdc.gov/nchs/data/nvsr/nvsr61/nvsr61_06.pdf (accessed December 23, 2013)

These treatments prolong life, but they can also prolong the process of dying. In many cases, moreover, they may even add to a patient's suffering.

The following sections describe the types of life-sustaining medical interventions used in end-of-life care.

Cardiopulmonary Resuscitation

Traditional cardiopulmonary resuscitation (CPR) consists of two basic life-support skills that are administered in the event of cardiac or respiratory arrest: artificial circulation and artificial respiration. Cardiac arrest may be caused by a heart attack, which occurs when the blood flow to the heart is interrupted. A coronary artery that is clogged with an accumulation of fatty deposits is a common cause of interrupted blood flow to the heart. By contrast, respiratory arrest may be the result of an accident (such as drowning) or the final stages of a pulmonary disease (such as emphysema—a disease in which the alveoli [microscopic air sacs] of the lungs are destroyed).

In CPR, artificial circulation is accomplished by compressing the chest rhythmically to cause blood to flow sufficiently to give a person a chance for survival. Artificial respiration (rescue breathing) is accomplished by breathing into the victim's mouth. Research indicates that in the case of cardiac arrest, providing chest compressions alone is more effective than providing chest compressions and rescue breathing. Medical researchers have determined that taking the time to give rescue breaths to heart attack victims reduces the effectiveness of chest compressions, and effective chest compressions are vital in helping the heart retain its ability to beat after being shocked with a defibrillator (a device that delivers an electrical shock to the heart, hopefully causing it to restart). Nevertheless, if someone has experienced respiratory arrest, rescue breathing must be performed to keep that person alive until an ambulance arrives.

The American Heart Association (AHA) states in "Cardiac Arrest Statistics" (December 17, 2013, http://www.heart.org/HEARTORG/General/Cardiac-Arrest-Statistics_UCM_448311_Article.jsp) that survival rates differ significantly depending on whether one experiences cardiac arrest in a hospital or away from a hospital. Among the 359,400 instances of out-of-hospital cardiac arrest the AHA counted in 2013, CPR was performed

TABLE 4.2

Deaths and death rates for the 10 leading causes of death, by age group, 2011

[Data are based on a continuous file of records received from the states. Rates are per 100,000 population in specified group. Figures for 2011 are based on weighted data rounded to the nearest individual, so categories may not add to totals or subtotals.]

Rank[a]	Cause of death	Number	Rate
All ages[b]			
—	All causes	2,512,873	806.5
1	Diseases of heart	596,339	191.4
2	Malignant neoplasms	575,313	184.6
3	Chronic lower respiratory diseases	143,382	46.0
4	Cerebrovascular diseases	128,931	41.4
5	Accidents (unintentional injuries)	122,777	39.4
—	Motor vehicle accidents	34,676	11.1
—	All other accidents	88,101	28.3
6	Alzheimer's disease	84,691	27.2
7	Diabetes mellitus	73,282	23.5
8	Influenza and pneumonia	53,667	17.2
9	Nephritis, nephrotic syndrome and nephrosis	45,731	14.7
10	Intentional self-harm (suicide)	38,285	12.3
—	All other causes		208.8
1–4 years			
—	All causes	4,214	26.1
1	Accidents (unintentional injuries)	1,346	8.3
—	Motor vehicle accidents	416	2.6
—	All other accidents	930	5.8
2	Congenital malformations, deformations and chromosomal abnormalities	483	3.0
3	Assault (homicide)	370	2.3
4	Malignant neoplasms	352	2.2
5	Diseases of heart	158	1.0
6	Influenza and pneumonia	96	0.6
7	Septicemia	59	0.4
8	Chronic lower respiratory diseases	44	0.3
9	In situ neoplasms, benign neoplasms and neoplasms of uncertain or unknown behavior	43	0.3
9	Cerebrovascular diseases	43	0.3
—	All other causes	1,220	7.5
5–14 years			
—	All causes	5,395	13.1
1	Accidents (unintentional injuries)	1,613	3.9
—	Motor vehicle accidents	867	2.1
—	All other accidents	746	1.8
2	Malignant neoplasms	865	2.1
3	Congenital malformations, deformations and chromosomal abnormalities	356	0.9
4	Intentional self harm (suicide)	281	0.7
5	Assault (homicide)	269	0.7
6	Diseases of heart	185	0.5
7	Chronic lower respiratory diseases	134	0.3
8	Influenza and pneumonia	112	0.3
9	Cerebrovascular diseases	83	0.2
10	In situ neoplasms, benign neoplasms and neoplasms of uncertain or unknown behavior	72	0.2
—	All other causes	1,425	3.5
15–24 years			
—	All causes	29,605	67.6
1	Accidents (unintentional injuries)	12,032	27.5
—	Motor vehicle accidents	6,984	15.9
—	All other accidents	5,048	11.5
2	Intentional self harm (suicide)	4,688	10.7
3	Assault (homicide)	4,508	10.3
4	Malignant neoplasms	1,609	3.7
5	Diseases of heart	948	2.2
6	Congenital malformations, deformations and chromosomal abnormalities	429	1.0
7	Influenza and pneumonia	213	0.5
8	Cerebrovascular diseases	186	0.4
9	Pregnancy, childbirth and the puerperium	166	0.4
10	Chronic lower respiratory diseases	160	0.4
—	All other causes	4,666	10.7

by bystanders in 40.1% of cases and the overall survival rate was 9.5%. By comparison, among the 209,000 instances of cardiac arrest that occurred in hospitals (where CPR and other life-saving techniques were routinely used), the overall survival rate was 23.9% for adults and 40.2% for children.

The low survival rate for those who experience cardiac arrest away from a hospital is to a substantial degree attributable to the fact that less than half of all such people receive CPR. Steven M. Bradley and Tom D. Rea suggest in "Improving Bystander

TABLE 4.2

Deaths and death rates for the 10 leading causes of death, by age group, 2011 [CONTINUED]

[Data are based on a continuous file of records received from the states. Rates are per 100,000 population in specified group. Figures for 2011 are based on weighted data rounded to the nearest individual, so categories may not add to totals or subtotals.]

Rank[a]	Cause of death	Number	Rate
25–44 years			
—	All causes	113,341	137.5
1	Accidents (unintentional injuries)	29,424	35.7
—	Motor vehicle accidents	10,181	12.4
—	All other accidents	19,243	23.3
2	Malignant neoplasms	15,210	18.5
3	Diseases of heart	13,479	16.4
4	Intentional self harm (suicide)	12,269	14.9
5	Assault (homicide)	6,639	8.1
6	Chronic liver disease and cirrhosis	2,919	3.5
7	Diabetes mellitus	2,474	3.0
8	Human immunodeficiency virus (HIV) disease	2,262	2.7
9	Cerebrovascular diseases	2,245	2.7
10	Influenza and pneumonia	1,341	1.6
—	All other causes	25,079	30.4
45–64 years			
—	All causes	505,730	610.9
1	Malignant neoplasms	161,072	194.6
2	Diseases of heart	105,013	126.9
3	Accidents (unintentional injuries)	34,621	41.8
—	Motor vehicle accidents	9,701	11.7
—	All other accidents	24,920	30.1
4	Chronic lower respiratory diseases	19,646	23.7
5	Chronic liver disease and cirrhosis	19,551	23.6
6	Diabetes mellitus	18,548	22.4
7	Cerebrovascular diseases	16,848	20.4
8	Intentional self harm (suicide)	14,852	17.9
9	Septicemia	7,365	8.9
10	Nephritis, nephrotic syndrome and nephrosis	6,758	8.2
—	All other causes	101,456	122.6
65 years and over			
—	All causes	1,830,553	4,422.3
1	Diseases of heart	476,220	1,150.5
2	Malignant neoplasms	396,126	957.0
3	Chronic lower respiratory diseases	122,381	295.6
4	Cerebrovascular diseases	109,393	264.3
5	Alzheimer's disease	83,746	202.3
6	Diabetes mellitus	52,068	125.8
7	Influenza and pneumonia	45,321	109.5
8	Accidents (unintentional injuries)	42,635	103.0
	Motor vehicle accidents	6,432	15.5
—	All other accidents	36,203	87.5
9	Nephritis, nephrotic syndrome and nephrosis	37,927	91.6
10	Septicemia	26,596	64.3
—	All other causes	438,140	1,058.5

—Category not applicable.
[a]Rank based on number of deaths.
[b]Includes deaths under age 1 year.
Notes: For certain causes of death such as unintentional injuries, homicides, suicides, and respiratory diseases, preliminary and final data differ because of the truncated nature of the preliminary file. Data are subject to sampling or random variation.

SOURCE: Donna L. Hoyert and Jiaquan Xu, "Table 7. Deaths and Death Rates for the 10 Leading Causes of Death in Specified Age Groups: United States, Preliminary 2011," in "Deaths: Preliminary Data for 2011," *National Vital Statistics Reports*, vol. 61, no. 6, October 10, 2012, http://www.cdc.gov/nchs/data/nvsr/nvsr61/nvsr61_06.pdf (accessed December 23, 2013)

Cardiopulmonary Resuscitation" (*Current Opinion in Critical Care*, vol. 17, no. 3, June 2011) that changing the emphasis in CPR education to focus on chest compressions alone in cases of heart attack would likely save lives, since it is easier for a bystander to administer chest compressions without rescue breathing when he or she notices a person who is unconscious and not breathing normally.

REFUSAL OF CPR WITH A DO-NOT-RESUSCITATE ORDER. CPR is intended for generally healthy individuals who unexpectedly suffer a heart attack or other trauma, such as drowning. Usually, following CPR, survivors eventually resume a normal life. Outcomes are quite different, understandably, for patients who suffer cardiac arrest in the final stages of a terminal illness. In "Life-Support Interventions at the End of Life: Unintended

TABLE 4.3

Deaths, death rates, and life expectancy at birth by race and sex, and infant deaths and mortality rates by race, 2010–11

[Data are based on a continuous file of records received from the states. Figures for 2011 are based on weighted data rounded to the nearest individual, so categories may not add to totals.]

	All races[a]		White[b]		Black[b]	
Measure and sex	**2011**	**2010**	**2011**	**2010**	**2011**	**2010**
All deaths	2,513,171	2,468,435	2,153,864	2,114,749	290,135	286,959
Male	1,253,716	1,232,432	1,070,817	1,051,514	146,843	145,802
Female	1,259,456	1,236,003	1,083,046	1,063,235	143,292	141,157
Age-adjusted death rate[c]	740.6	747.0	738.1	741.8	877.4	898.2
Male	874.5	887.1	869.3	878.5	1,067.3	1,104.0
Female	631.9	634.9	629.7	630.8	740.1	752.5
Life expectancy at birth (in years)	78.7	78.7	79.0	78.9	75.3	75.1
Male	76.3	76.2	76.6	76.5	72.1	71.8
Female	81.1	81.0	81.3	81.3	78.2	78.0
All infant deaths	23,910	24,586	15,438	15,954	7,234	7,401
Infant mortality rate[d]	6.05	6.15	5.11	5.20	11.42	11.63

[a]Includes races other than white and black.
[b]Race categories are consistent with the 1977 Office of Management and Budget (OMB) standards. Multiple-race data were reported for deaths by 38 states and the District of Columbia in 2011 and by 37 states and the District of Columbia in 2010, and were reported for births (used as the denominator in computing infant mortality rates), by 40 states and the District of Columbia in 2011 and by 38 states and the District of Columbia in 2010. The multiple-race data for these reporting areas were bridged to the single-race categories of the 1977 OMB standards for comparability with other reporting areas.
[c]Age-adjusted death rates are per 100,000 U.S. standard population, based on the year 2000 standard.
[d]Infant mortality rates are deaths under age 1 year per 1,000 live births in specified group.

SOURCE: Donna L. Hoyert and Jiaquan Xu, "Table A. Deaths, Age-Adjusted Death Rates, and Life Expectancy at Birth, by Race and Sex; and Infant Deaths and Mortality Rates, by Race: United States, Final 2010 and Preliminary 2011," in "Deaths: Preliminary Data for 2011," *National Vital Statistics Reports*, vol. 61, no. 6, October 10, 2012, http://www.cdc.gov/nchs/data/nvsr/nvsr61/nvsr61_06.pdf (accessed December 23, 2013)

Consequences" (*American Journal of Nursing*, vol. 110, no. 1, January 2010), Shirley A. Scott of the Orlando Regional Medical Center in Orlando, Florida, notes that "fewer than 5% of terminally ill patients survive CPR to leave the hospital. Even if they do survive, they may require mechanical ventilation indefinitely. Depending on how long a patient's brain was deprived of oxygen, there may be brain damage significant enough to result in coma or leave the patient in a persistent vegetative state. Quality of life may be considerably diminished, and the prolonged dying process will likely add to the stress the family is already experiencing." Scott adds that during CPR a dying patient may experience a broken rib or ribs, which can puncture the lungs and necessitate the insertion of a chest tube. The chest tube is usually uncomfortable and is a common site of infection. CPR may also result in a ruptured liver or spleen, which would require surgery.

A terminally ill person not wishing to be resuscitated in case of cardiac or respiratory arrest may ask a physician to write a do-not-resuscitate (DNR) order on his or her medical chart. This written order instructs health care personnel not to initiate CPR. Even if a patient's living will (a written document outlining one's wishes regarding medical and end-of-life care and granting decision-making authority to others in the case that the patient becomes incapacitated) includes refusal of CPR, emergency personnel hurrying to respond to a heart attack or other incident may be unable to check a living will before initiating the procedure. This underscores the necessity of having the DNR order noted on the chart.

NONHOSPITAL DNR ORDERS. People who do not want CPR performed in case of an emergency that occurs away from a hospital can request a nonhospital DNR order from their physician. Also called a prehospital DNR order, it instructs emergency medical personnel to withhold CPR. The DNR order may be on a bracelet or necklace or on a wallet card. While this is the best method of ensuring that one's end-of-life wishes are carried out in a nonhospital setting, there is no guarantee that bystanders will not perform CPR in contravention of a DNR order. Laypeople cannot be held liable for performing CPR on an individual with a nonhospital DNR order.

Mechanical Ventilation

When a patient's lungs are not functioning properly, a ventilator (or respirator) can breath for the patient. Most ventilators are positive-pressure ventilators. That is, they deliver gas under pressure to the patient's lungs. The pressure is relieved when gas is exhaled via an exhalation pathway. Negative-pressure ventilators, known colloquially as iron lungs, were common prior to the 1960s. They are tank-shaped devices that enclose much of a patient's body. By lowering air pressure inside the machine a patient's chest could be made to expand, drawing air into their lungs. Increasing pressure in the iron lung would then force the lungs to compress and cause the air to be exhaled. Iron lungs were largely phased out with the rise of positive-pressure ventilators, which do not obstruct patients' movements, or doctors' and nurses' ability to examine their bodies, nearly as much. In positive-pressure ventilators, oxygen is supplied to the lungs via a tube that is inserted through the mouth or

FIGURE 4.2

Life expectancy at birth, by race, Hispanic origin, and sex, 2006–11

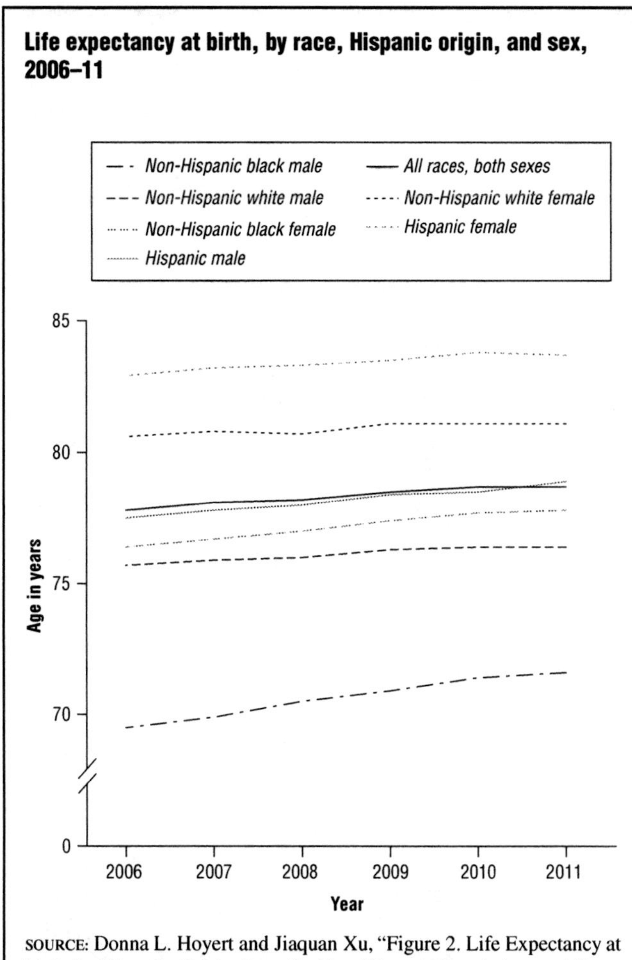

SOURCE: Donna L. Hoyert and Jiaquan Xu, "Figure 2. Life Expectancy at birth, by Hispanic Origin, Race for Non-Hispanic Population, and Sex: United States, 2006–2010 Final and 2011 Preliminary," in "Deaths: Preliminery Data for 2011," *National Vital Statistics Reports*, vol. 61, no. 6, October 10, 2012, http://www.cdc.gov/nchs/data/nvsr/nvsr61/nvsr61_06.pdf (accessed December 23, 2013)

nose into the windpipe. Mechanical ventilation is generally used to temporarily maintain normal breathing in those who have been in serious accidents or who suffer from a serious illness, such as pneumonia. In some cases, if the patient needs ventilation indefinitely, the physician might perform a tracheotomy to open a hole in the neck for placement of the breathing tube in the windpipe.

Ventilators are also used on terminally ill patients. In these cases the machine keeps the patient breathing but does nothing to cure the disease. Once ventilation is started, it raises the question of when ventilation will be stopped. Those preparing a living will are advised to give clear instructions about their desires regarding continued use of an artificial respirator that could prolong the process of dying.

Artificial Nutrition and Hydration

Artificial nutrition and hydration (ANH) is another medical technology that has complicated the dying process. It is a process where nutrients and fluids are supplied to a patient intravenously or through a stomach or intestinal tube, fully meeting the nutritional and hydration needs of people who are either not capable of, or interested in, eating and drinking normally. This can save the life of someone who is temporarily unable to eat or drink because of illness or injury; it can also meet the nutritional needs of permanently comatose or terminally ill patients who would otherwise die.

ANH has a strong emotional impact because it relates to basic sustenance. The prospect of withholding food and water from a loved one can be so powerful that even families who know that the patient would not want to be kept alive may still struggle to fulfill his or her wishes. However, as the National Hospital and Palliative Care Organization explains in "Artificial Nutrition (Food) and Hydration (Fluids) at the End of Life" (2010, http://www.caringinfo.org/files/public/brochures/Artificial NutritionAndHydration.pdf), it is often not as cruel as it might seem to stop ANH. The organization reports that appetite loss is common in dying patients and that the withdrawal of ANH does not prolong death or make it more painful. By contrast, continuing ANH for a patient whose body is shutting down in preparation for death can increase discomfort. The Academy of Nutrition and Dietetics supports this view of ANH, as Julie O'Sullivan Maillet, Denise Baird Schwartz, and Mary Ellen Posthauer write in "Position of the Academy of Nutrition and Dietetics: Ethical and Legal Issues in Feeding and Hydration" (*Journal of the Academy of Nutrition and Dietetics*, vol. 113, no. 6, June 2013). The researchers state that "loss of appetite is common with terminally ill individuals and it does not reduce quality of life except for reducing the enjoyment of food. Withholding or minimizing hydration can have the desirable effect of reducing disturbing oral and bronchial secretions, and reduced cough from diminished pulmonary congestion. Withholding nutrition has been studied closely and the majority of reports indicate that physiological adaptation allows individuals not to suffer from the absence of food."

ANH has traditionally been used in end-of-life care when patients experience a loss of appetite and difficulty swallowing. Health care practitioners use ANH to prolong life, prevent aspiration pneumonia (inflammation of the lungs due to inhaling food particles or fluid), maintain independence and physical function, and decrease suffering and discomfort. However, ANH does not always accomplish these goals. Tube feeding does not always prolong life, and insertion or placement of the tube can result in complications that themselves cause death. Neither does ANH always protect against aspiration pneumonia.

Kidney Dialysis

Kidney dialysis is a medical procedure in which a machine takes over the function of the kidneys, removing waste products from the bloodstream. Dialysis can be

TABLE 4.4

Deaths, death rates, and age-adjusted death rates, by state and territory, 2010–11

[By place of residence. Data are based on a continuous file of records received from the states. Rates are per 100,000 population. Age-adjusted rates are per 100,000 U.S. standard population. Figures for 2011 are based on weighted data rounded to the nearest individual, so categories may not add to totals.]

	2011			2010		
Area	Number	Rate	Age-adjusted rate	Number	Rate	Age-adjusted rate
United States*	2,513,171	806.6	740.6	2,468,435	799.5	747.0
Alabama	48,683	1,013.7	933.7	48,038	1,005.0	939.7
Alaska	3,849	532.6	747.9	3,728	524.9	771.5
Arizona	48,381	746.3	688.9	46,762	731.6	693.1
Arkansas	29,632	1,008.6	894.6	28,916	991.7	892.7
California	238,993	634.1	638.8	234,012	628.2	646.7
Colorado	32,563	636.4	677.8	31,465	625.6	682.7
Connecticut	29,548	825.2	660.9	28,692	802.8	652.9
Delaware	7,840	864.3	763.4	7,706	858.2	769.9
District of Columbia	4,589	742.6	756.0	4,672	776.4	792.4
Florida	173,961	912.8	677.1	173,791	924.4	701.1
Georgia	70,401	717.3	806.2	71,263	735.6	845.4
Hawaii	9,921	721.6	584.8	9,617	707.0	589.6
Idaho	12,026	758.7	744.9	11,429	729.1	731.6
Illinois	101,898	791.8	737.3	99,931	778.8	736.9
Indiana	58,195	893.0	825.0	56,743	875.2	820.6
Iowa	28,184	920.4	722.7	27,745	910.8	721.7
Kansas	25,119	874.8	767.2	24,502	858.8	762.2
Kentucky	42,624	975.5	910.3	41,983	967.5	915.0
Louisiana	40,680	889.2	882.1	40,667	897.1	903.8
Maine	13,031	981.1	749.5	12,750	959.8	749.6
Maryland	43,750	750.6	715.9	43,325	750.4	728.6
Massachusetts	53,699	815.2	676.1	52,583	803.1	675.0
Michigan	89,496	906.2	784.2	88,021	890.6	786.2
Minnesota	39,822	745.1	659.2	38,972	734.8	661.5
Mississippi	29,278	983.0	956.2	28,965	976.1	962.0
Missouri	55,813	928.6	811.4	55,281	923.1	819.5
Montana	9,117	913.3	760.7	8,827	892.1	754.7
Nebraska	15,477	839.9	719.8	15,171	830.7	717.8
Nevada	20,340	746.9	789.6	19,623	726.6	795.4
New Hampshire	10,821	820.9	710.0	10,201	774.9	690.4
New Jersey	70,553	799.8	690.6	69,495	790.4	691.1
New Mexico	16,434	789.3	748.0	15,931	773.7	749.0
New York	148,903	765.0	664.2	146,432	755.7	665.5
North Carolina	79,875	827.2	790.8	78,773	826.1	804.9
North Dakota	5,964	872.0	697.3	5,944	883.7	704.3
Ohio	111,444	965.3	822.0	108,711	942.3	815.7
Oklahoma	37,142	979.6	910.1	36,529	973.8	915.5
Oregon	32,786	846.8	724.1	31,890	832.4	723.1
Pennsylvania	128,290	1,006.8	776.1	124,596	980.9	765.9
Rhode Island	9,585	911.7	707.6	9,579	910.1	721.7
South Carolina	42,093	899.6	839.9	41,614	899.7	854.8
South Dakota	7,313	887.4	720.4	7,100	872.0	715.1
Tennessee	60,544	945.5	879.1	59,578	938.8	890.8
Texas	168,643	656.8	751.6	166,527	662.3	772.3
Utah	15,265	541.8	699.0	14,776	534.6	703.2
Vermont	5,434	867.5	711.0	5,380	859.8	718.7
Virginia	60,807	751.0	741.6	59,032	737.8	741.6
Washington	49,692	727.6	690.4	48,146	716.0	692.3
West Virginia	21,868	1,178.6	953.3	21,275	1,148.1	933.6
Wisconsin	48,419	847.7	721.3	47,308	831.9	719.0
Wyoming	4,387	772.1	754.6	4,438	787.4	778.8
Puerto Rico	29,641	799.7	708.7	29,153	783.3	712.8
Virgin Islands	—	—	—	715	672.8	663.2
Guam	825	516.9	756.1	857	537.5	810.6
American Samoa	276	500.0	1,090.3	224	403.8	932.9
Northern Marianas	—	—	—	174	325.1	863.3

—Data not available.
*Excludes data for Puerto Rico, Virgin Islands, Guam, American Samoa, and Northern Marianas.
Note: Data are subject to sampling or random variation.

SOURCE: Donna L. Hoyert and Jiaquan Xu, "Table 3. Deaths, Death Rates, and Age-Adjusted Death Rates: United States, and Each State and Territory, Final 2010 and Preliminary 2011," in "Deaths: Preliminary Data for 2011," *National Vital Statistics Reports*, vol. 61, no. 6, October 10, 2012, http://www.cdc.gov/nchs/data/nvsr/nvsr61/nvsr61_06.pdf (accessed December 23, 2013)

used when an illness or injury temporarily impairs kidney function. It may also be used by patients with irreversibly damaged kidneys who are awaiting organ transplantation.

Kidney failure may also occur as an end stage of a terminal illness. In such cases, dialysis may cleanse the body of waste products, but it cannot cure the disease.

Dialysis patients may suffer from various side effects, including chemical imbalances in the body, low blood pressure, nausea and vomiting, headache, itching, and fatigue. Dialysis must be performed several times a week in the absence of functioning kidneys. Those terminally ill patients who wish to let their illness take its course may choose to stop dialysis. Death might follow within a day, or the patient might live for several weeks more, depending on the state of the kidneys and the patient's underlying health. As waste products build up in the body, the patient may experience drowsiness, difficulty breathing, and fluid weight gain. In most cases doctors can help such patients manage their discomfort as the body approaches death.

DISORDERS OF CONSCIOUSNESS

A coma is a deep state of unconsciousness that is caused by damage to the brain, often from illness or trauma. The patient is neither awake nor aware; his or her eyes are always closed. A coma rarely lasts for more than one month, and most people in a coma recover quickly, die, or progress to a vegetative state within that time.

Most often, patients who do not recover quickly from a coma progress to a vegetative/unresponsive state: they experience periods of wakefulness (eyes open) but without awareness. Those in a vegetative/unresponsive state for one month are then considered to be in a persistent vegetative state, and eventually, if they remain unresponsive, they are considered to be in a permanent vegetative state/unresponsive wakefulness state (PVS/UWS). The word *permanent* intentionally refers to the absence of any medical grounds for believing that there is a chance of recovery.

PVS/UWS patients are unaware of themselves or their surroundings. They do not respond to stimuli, understand language, or have control of bowel and bladder functions. They may intermittently open their eyes but are not conscious—a condition often referred to as eyes-open unconsciousness.

Some PVS/UWS patients do recover and regain partial consciousness. This condition is called a minimally conscious state (MCS). The perception of the minimally conscious patient is severely altered, but the patient is awake and shows an awareness of self or the environment, exhibiting behaviors such as following simple commands and smiling or crying at appropriate times. Some patients eventually emerge from an MCS, while some remain in an MCS permanently. Table 4.5 lists the criteria for the diagnosis of an MCS.

Locked-in syndrome is another disorder of consciousness that can occur after a coma. In this rare condition, the patient is awake and has full consciousness, but all the voluntary muscles of the body are paralyzed except (usually) for those that control vertical eye movement and blinking. People with locked-in syndrome communicate primarily with eye or eyelid movements.

TABLE 4.5

Criteria for a minimally conscious state (MCS)

Impaired responsiveness
Limited by perceptible awareness of surroundings or self evidenced by one or more of the following:

MCS−	MCS+
Following someone with the eyes	Following commands
Crying or smiling appropriately to emotional stimuli	Using words understandably
Localization of unpleasant stimuli	Non-functional communication

MCS− = low-level behavioral responses.
MCS+ = high-level behavioral responses.

SOURCE: Created by Sandra Alters for Gale, © 2014

In "From Unresponsive Wakefulness to Minimally Conscious PLUS and Functional Locked-In Syndromes: Recent Advances in Our Understanding of Disorders of Consciousness" (*Journal of Neurology*, vol. 258, no. 7, July 2011), Marie-Aurélie Bruno et al. propose splitting the category of MCS into MCS+ (high-level behavioral responses) and MCS− (low-level behavioral responses). High-level behavioral responses include following commands and saying words that are understandable. (See Table 4.5.) Low-level behavioral responses include following someone with the eyes and smiling or crying appropriately to emotional stimuli. A person with MCS+ can exhibit lower-level behaviors as well as higher-level behaviors.

PVS/UWS and MCS patients cannot, of course, make decisions about their own health care. Many of the highest-profile court cases and public controversies surrounding end-of-life care have involved individuals with these conditions, in some cases pitting different family members against one another in their attempts to determine what is best for their loved one, and in other cases pitting family members against the state or politicians. One of the reasons that most health care professionals urge individuals to create a living will or advance directive is to spare their loved ones the heartache and stress associated with making life-and-death decisions in cases like these.

ORGAN TRANSPLANTATION

Most organ and tissue donations are from the bodies of people who are deceased. In particular, people who have suffered a brain injury and subsequent brain death often have other healthy bodily organs that may be successfully donated to patients in need. In these cases, once death is pronounced the body is kept on mechanical support (if possible) to maintain the organs until it is determined whether the person will be a donor. In addition, living people may donate a kidney; parts of a lung, liver, or pancreas; or bone marrow. Most living donors make their donations to help a family member or close friend. Whatever their source, donated organs must usually be transplanted within six to 48 hours of harvest, although some tissue may be stored for future use.

Organ transplantation has come a long way since the first kidney was transplanted from one identical twin to another in 1954. The introduction in 1983 of cyclosporine, an immunosuppressant drug that helps prevent the body's immune system from rejecting a donated organ, made it possible to successfully transplant a variety of organs and tissues.

Figure 4.3 shows the organs and tissues that are transplantable with 21st-century immunosuppressant drugs and technologies. The organs that may be donated and transplanted include the heart, intestines, kidneys, liver, lungs, and pancreas. One person who dies in conditions conducive to organ donation can save the lives of up to eight people. Transplantable tissues include blood vessels, bone, cartilage, corneas, heart valves, ligaments, middle ears, skin, and tendons. These tissues can be used in a variety of ways, such as the repair of hearts or connective tissues, or the restoration of sight or hearing.

FIGURE 4.3

Transplantable organs and tissue

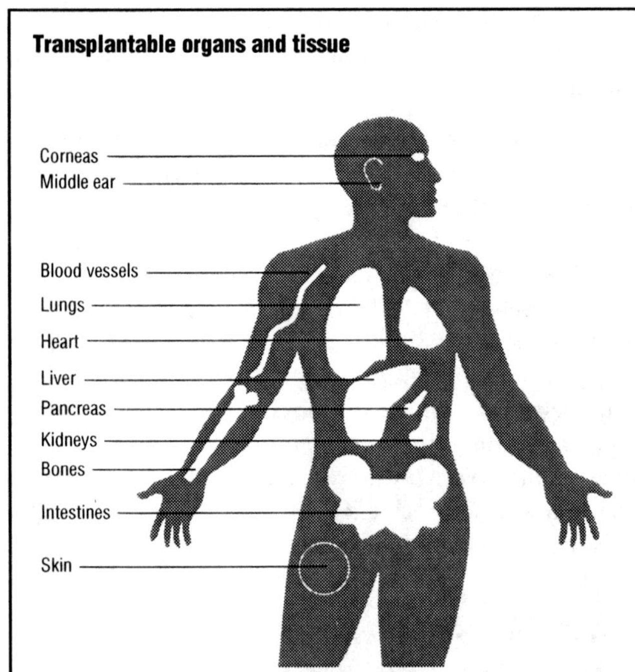

SOURCE: "Through Organ Donation, One Person Can Save up to Eight Lives. Those Who Donate Tissue Can Enhance the Lives of Many More," in "The Gift of Life," U.S. Department of Health and Human Services, Health Resources and Services Administration, October 2012, http://organdonor.gov/images/pdfs/giftoflifegeneralbrochure.pdf (accessed December 27, 2013)

TABLE 4.6

Median wait time for organ donation, by organ needed, 2013

Organ	Median national waiting time
Hearts	113 days
Lungs	141 days
Livers	361 days
Kidneys	1,219 days
Pancreata	260 days
Intestine	159 days

SOURCE: "Organ Transplantation: The Process," in *Organdonor.gov*, U.S. Department of Health and Human Services, 2013, http://organdonor.gov/about/transplantationprocess.html (accessed December 27, 2013)

While tissue donation does not save lives, it can immeasurably improve life for many people in addition to the recipients of organs.

Soon after organ transplantation began, the demand for donor organs exceeded the supply. In 1984 Congress passed the National Organ Transplant Act to create "a centralized network to match scarce donated organs with critically ill patients." In the 21st century organ transplant is an accepted medical treatment for a number of end-stage illnesses, but many people who might see their lives extended through transplants do not live long enough to receive the organs that they need. As Table 4.6 shows, the median time spent on waiting lists varies by the organ needed. Those in need of heart transplants typically see the shortest wait times, followed by those in need of lung and intestines transplants. The median wait time for recipients of pancreas transplants was 260 days as of 2013, and the median wait time for those in need of liver transplants was almost a year. Kidneys were the organs in most demand nationally, with the median wait time for a new kidney surpassing three years.

The U.S. Department of Health and Human Services (HHS) reports in "The Gift of Life" (2012, http://organdonor.gov/images/pdfs/giftoflifegeneralbrochure.pdf) that in 2012 more than 100 million people in the United States were registered organ donors. Very few people die from brain injuries or from other causes that make donation possible, however. The number of people in need of transplanted organs has for decades grown faster than the number of donors, creating conditions of permanent shortage and long waiting lists for those who need transplants. Figure 4.4 shows the widening gap between the number of people in need of transplants and the number of donors between 1989 and 2011. In 2011 there were 14,147 donors, who accounted for 28,535 transplants. That same year 113,754 people in need of transplants remained on waiting lists. HHS's Organ Procurement and Transplantation Network reports on its website (http://optn.transplant.hrsa.gov/latestData/rptData.asp) that as of January 2014 there were 120,839 people on the

FIGURE 4.4

The number of transplant donors, recipients, and people on transplant waiting list, 1989–2011

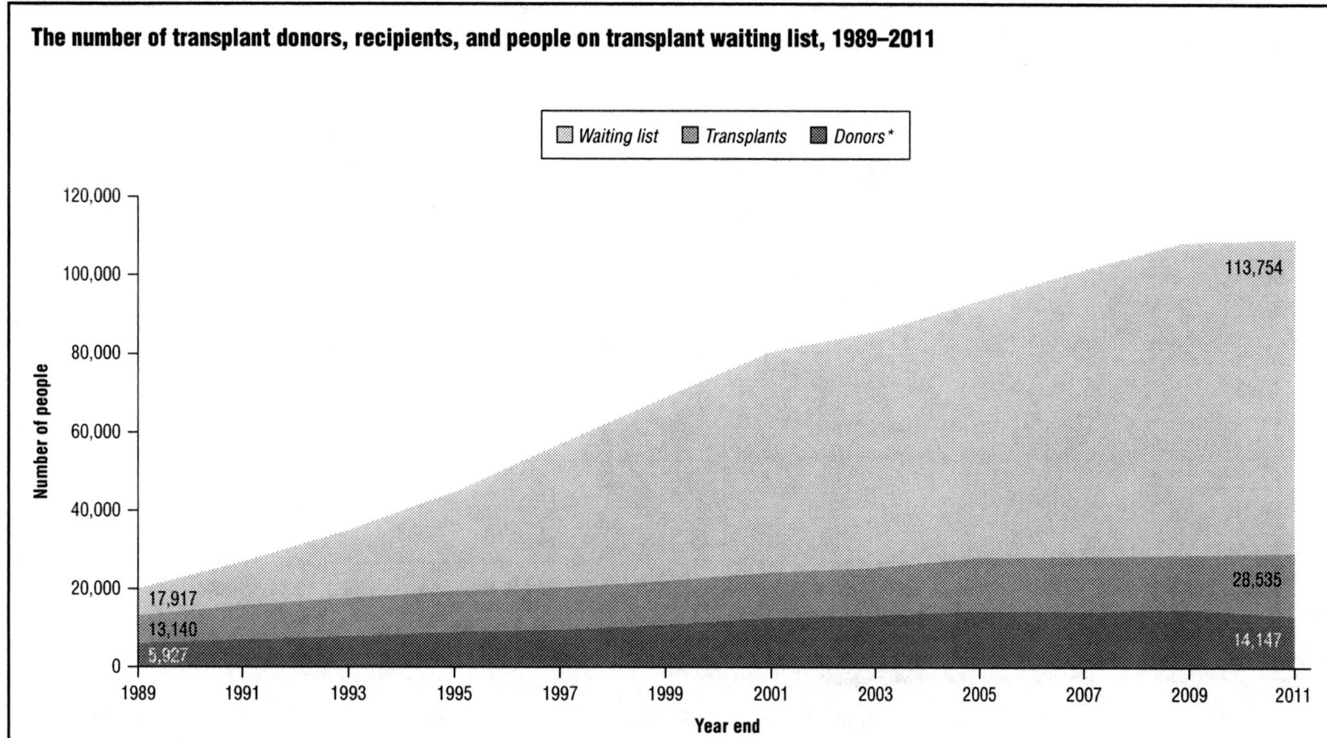

*Data include deceased and living donors. A donor may be able to donate more than one organ.

SOURCE: "The Gap Continues to Widen," in *The Gift of Life*, U.S. Department of Health and Human Services, Health Resources and Services Administration, October 2012, http://organdonor.gov/images/pdfs/giftoflifegeneralbrochure.pdf (accessed December 27, 2013)

TABLE 4.7

Transplant candidates on waiting list for organs, by organ needed, January 2014*

All*	**120,856**
Kidney	98,983
Pancreas	1,165
Kidney/pancreas	2,026
Liver	15,666
Intestine	249
Heart	3,720
Lung	1,595
Heart/lung	46

*All candidates will be less than the sum due to candidates waiting for multiple organs.
Note: Data current as of January 20, 2014.

SOURCE: "Waiting List Candidates as of Today 8:09 p.m.," in *Data*, U.S. Department of Health and Human Services, Health Resources and Services Administration, Organ Procurement and Transplantation Network, January 20, 2014, http://optn.transplant.hrsa.gov/data/default.asp (accessed December 27, 2013)

transplant waiting list in the United States. As Table 4.7 shows, 98,983 (81.9%) of these people were waiting for kidney transplants. Another 13% (15,666) of those on the waiting list were in need of liver transplants, and 3.1% (1,595) were waiting for heart transplants. Smaller numbers of people needed lung, pancreas, or intestines transplants, or a combination of kidney/pancreas or heart/lung transplants.

Although people in need of donated kidneys and livers typically spent the longest time on transplant waiting lists, as of 2011 these were also the types of transplant that were performed most often. (See Figure 4.5.) The number of kidney transplants performed annually grew significantly between 1998 and 2011, from approximately 13,000 to over 17,000, while the number of liver transplants performed grew more gradually, from just under 5,000 to just over 6,000. The number of heart transplants fluctuated during this period and remained flat overall, as did the number of pancreas and intestine transplants. Lung transplants became significantly more common.

As Table 4.8 shows, the total number of organ donors fluctuated only slightly between 2003 and 2012, from a low of 13,285 in 2003 to a high of 14,750 in 2006. The total for 2012, 14,010, was the second lowest during this period. The number of living donors—almost all of whom donated kidneys in each year for which data were available—dropped during this period, from 6,828 in 2003 to 5,867 in 2012. The number of deceased donors increased from 6,457 in 2003 to 8,143 in 2012.

Among the 8,143 deceased donors in 2012, the most common causes of death were stroke or aneurysm (2,833), head trauma (2,627), and anoxia (lack of oxygen, 2,436 deaths). (See Table 4.9.) The numbers of donors

FIGURE 4.5

Transplants performed during the year, by organ, 1998–2011

[All ages.]

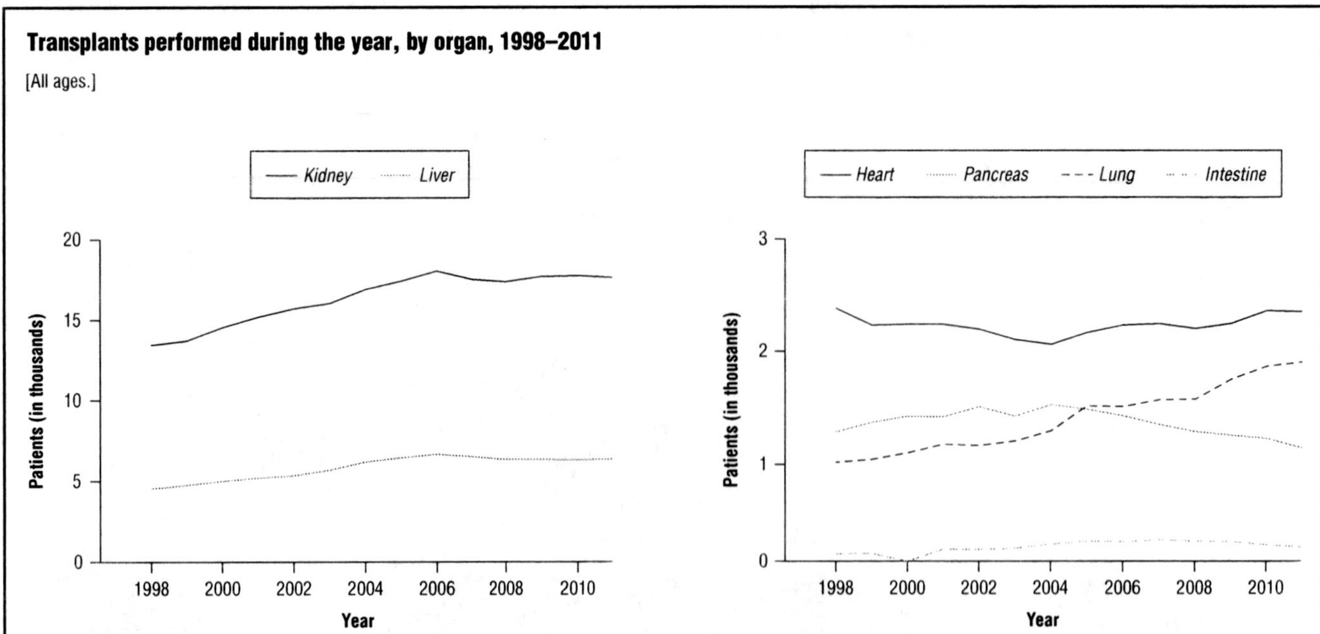

Notes: Kidney: Patients receiving a kidney-alone or simultaneous kidney-pancreas transplant. Lung: Patients receiving a lung-alone or simultaneous heart-lung transplant. Other organs: Patients receiving a transplant. Retransplants are counted.

SOURCE: "INT 2. Transplants Performed during the Year (Adult & Pediatric Combined)," in *United States Organ Transplantation: OPTN & SRTR Annual Data Report 2011*, U.S. Department of Health and Human Services, Health Resources and Services Administration, December 2012, http://srtr.transplant .hrsa.gov/annual_reports/2011/pdf/2011_SRTR_ADR.pdf (accessed December 27, 2013)

whose deaths were caused by stroke or head trauma remained relatively consistent between 2003 and 2012, whereas the number of donors who died from anoxia grew significantly during this period. Many anoxia deaths are likely caused by either drowning or by heart attacks in which the victims were revived after a lack of circulation or respiration had caused brain death. Motor vehicle accidents, gunshot wounds, and falls or blows to the head are common causes of fatal head trauma. Strokes and aneurysms can occur for a variety of reasons. People who die as a result of these causes frequently experience brain death although much of the body remains functional, making them good prospects for organ donation.

In spite of the tremendous good that deceased organ donors do for those in need of transplants, the fact that these deaths often occur by accident or are otherwise unforeseen makes the decision to donate organs a difficult one. As with determinations about other end-of-life issues, grieving family members often find the added decision making a burden for which they are unprepared. It is vitally important, therefore, for those adults who know they want to donate organs to make their wishes known.

The Uniform Anatomical Gift Act of 1968 established a person's right to sign a donor card indicating a desire to donate organs or tissue after death. (See Figure 4.6.) People who wish to be donors can complete a donor card and, provided they carry it at all times, health care professionals will consult it in the event of unforeseen death. Alternatively, the wish to be a donor can be indicated on a driver's license or in a living will, or prospective donors may sign up for their state's registry online at http://www.organdonor.gov/becoming donor/ stateregistries.html. Prospective donors should inform their family and physician of their decision. At the time of death, hospitals always ask for the family's consent, even if a donor has already indicated his or her wish to donate organs. Should the family refuse, doctors will not take the organs, regardless of the deceased's wish.

HOSPICE CARE

The modern hospice movement developed in response to the need to provide humane care to terminally ill patients, while at the same time lending support to their families. The British physician Cicely Saunders (1918–2005) is considered to be the founder of the modern hospice movement—first in England in 1967 and later in Canada and the United States. The soothing, calming care provided by hospice workers is called palliative care, and it aims to relieve patients' pain and the accompanying symptoms of terminal illness, while providing comfort to patients and their families.

Hospice may refer to a place—a freestanding facility or designated floor in a hospital or nursing home—or to a program such as hospice home care, in

TABLE 4.8

Organ donors by donor type, 2003–12

[Donors recovered: January 1, 1988–September 30, 2013. Based on Organ Procurement and Transplantation Network (OPTN) data as of December 20, 2013.]

	All donor types	Deceased donor	Living donor
2012			
All donors	14,010	8,143	5,867
Kidney	13,040	7,421	5,619
Liver	6,876	6,630	246
Heart	2,451	2,451	0
Pancreas	1,451	1,451	0
Lung	1,710	1,708	2
Intestine	114	114	0
2011			
All donors	14,147	8,126	6,021
Kidney	13,205	7,434	5,771
Liver	6,931	6,684	247
Heart	2,380	2,380	0
Pancreas	1,562	1,562	0
Lung	1,758	1,756	2
Intestine	136	135	1
2010			
All donors	14,504	7,943	6,561
Kidney	13,519	7,241	6,278
Liver	6,893	6,611	282
Heart	2,406	2,406	0
Pancreas	1,660	1,660	0
Lung	1,697	1,697	0
Intestine	160	159	1
2009			
All donors	14,631	8,022	6,609
Kidney	13,635	7,248	6,387
Liver	6,958	6,739	219
Heart	2,281	2,281	0
Pancreas	1,740	1,740	0
Lung	1,569	1,568	1
Intestine	189	187	2
2008			
All donors	14,207	7,989	6,218
Kidney	13,156	7,188	5,968
Liver	7,000	6,751	249
Heart	2,222	2,222	0
Pancreas	1,830	1,829	1
Lung	1,388	1,388	0
Intestine	197	197	0
2007			
All donors	14,400	8,085	6,315
Kidney	13,283	7,240	6,043
Liver	7,202	6,936	266
Heart	2,286	2,286	0
Pancreas	1,924	1,924	0
Lung	1,388	1,382	6
Intestine	206	205	1
2006			
All donors	14,750	8,017	6,733
Kidney	13,612	7,176	6,436
Liver	7,303	7,015	288
Heart	2,277	2,276	1
Pancreas	2,031	2,030	1
Lung	1,330	1,325	5
Intestine	188	184	4
2005			
All donors	14,497	7,593	6,904
Kidney	13,273	6,700	6,573
Liver	7,016	6,693	323
Heart	2,220	2,220	0
Pancreas	2,050	2,048	2
Lung	1,287	1,285	2
Intestine	191	184	7
2004			
All donors	14,154	7,150	7,004
Kidney	12,972	6,325	6,647
Liver	6,642	6,319	323
Heart	2,096	2,096	0
Pancreas	2,022	2,022	0
Lung	1,092	1,064	28
Intestine	172	166	6
2003			
All donors	13,285	6,457	6,828
Kidney	12,226	5,753	6,473
Liver	6,004	5,682	322
Heart	2,120	2,120	0
Pancreas	1,779	1,776	3
Lung	990	961	29

TABLE 4.8

Organ donors by donor type, 2003–12 [CONTINUED]

[Donors recovered: January 1, 1988–September 30, 2013. Based on Organ Procurement and Transplantation Network (OPTN) data as of December 20, 2013.]

SOURCE: "Donors Recovered in the U.S. by Donor Type," in *Data*, U.S. Department of Health and Human Services, Health Resources and Services Administration, Organ Procurement and Transplantation Network, December 27, 2013, http://optn.transplant.hrsa.gov/data/default.asp (accessed December 27, 2013)

which a team of health care professionals helps the dying patient and family at home. Hospice teams may involve physicians, nurses, social workers, pastoral counselors, and trained volunteers. In the United States hospice care generally begins when a terminally ill individual has been given a prognosis of six months or less to live.

Hospice workers consider the patient and family to be the "unit of care" and focus their efforts on attending to emotional, psychological, and spiritual needs as well as to physical comfort and well-being. With hospice care, as a patient nears death, medical details move to the background as personal details move to the foreground to avoid providing care that is not wanted by the patient, even if some clinical benefit might be expected.

The Population Served

According to the National Hospice and Palliative Care Organization (NHPCO) report *NHPCO's Facts and Figures: Hospice Care in America, 2013 Edition* (2013, http://www.nhpco.org/sites/default/files/public/Statistics_Research/2013_Facts_Figures.pdf), an estimated 1.5 million to 1.6 million Americans received hospice care in 2012. This included those who died in hospice care, those who began receiving care in 2011 and were still receiving care in 2013, and those who left hospice care prior to death. The number of hospice patients nationally has been steadily increasing since 2008, when 1.3 million people were served by hospice providers. Much of this growth in the hospice population has corresponded with increasing use of Medicare's hospice coverage provisions.

TABLE 4.9

Deceased organ donors by cause of death, 2003–12

	All causes	Not reported	Anoxia	Cerebro-vascular/ stroke	Head trauma	CNS tumor	Not collected prior to 4/1/94	Other specify
2012	8,143	0	2,436	2,833	2,627	41	0	206
2011	8,126	0	2,278	2,932	2,685	41	0	190
2010	7,943	0	1,942	3,049	2,720	35	0	197
2009	8,022	0	1,893	3,178	2,670	43	0	238
2008	7,989	0	1,732	3,206	2,793	42	0	216
2007	8,085	0	1,489	3,308	3,026	46	0	216
2006	8,017	0	1,348	3,355	3,058	57	0	199
2005	7,593	0	1,147	3,336	2,908	57	0	145
2004	7,150	1	1,024	3,127	2,794	60	0	144
2003	6,457	0	855	2,767	2,617	49	0	169

Notes: CNS = Central nervous system.
Data subject to change based on future data submission or correction.

SOURCE: "Deceased Donors Recovered in the U.S. by Cause of Death," in *Data*, U.S. Department of Health and Human Services, Health Resources and Services Administration, Organ Procurement and Transplantation Network, December 27, 2013, http://optn.transplant.hrsa.gov/data/default.asp (accessed December 27, 2013)

FIGURE 4.6

Organ/tissue donor card

Donate Life

Organ/Tissue Donor Card

I wish to donate my organs and tissues. I wish to give:

☐ any needed organs and tissues ☐ only the following organs and tissues:

____

Donor Signature ________________ Date ________

Witness ____________________

Witness ____________________

SOURCE: Organ/Tissue Donor Card, U.S. Department of Health and Human Services, undated

Females accounted for more than half (56.4%) of hospice patients in 2012. More than eight in 10 (84.5%) hospice patients were aged 65 years and older, according to the NHPCO. Pediatric and young adult hospice patients under the age of 34 years accounted for less than 1% of the total hospice population, and adults aged 35 to 64 years accounted for 15.7% of the total. Cancer was the most common primary diagnosis among hospice patients, 36.9% of whom had some form of the disease. Dementia was the primary diagnosis of 12.8% of patients, heart disease the primary diagnosis of 11.2%, and lung disease the primary diagnosis of 8.2%. A range of other conditions accounted for smaller proportions of hospice patients, and substantial numbers (14.2%) had an unspecified debility.

A majority (66%) of hospice patients who died in 2012 did so in their place of residence, according to the NHPCO. For 41.5% of deceased hospice patients, that place of residence was a private home; for 17.2%, it was a nursing home; and for 7.3%, it was a residential facility other than a nursing home. Another 33% of hospice patients who died in 2012 passed away somewhere other than their home: 27.6% in a hospice inpatient facility and 6.6% in an acute care hospital setting.

In "Change in End-of-Life Care for Medicare Beneficiaries: Site of Death, Place of Care, and Health Care Transitions in 2000, 2005, and 2009" (*Journal of the American Medical Association*, vol. 309, no. 5, February 6, 2013), a comprehensive study of the shift toward increased utilization of hospice care (and of other early 21st-century changes in end-of-life care), J. M. Teno et al. find that although hospice use rapidly increased during the first decade of the 21st century, fully 28.4% of Medicare beneficiaries who died in hospice care in 2009 received such care for three days or less. Moreover, in 40% of these cases the shift to hospice care only occurred after a stay in a hospital's intensive care unit. This finding suggests that many people who might benefit from hospice care's focus on quality of life were not obtaining those benefits. Instead, many people appeared to be using hospice care as a last resort, once all medical interventions had been tried, rather than as a means of improving the end-of-life experience.

CHAPTER 5
OLDER ADULTS

THE LONGEVITY REVOLUTION

The increase in life expectancy brought about by the combination of improved sanitation, medical advances, and reduced mortality rates for infants and children has fundamentally changed the nature of U.S. society. As Table 5.1 shows, the average life expectancy for all U.S. residents increased dramatically between 1900 and 1950 and continued on its pronounced upward trajectory through 2010. A society in which most people expect to live to the age of 47.3 (the average U.S. life expectancy in 1900) is necessarily different from a society in which most people can expect to live to the age of 78.7 (the average U.S. life expectancy in 2010). As noted in Chapter 1, adults aged 65 years and older constituted 13% of the total U.S. population in 2010 (up from 4% in 1900) and were projected to account for more than one out of five Americans (21.9%) in 2060.

The full implications of this "longevity revolution," as the aging of the U.S. population is sometimes called, have only begun to be understood. Although the personal benefits of a long life may be obvious, many older people struggle to redefine their goals and hopes once their working lives draw to a close and their children are grown. Other older adults welcome these changes and report higher levels of life satisfaction in their later years than at any other time of life. As more middle-aged adults find themselves caring for their aged parents for longer periods, changes in family and social life are likely. Adults who must be able to afford care both for children and for parents may be forced to extend their own careers into old age or to make other changes in household finances and family structures. As businesses and social institutions respond to the needs and desires of an older population, daily life in U.S. cities and towns will undoubtedly change.

The longevity revolution has many possible implications for the U.S. economy as well. Some economists predict a sustained economic slowdown as the population of working-age adults shrinks relative to the population as a whole. Likewise, in the absence of reform or a reallocation of resources, many economists and government officials expect the burgeoning of the elderly population to strain the public benefit programs that together provide a safety net for those aged 65 years and older. Programs such as Social Security, which provides those aged 65 years and older with pensions, and Medicare, which provides older people with universal health care coverage, are funded through contributions from working-age people. With a smaller working-age population attempting to support a greatly expanded population of retirees, there are widespread concerns about how these programs will continue to be funded.

Additionally, end-of-life controversies such as those addressed throughout this book are directly related to the social and political effects of the longevity revolution. How the country's institutions—from churches and medical facilities to the courts and government—respond to the many dilemmas raised at the end of life in the 21st century will undoubtedly be determined in large part by the needs and desires of an increasingly influential population of older Americans.

CHARACTERISTICS OF AGING AMERICANS

Although the population of Americans aged 65 years and older has been growing steadily since the early 20th century, an unprecedented acceleration in this group's rate of growth began in 2011, when the first Baby Boomers began turning 65. The Federal Interagency Forum on Aging-Related Statistics notes in *Older Americans 2012: Key Indicators of Well-Being* (June 2012, http://www.agingstats.gov/agingstatsdotnet/Main_Site/Data/2012_Documents/Docs/EntireChartbook.pdf) that the number of older Americans is projected to expand dramatically between 2011 and 2030. After 2030, this group's rate of

TABLE 5.1

Life expectancy at birth, at age 65, and at age 75, by sex, race, and Hispanic origin, selected years 1900–2010

[Data are based on death certificates]

Specified age and year	All races			White			Black or African American[a]		
	Both sexes	Male	Female	Both sexes	Male	Female	Both sexes	Male	Female
	Life expectancy, in years								
At birth									
1900[b, c]	47.3	46.3	48.3	47.6	46.6	48.7	33.0	32.5	33.5
1950[c]	68.2	65.6	71.1	69.1	66.5	72.2	60.8	59.1	62.9
1960[c]	69.7	66.6	73.1	70.6	67.4	74.1	63.6	61.1	66.3
1970	70.8	67.1	74.7	71.7	68.0	75.6	64.1	60.0	68.3
1980	73.7	70.0	77.4	74.4	70.7	78.1	68.1	63.8	72.5
1990	75.4	71.8	78.8	76.1	72.7	79.4	69.1	64.5	73.6
1995	75.8	72.5	78.9	76.5	73.4	79.6	69.6	65.2	73.9
2000	76.8	74.1	79.3	77.3	74.7	79.9	71.8	68.2	75.1
2001	77.0	74.3	79.5	77.5	74.9	80.0	72.0	68.5	75.3
2002	77.0	74.4	79.6	77.5	74.9	80.1	72.2	68.7	75.4
2003	77.2	74.5	79.7	77.7	75.1	80.2	72.4	68.9	75.7
2004	77.6	75.0	80.1	78.1	75.5	80.5	72.9	69.4	76.1
2005	77.6	75.0	80.1	78.0	75.5	80.5	73.0	69.5	76.2
2006	77.8	75.2	80.3	78.3	75.8	80.7	73.4	69.9	76.7
2007	78.1	75.5	80.6	78.5	76.0	80.9	73.8	70.3	77.0
2008	78.2	75.6	80.6	78.5	76.1	80.9	74.3	70.9	77.3
2009	78.5	76.0	80.9	78.8	76.4	81.2	74.7	71.4	77.7
2010	78.7	76.2	81.0	78.9	76.5	81.3	75.1	71.8	78.0
At 65 years									
1950[c]	13.9	12.8	15.0	14.1	12.8	15.1	13.9	12.9	14.9
1960[c]	14.3	12.8	15.8	14.4	12.9	15.9	13.9	12.7	15.1
1970	15.2	13.1	17.0	15.2	13.1	17.1	14.2	12.5	15.7
1980	16.4	14.1	18.3	16.5	14.2	18.4	15.1	13.0	16.8
1990	17.2	15.1	18.9	17.3	15.2	19.1	15.4	13.2	17.2
1995	17.4	15.6	18.9	17.6	15.7	19.1	15.6	13.6	17.1
2000	17.6	16.0	19.0	17.7	16.1	19.1	16.1	14.1	17.5
2001	17.9	16.2	19.2	18.0	16.3	19.3	16.2	14.2	17.7
2002	17.9	16.3	19.2	18.0	16.4	19.3	16.3	14.4	17.8
2003	18.1	16.5	19.3	18.2	16.6	19.4	16.5	14.5	18.0
2004	18.4	16.9	19.6	18.5	17.0	19.7	16.8	14.9	18.3
2005	18.4	16.9	19.6	18.5	17.0	19.7	16.9	15.0	18.3
2006	18.7	17.2	19.9	18.7	17.3	19.9	17.2	15.2	18.6
2007	18.8	17.4	20.0	18.9	17.4	20.1	17.3	15.4	18.8
2008	18.8	17.4	20.0	18.9	17.5	20.0	17.5	15.5	18.9
2009	19.1	17.7	20.3	19.2	17.7	20.3	17.8	15.9	19.2
2010	19.1	17.7	20.3	19.2	17.8	20.3	17.8	15.9	19.3
At 75 years									
1980	10.4	8.8	11.5	10.4	8.8	11.5	9.7	8.3	10.7
1990	10.9	9.4	12.0	11.0	9.4	12.0	10.2	8.6	11.2
1995	11.0	9.7	11.9	11.1	9.7	12.0	10.2	8.8	11.1
2000	11.0	9.8	11.8	11.0	9.8	11.9	10.4	9.0	11.3
2001	11.2	9.9	12.0	11.2	10.0	12.1	10.5	9.0	11.5
2002	11.2	10.0	12.0	11.2	10.0	12.1	10.5	9.1	11.5
2003	11.3	10.1	12.1	11.3	10.2	12.1	10.7	8.7	11.6
2004	11.5	10.4	12.4	11.6	10.4	12.4	10.9	9.4	11.2
2005	11.5	10.4	12.3	11.5	10.4	12.3	10.9	9.4	11.2
2006	11.7	10.6	12.5	11.1	10.6	12.5	11.1	9.1	12.0
2007	11.9	10.7	12.6	11.9	10.8	12.6	11.2	9.8	12.1
2008	11.8	10.7	12.6	11.8	10.7	12.6	11.3	9.8	12.2
2009	12.1	11.0	12.9	12.1	10.4	12.9	11.6	10.2	12.5
2010	12.1	11.0	12.9	12.1	11.0	12.8	11.6	10.2	12.5

growth is expected to slow. However, although the absolute number of older Americans will continue growing, the proportion of 65-and-older adults relative to the population as a whole is expected to remain steady at just over 20% through the middle of the 21st century.

The Oldest-Old

The "oldest-old" subset of the population (those aged 85 years and older) grew even more rapidly than the 65-and-older population between 1970 and 2010. According to the Federal Interagency Forum on Aging-Related Statistics, in *Older Americans 2012*, although the 65-and-older population doubled between 1970 and 2010, growing from 20.1 million to 40.3 million, the 85-and-older population nearly quadrupled, growing from 1.5 million in 1970 to 5.5 million in 2010. The 65-and-older population is expected to double again between 2010 and 2040, reaching 88.5 million in 2050, whereas the 85-and-older population is expected to nearly quadruple again by 2050, growing to 19 million.

TABLE 5.1

Life expectancy at birth, at age 65, and at age 75, by sex, race, and Hispanic origin, selected years 1900–2010 [CONTINUED]

[Data are based on death certificates]

Specified age and year	White, not Hispanic			Black, not Hispanic			Hispanic[d]		
	Both sexes	Male	Female	Both sexes	Male	Female	Both sexes	Male	Female
At birth				Life expectancy, in years					
2006	78.2	75.7	80.6	73.1	69.5	76.4	80.3	77.5	82.9
2007	78.4	75.9	80.8	73.5	69.9	76.7	80.7	77.8	83.2
2008	78.4	76.0	80.7	73.9	70.5	77.0	80.8	78.0	83.3
2009	78.7	76.3	81.1	74.3	70.9	77.4	81.1	78.4	83.5
2010	78.8	76.4	81.1	74.7	71.4	77.7	81.2	78.5	83.8
At 65 years									
2006	18.7	17.2	19.9	17.1	15.1	18.5	20.2	18.5	21.5
2007	18.8	17.4	20.0	17.2	15.3	18.7	20.5	18.7	21.7
2008	18.8	17.4	20.0	17.4	15.4	18.8	20.4	18.7	21.6
2009	19.1	17.7	19.5	17.7	15.8	19.1	20.7	19.0	21.9
2010	19.1	17.7	20.3	17.7	15.8	19.1	20.6	18.8	22.0
At 75 years									
2006	11.7	10.6	12.5	11.1	9.6	12.0	13.0	11.7	13.7
2007	11.8	10.7	12.6	11.2	9.7	12.1	13.1	11.8	13.8
2008	11.8	10.7	12.6	11.3	9.8	12.2	13.0	11.7	13.8
2009	12.0	11.0	12.9	11.6	10.1	12.4	13.3	12.0	13.8
2010	12.0	11.0	12.8	11.6	10.1	12.5	13.2	11.7	14.1

[a]Data shown for 1900–1960 are for the nonwhite population.
[b]Death registration area only. The death registration area increased from 10 states and the District of Columbia (D.C.) in 1900 to the coterminous United States in 1933.
[c]Includes deaths of persons who were not residents of the 50 states and D.C.
[d]Hispanic origin was added to the U.S. standard death certificate in 1989 and was adopted by every state in 1997. To estimate life expectancy, age-specific death rates were corrected to address racial and ethnic misclassification, which underestimates deaths in the Hispanic population. To address the effects of age misstatement at the oldest ages, the probability of death for Hispanic persons older than 80 years is estimated as a function of non-Hispanic white mortality with the use of the Brass relational logit model.
Notes: Populations for computing life expectancy for 1991–1999 are 1990-based postcensal estimates of the U.S. resident population. Starting with *Health, United States, 2012*, populations for computing life expectancy for 2001–2009 were based on intercensal population estimates of the U.S. resident population. Populations for computing life expectancy for 2010 were based on 2010 census counts. In 1997, life table methodology was revised to construct complete life tables by single years of age that extend to age 100. (Anderson RN. Method for constructing complete annual U.S. life tables. NCHS. Vital Health Stat 2(129). 1999.) Previously, abridged life tables were constructed for 5-year age groups ending with 85 years and over. In 2000, the life table methodology was revised. The revised methodology is similar to that developed for the 1999–2001 decennial life tables. In 2008, the life table methodology was further refined. Starting with 2003 data, some states allowed the reporting of more than one race on the death certificate. The multiple-race data for these states were bridged to the single-race categories of the 1977 Office of Management and Budget standards, for comparability with other states. The race groups, white and black include persons of Hispanic and non-Hispanic origin. Persons of Hispanic origin may be of any race. Data for additional years are available. NCHS = National Center for Health Statistics.

SOURCE: "Table 18. Life Expectancy at Birth, at Age 65, and at Age 75, by Sex, Race, and Hispanic Origin: United States, Selected Years 1900–2010," in *Health, United States, 2012: With Special Feature on Emergency Care*, Centers for Disease Control and Prevention, National Center for Health Statistics, 2013, http://www.cdc.gov/nchs/data/hus/hus12.pdf (accessed December 27, 2013)

The population of centenarians (people who are aged 100 years old and older) has also increased rapidly since the late 20th century. In *A Profile of Older Americans: 2012* (April 2013, http://www.aoa.gov/AoARoot/(S(2ch3qw55k1qylo45dbihar2u))/Aging_Statistics/Profile/2012/docs/2012profile.pdf), the U.S. Department of Health and Human Services' Administration on Aging indicates that the centenarian population increased 66% between 1980 to 2010, from 32,194 to 53,364.

Although medical advances and lifestyle choices can explain increases in longevity in the aggregate, centenarians represent a special case within the larger story of the longevity revolution. The most comprehensive study of centenarians ever undertaken, the long-running New England Centenarian Study (http://www.bumc.bu.edu/centenarian/), which began in 1995 and was ongoing as of April 2014, involves research into the genetic makeup and lifestyles of more than 1,600 centenarians, including more than 100 supercentenarians (people who are aged 110 years and older). The researchers have found that people who live more than 100 years are typically characterized by very specific genetic patterns not shared by those who die at younger ages. However, the researchers have also found evidence suggesting that lifestyle may play a role in activating or suppressing certain genetic components of extreme longevity. Centenarians are united by their ability to escape, delay, or survive the chronic conditions that are the primary causes of death for most people who reach old age. Among the study's population of centenarians, 15% have been classified as "escapers," people who have no evidence of serious disease at all; 43% have been classified as "delayers," people who succumb to chronic conditions like most other elderly people but who do not exhibit symptoms prior to the age of 80; and 42% have been classified as "survivors," people who had serious diseases prior to the age of 80 but were able to recover their health.

Geographic Distribution

The aging of the U.S. population has not occurred at the same rate in all parts of the country. Figure 5.1 shows the variation in the 65-and-older population as a

FIGURE 5.1

Adults 65 years and over as a percentage of total population, by state, 2011

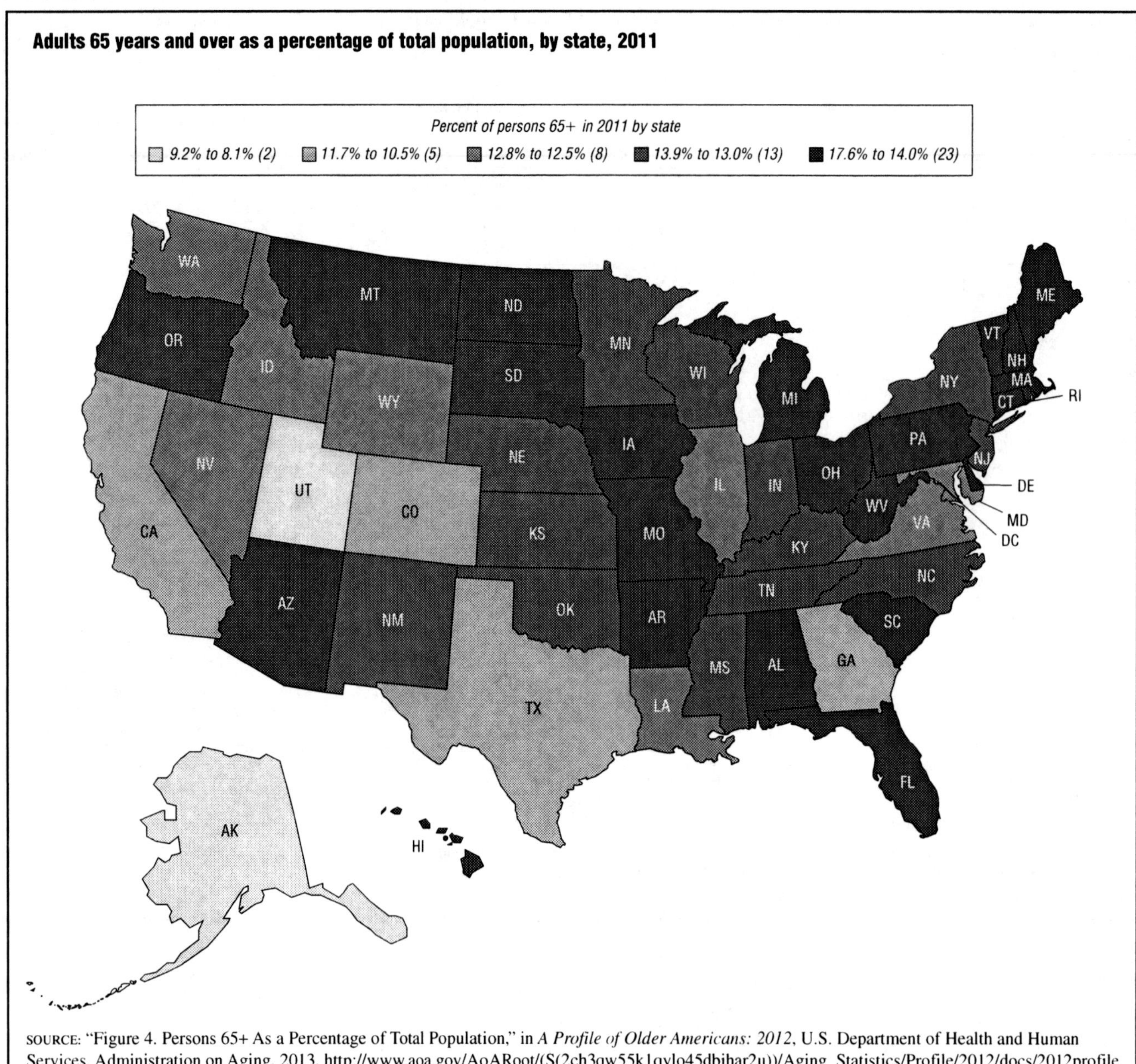

SOURCE: "Figure 4. Persons 65+ As a Percentage of Total Population," in *A Profile of Older Americans: 2012*, U.S. Department of Health and Human Services, Administration on Aging, 2013, http://www.aoa.gov/AoARoot/(S(2ch3qw55k1qylo45dbihar2u))/Aging_Statistics/Profile/2012/docs/2012profile.pdf (accessed February 6, 2014)

proportion of total population in each state as of 2011. People aged 65 years and older accounted for 15% or more of the total population in 11 states: Arkansas, Delaware, Florida, Hawaii, Iowa, Maine, Montana, Pennsylvania, Rhode Island, Vermont, and West Virginia. The youngest states were Utah and Alaska, where between 8.1% and 9.2% of the population was aged 65 years and older. Other states with relatively low proportions of older residents were California, Colorado, Georgia, and Texas, in each of which between 10.5% and 11.7% of the population was elderly.

In terms of absolute numbers, however, the elderly population tended to be largest in the states with the largest overall populations, although some of these states were not among those with the highest percentages of elderly residents. According to the Administration on Aging, in *A Profile of Older Americans*, more than half of all people aged 65 years and older lived in nine states in 2011: California, Florida, Illinois, Michigan, New York, North Carolina, Ohio, Pennsylvania, and Texas.

Demographic Characteristics

Besides growing larger, the older population in the United States is growing more diverse, which is a reflection of the increased diversity in the population at large. This trend is expected to accelerate considerably in the 21st century. As Figure 5.2 shows, in 2010, 80% of 65-and-older adults were non-Hispanic white, 9% were African American, 7% were Hispanic, and 3% were

FIGURE 5.2

65 and over population, by race and Hispanic origin, 2010 and projected 2050

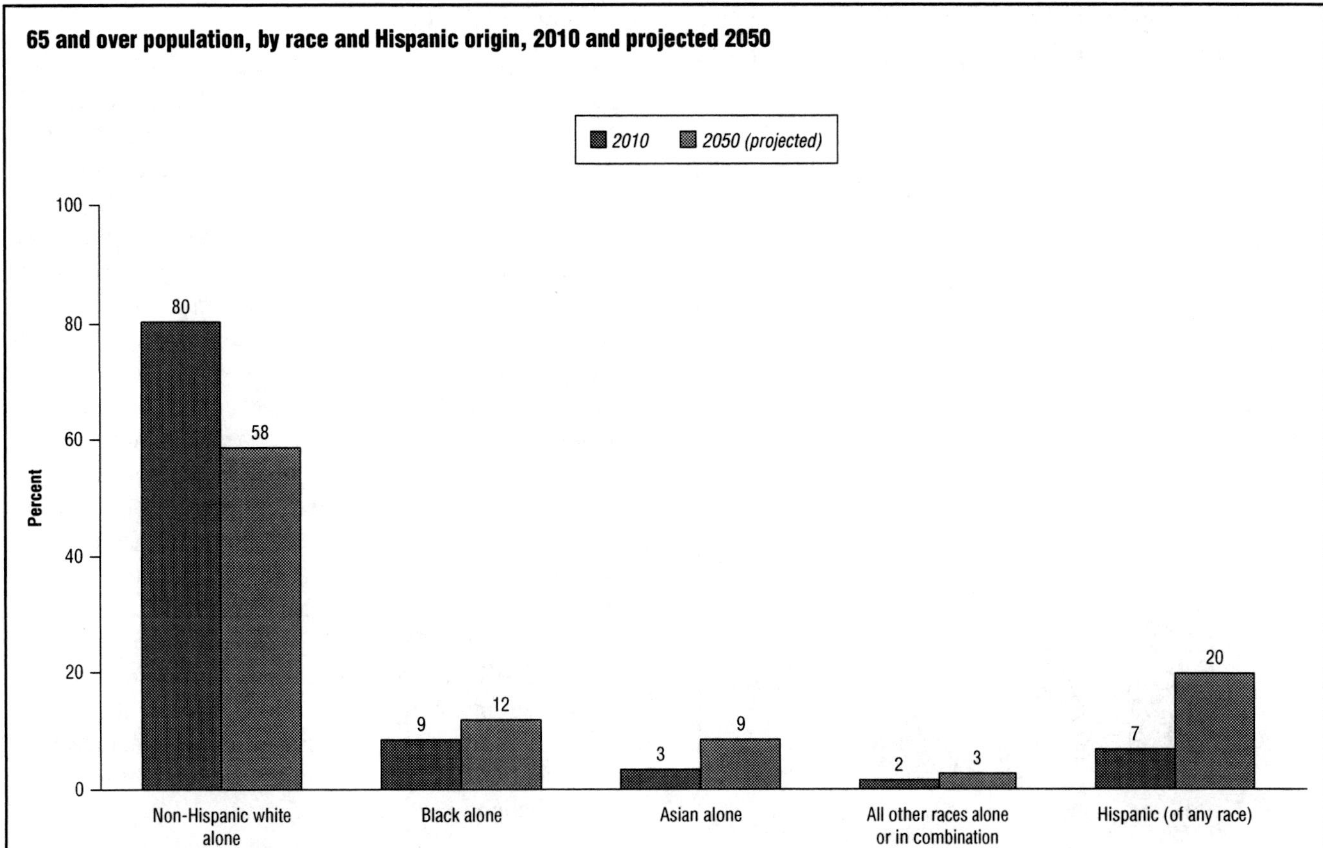

Notes: These projections are based on Census 2000 and are not consistent with the 2010 Census results. Projections based on the 2010 Census will be released in late 2012. The term "non-Hispanic white alone" is used to refer to people who reported being white and no other race and who are not Hispanic. The term "black alone" is used to refer to people who reported being black or African American and no other race, and the term "Asian alone" is used to refer to people who reported only Asian as their race. The use of single-race populations in this chart does not imply that this is the preferred method of presenting or analyzing data. The U.S. Census Bureau uses a variety of approaches. The race group "All other races alone or in combination" includes American Indian and Alaska Native alone; Native Hawaiian and other Pacific Islander alone; and all people who reported two or more races. Reference population: These data refer to the resident population.

SOURCE: "Population Age 65 and over, by Race and Hispanic Origin, 2010 and Projected 2050," in *Older Americans 2012: Key Indicators of Well-Being*, Federal Interagency Forum on Aging Related Statistics, 2012, http://www.agingstats.gov/agingstatsdotnet/Main_Site/Data/2012_Documents/Docs/EntireChartbook.pdf (accessed February 7, 2014)

Asian American. By 2050 the 65-and-older population is expected to be 58% white, 20% Hispanic, 12% African American, and 9% Asian American.

The marital status and living arrangements of the 65-and-older population vary significantly by sex. In 2012, 72% of older men were married, compared with only 45% of older women, although roughly equal percentages of women and men were divorced or separated (14% of women and 12% of men) or single or never married (4% of women and 5% of men). (See Figure 5.3.) There are two primary reasons for this disparity: women live longer than men, on average, and therefore are more likely to survive their husbands; and men are more likely than women to remarry after divorce or the death of a spouse. In 2012, 37% of 65-and-older women were widows, compared with only 12% of 65-and-older men. Accordingly, older women were much more likely than older men to live alone. While 19% of older men lived alone in 2012, 36% of older women did. (See Figure 5.4.)

Besides growing and becoming more diverse, the older population has become steadily more educated since the start of the 21st century. In 1965 only 23.5% of 65-and-older adults had a high school diploma and only 5% had a bachelor's degree or higher. (See Figure 5.5.) By 2010, 79.5% of 65-and-older adults had at least a high school diploma and 22.5% had a bachelor's degree or higher.

Education levels are positively correlated with income levels and standard of living, and indeed, as Figure 5.6 shows, the period between 1974 and 2010 saw the older population's income distribution shift. In 1974, 14.6% of Americans aged 65 years and older lived below the federal poverty line, and another 34.6% were considered low-income (i.e., their incomes represented between 100% and 199% of the poverty line). By 2010 only 9% of older people lived below the poverty line, and 25.6% were in the low-income group. The proportion of older Americans in the middle-income group (200% to 399% of poverty) remained relatively steady over this period, rising from 32.6% to 34%, while the proportion of older Americans in the high-income group (400% of poverty or higher) grew dramatically, rising from 18.2% to 31.4%.

FIGURE 5.3

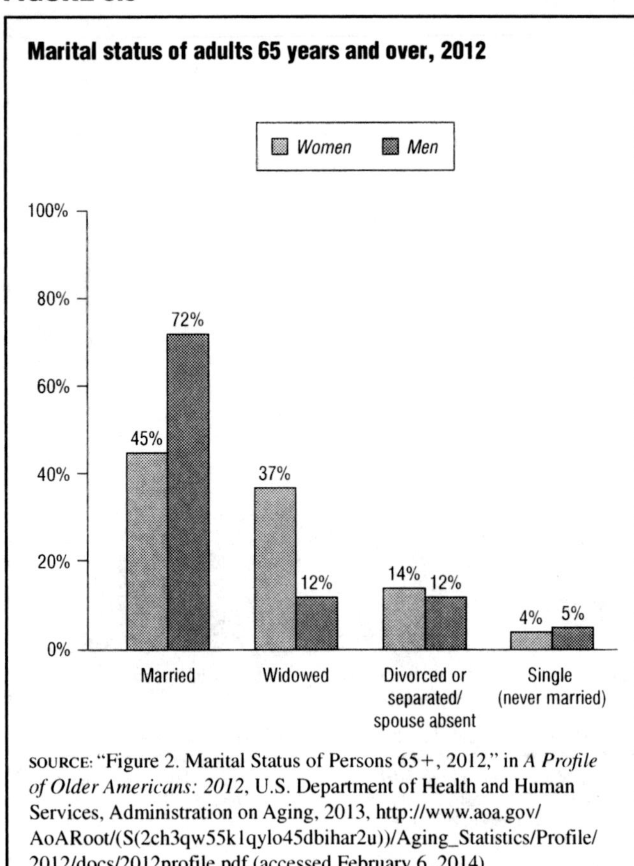

SOURCE: "Figure 2. Marital Status of Persons 65+, 2012," in *A Profile of Older Americans: 2012*, U.S. Department of Health and Human Services, Administration on Aging, 2013, http://www.aoa.gov/AoARoot/(S(2ch3qw55k1qylo45dbihar2u))/Aging_Statistics/Profile/2012/docs/2012profile.pdf (accessed February 6, 2014)

Since the 1960s, Social Security has been the most important source of income for 65-and-older individuals and couples. In 1962 Social Security accounted for 31% of older Americans' income, assets accounted for 16%, pensions for 9%, and earnings for 28%. (See Table 5.2.) Older Americans' reliance on Social Security increased over the following 14 years, accounting for 39% of 65-and-older income by 1976. Reliance on Social Security remained relatively steady through 2010, when the program accounted for 37% of 65-and-older income. Between 1962 and 2010 the proportion of 65-and-older incomes supplied by the other categories of funding varied. The relative contribution of asset income declined from 16% to 11%, and income from pensions (retirement plans administered by employers) increased from 9% to 19%. Meanwhile, the relative importance of earnings (typically from part-time employment) fluctuated during these five decades, falling from 28% of income in 1962 to a low of 16% in 1984. Earnings as a proportion of total 65-and-older income remained low through the 1990s, before becoming a more crucial source of income than ever before by 2010, when earnings accounted for 30% of income, second only to Social Security.

HEALTH AND MORBIDITY AMONG OLDER ADULTS

Heart disease has historically been the leading cause of death for the 65-and-older population in the United States, and it remained so in the early 21st century. The

FIGURE 5.4

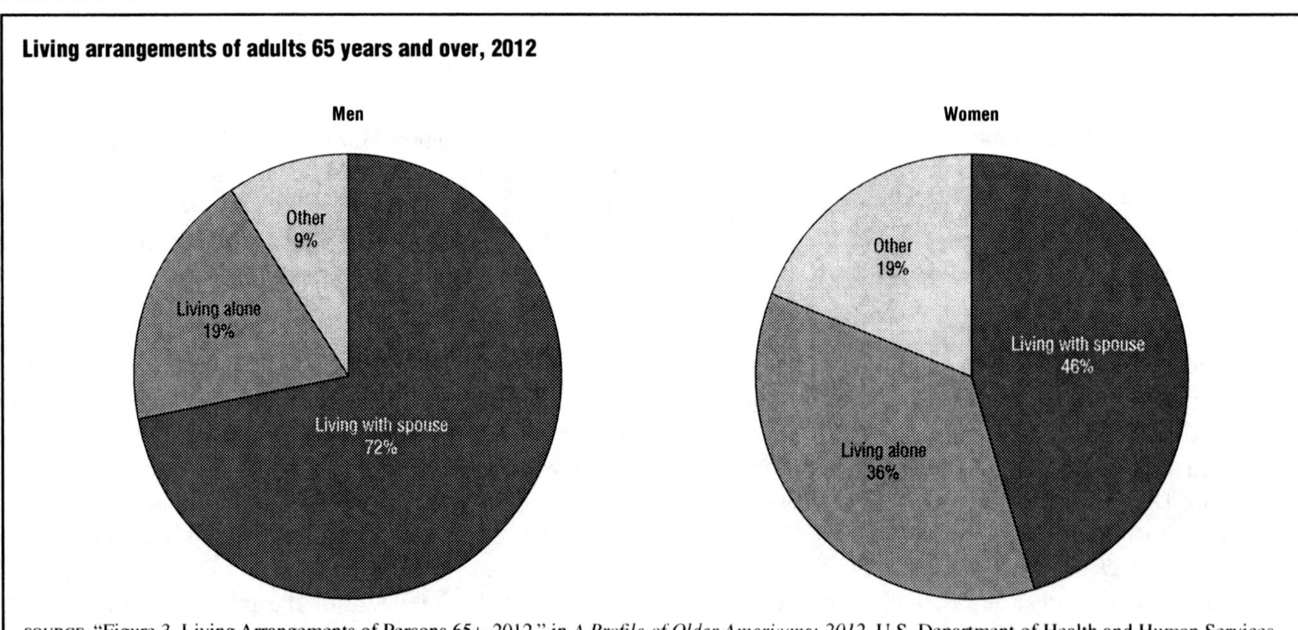

SOURCE: "Figure 3. Living Arrangements of Persons 65+, 2012," in *A Profile of Older Americans: 2012*, U.S. Department of Health and Human Services, Administration on Aging, 2013, http://www.aoa.gov/AoARoot/(S(2ch3qw55k1qylo45dbihar2u))/Aging_Statistics/Profile/2012/docs/2012profile.pdf (accessed February 6, 2014)

FIGURE 5.5

Educational attainment of the 65 and over population, 1965–2010

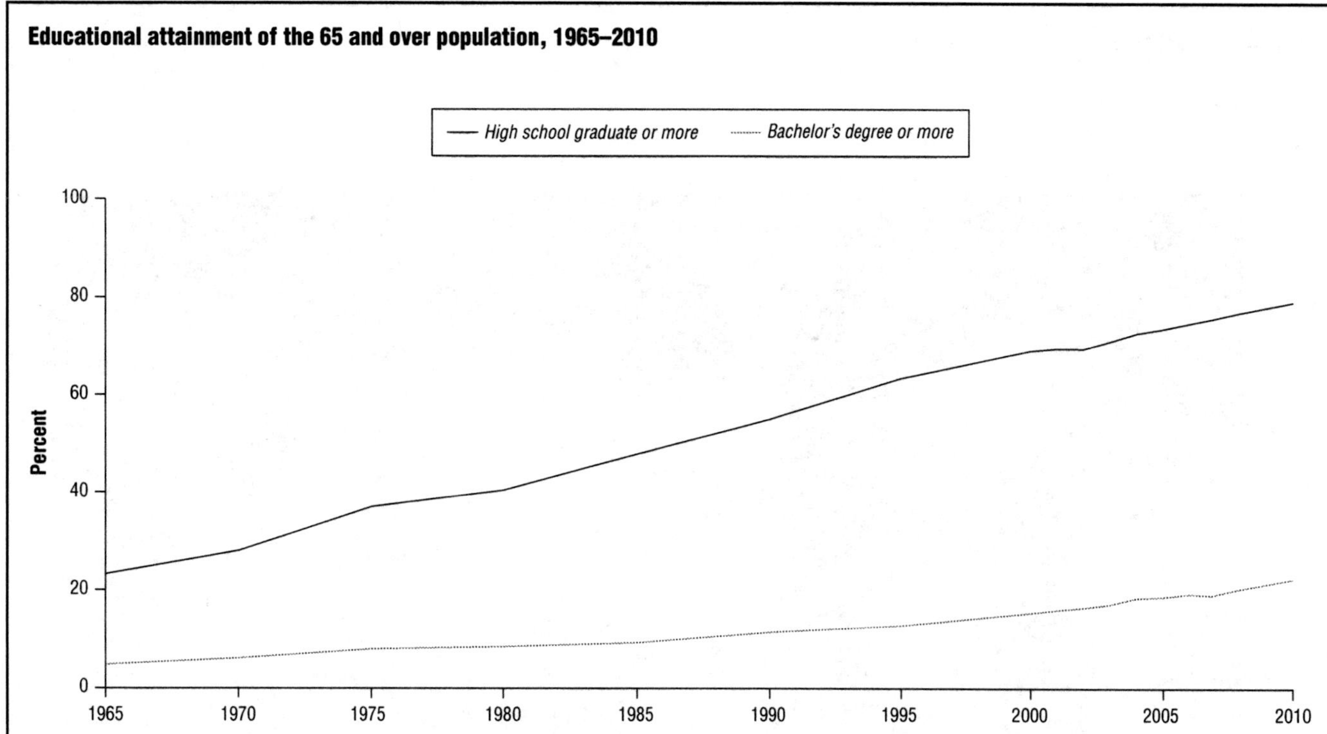

Note: A single question which asks for the highest grade or degree completed is now used to determine educational attainment. Prior to 1995, educational attainment was measured using data on years of school completed. Reference population: These data refer to the civilian noninstitutionalized population.

SOURCE: "Educational Attainment of the Population Age 65 and over, Selected Years 1965–2010," in *Older Americans 2012: Key Indicators of Well-Being*, Federal Interagency Forum on Aging Related Statistics, 2012, http://www.agingstats.gov/agingstatsdotnet/Main_Site/Data/2012_Documents/Docs/Entire Chartbook.pdf (accessed February 7, 2014)

rate of death from heart disease among older people has declined dramatically, however, from 2,547 deaths per 100,000 people in 1981 to 1,156 deaths per 100,000 people in 2009—a decrease of 54.6%. (See Figure 5.7.) Cancer remained the second-leading cause of death for older Americans during these decades, at 982 deaths per 100,000 in 2009, only 7% lower than the 1981 rate of 1,056. Between 1981 and 2009 the death rate from stroke fell even further than that of heart disease, from 624 to 264, a decrease of 57.7%. The death rate from influenza and pneumonia also fell significantly during this period, from 207 to 104. By contrast, older Americans in 2009 were more likely than their counterparts in 1981 to die from chronic lower respiratory diseases, diabetes, and Alzheimer's disease. Among these causes of death, the rate for Alzheimer's had risen by far the most, from 6 per 100,000 in 1981 to 184 per 100,000 in 2009. This is in large part because the risk of being diagnosed with Alzheimer's rises with age. As more people live longer into old age, the prevalence of Alzheimer's inevitably increases, and there is no cure for the disease.

Significant proportions of the elderly population were living with chronic conditions as of 2009–10, with significant variations by sex evident in certain conditions. (See Figure 5.8.) Older men were substantially more likely to have heart disease, cancer, and diabetes than were older women; and women were considerably more likely to have arthritis and slightly more likely to have hypertension (high blood pressure). Smaller numbers of both men and women reported having had a stroke, asthma, or chronic bronchitis or emphysema, and disparities by sex were less pronounced for these conditions.

According to the Federal Interagency Forum on Aging-Related Statistics, in *Older Americans 2012*, nearly eight out of 10 (75.6%) elderly adults reported being in good to excellent health between 2008 and 2010. There were significant differences in reported health status by race and Hispanic origin, however: whereas 78% of non-Hispanic whites aged 65 years and older reported being in good to excellent health, only 63% each of non-Hispanic African Americans and Hispanics assessed their own health as good to excellent. (See Figure 5.9.) Similar disparities occurred across all subgroups of the elderly population, with non-Hispanic whites being significantly more likely than their African American and Hispanic counterparts to characterize their health as good to excellent between the ages of 65 and 74 years, 75 and 84 years, and over the age of 85 years.

As Figure 5.10 shows, the likelihood that an elderly person will experience limitations in the ability to carry

FIGURE 5.6

Income distribution of 65 and over population, 1974–2010

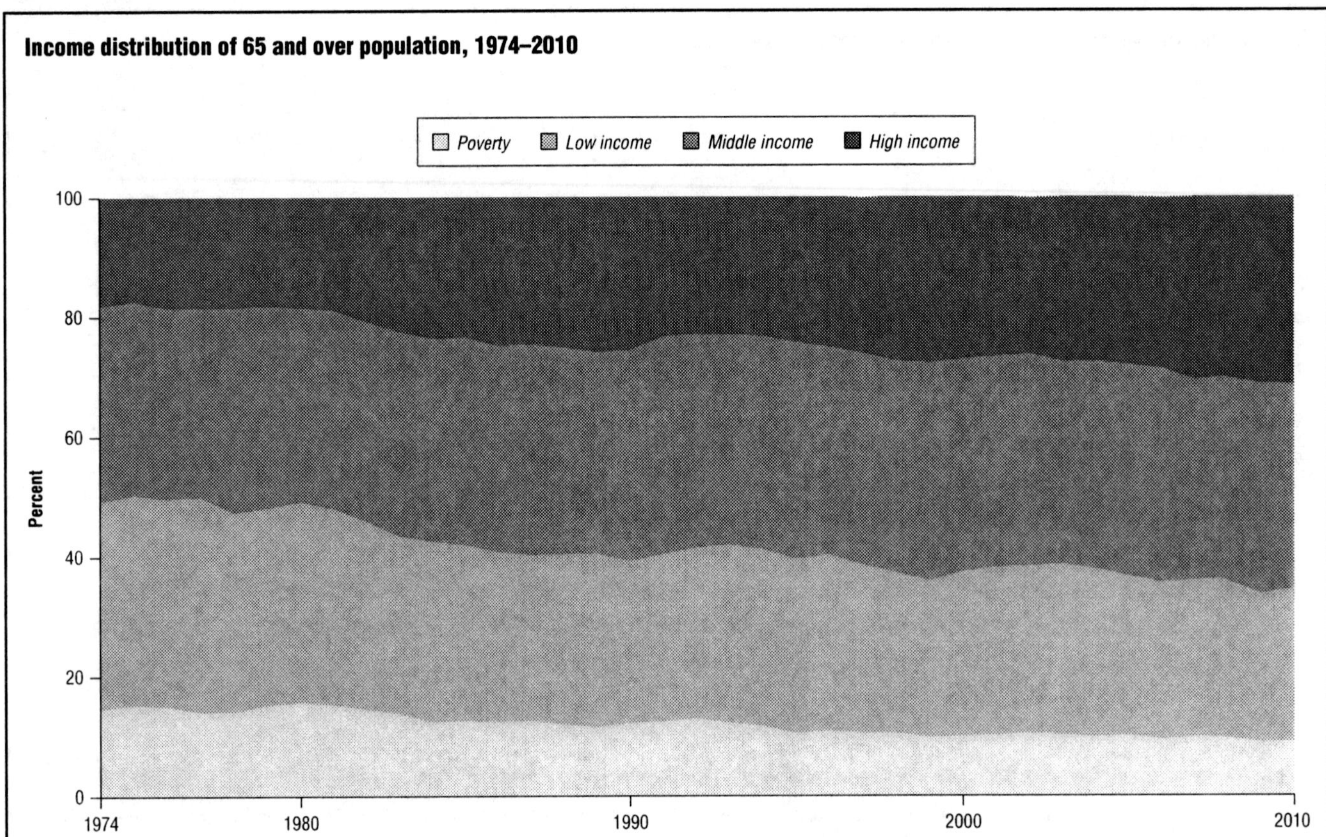

Notes: The income categories are derived from the ratio of the family's income (or an unrelated individual's income) to the corresponding poverty threshold. Being in poverty is measured as income less than 100 percent of the poverty threshold. Low income is between 100 percent and 199 percent of the poverty threshold. Middle income is between 200 percent and 399 percent of the poverty threshold. High income is 400 percent or more of the poverty threshold. Income distribution in the Current Population Survey is based on prior year income. Reference population: These data refer to the civilian noninstitutionalized population.

SOURCE: "Income Distribution of the Population Age 65 and over, 1974–2010," in *Older Americans 2012: Key Indicators of Well-Being*, Federal Interagency Forum on Aging Related Statistics, 2012, http://www.agingstats.gov/agingstatsdotnet/Main_Site/Data/2012_Documents/Docs/EntireChartbook.pdf (accessed February 7, 2014)

out the routine activities of daily life increases significantly with age. In 2010, 6% of adults between the ages of 65 and 74 years experienced limitations in their ability to bathe or shower themselves, compared with 11% of those between the ages of 75 and 84 years and 24% of those over the age of 85 years. Similar patterns prevailed for other daily activities, including dressing, eating, getting in and out of bed or in and out of chairs, and using the toilet. Among all daily activities, walking proved the most troublesome for all subsets of the elderly population. Nearly two out of 10 (17%) adults between the ages of 65 and 74 years, nearly three out of 10 (28%) adults between the ages of 75 and 84 years, and almost half (46%) of adults aged 85 years and older found themselves unable to walk freely.

The near-universality of health and wellness challenges among the elderly is the primary reason for the existence of Medicare, the subsidized health insurance coverage that is universally available to U.S. citizens and permanent residents aged 65 years and older. Indeed, although the uninsured rate for people under the age of 65 years was 17.7% in 2012, the uninsured rate for people aged 65 years and older was only 1.5%. (See Table 5.3.) Among all age groups, the elderly were by far the most likely to be insured, and the reason for this was the comprehensiveness of coverage under Medicare. As Figure 5.11 shows, 93% of those aged 65 years and older had health coverage through Medicare in 2011. Some older Americans had other forms of coverage that supplanted or supplemented Medicare, including either employer-based or directly purchased individual private coverage (which 58% of older people had), Medicaid (the federal program providing health coverage to impoverished children and adults of all ages; 9%), or coverage based on military service (9%). Medicare is thus a primary source of funding for end-of-life care.

As discussed in Chapter 1, in the 20th and 21st centuries it is more common for people to die in hospitals or other institutional settings than in the home, as was the norm through the 19th century. End-of-life care often takes one of two forms: aggressive

TABLE 5.2

Percentage distribution of sources of income for 65 and over couples and individuals, 1962–2010

Year	Total	Social Security	Asset Income	Pensions	Earnings	Other
1962	100	31	16	9	28	16
1967	100	34	15	12	29	10
1976	100	39	18	16	23	4
1978	100	38	19	16	23	4
1980	100	39	22	16	19	4
1982	100	39	25	15	18	3
1984	100	38	28	15	16	3
1986	100	38	26	16	17	3
1988	100	38	25	17	17	3
1990	100	36	24	18	18	4
1992	100	40	21	20	17	2
1994	100	42	18	19	18	3
1996	100	40	18	19	20	3
1998	100	38	20	19	21	2
1999	100	38	19	19	21	3
2000	100	38	18	18	23	3
2001	100	39	16	18	24	3
2002	100	39	14	19	25	3
2003	100	39	14	19	25	2
2004	100	39	13	20	26	2
2005	100	37	13	19	28	3
2006	100	37	15	18	28	3
2008	100	37	13	19	30	3
2009	100	37	11	19	30	3
2010	100	37	11	19	30	3

Notes: A married couple is age 65 and over if the husband is age 65 and over or the husband is younger than age 55 and the wife is age 65 and over. The definition of "other" includes, but is not limited to, unemployment compensation, workers compensation, alimony, child support, and personal contributors.
Reference population: These data refer to the civilian noninstitutionalized population.

SOURCE: "Percentage Distribution of Sources of Income for Married Couples and Nonmarried Persons Age 65 and over, 1962–2010," in *Older Americans 2012: Key Indicators of Well-Being*, Federal Interagency Forum on Aging Related Statistics, 2012, http://www.agingstats.gov/agingstatsdotnet/Main_Site/Data/2012_Documents/Docs/EntireChartbook.pdf (accessed February 7, 2014)

treatment intended to prolong life, which is commonly carried out in the intensive care units (ICUs) or critical care units (CCUs) of hospitals; and palliative and emotional support focusing on quality of life, which is commonly carried out by hospice care providers either in the home or in hospice centers. Many elderly people receive both types of care at the end of life, and Medicare covers both. As Figure 5.12 shows, 42.6% of Medicare recipients who died in 2009 used hospice care in the final month of life. This represents a dramatic increase since 1999, when only 19.2% of those who received end-of-life care through Medicare were in hospice care. By contrast, the proportion of Medicare recipients who received ICU or CCU care at the end of life was steadier throughout this period, rising from 22% in 1999 to 27.1% in 2009.

Hospitals remain the most common site of death for the elderly in the early 21st century, as in the late 20th century, but elderly people are becoming, on average, more likely to end their life outside of hospitals, perhaps in response to the broader cultural shift emphasizing palliative care and quality of life. (See Figure 5.13.) Nearly one-third (32.4%) of 65-and-older deaths occurred in hospitals in 2009, compared with 48.7% in 1989. Meanwhile, the proportion of 65-and-older deaths occurring in nursing homes or other long-term care facilities (26.7%) had risen slightly since 1989 (from 21.3%), and the proportion of 65-and-older deaths occurring in the home (24.3%) had risen more significantly (from 14.9%).

GERIATRICS

Geriatrics, the medical subspecialty that is concerned with the prevention and treatment of diseases in the elderly, has evolved alongside the public-health advances that have extended life expectancy in the developed world. Geriatricians are physicians trained in internal medicine or family practice who obtain additional training and certification in the diagnosis and treatment of older adults. Geriatricians rely on the findings of researchers and gerontologists (nonphysician professionals who conduct scientific studies of aging and older adults) to help older adults maintain function and independence.

Gerontology was unheard of before the 19th century, when most people died at an early age. Those who reached old age accepted their deteriorating health as a part of aging. The field of research was born during the early 20th century, when scientists began investigating the pathological changes that accompany the aging

FIGURE 5.7

Death rates for selected leading causes of death among 65 and over population, 1981–2009

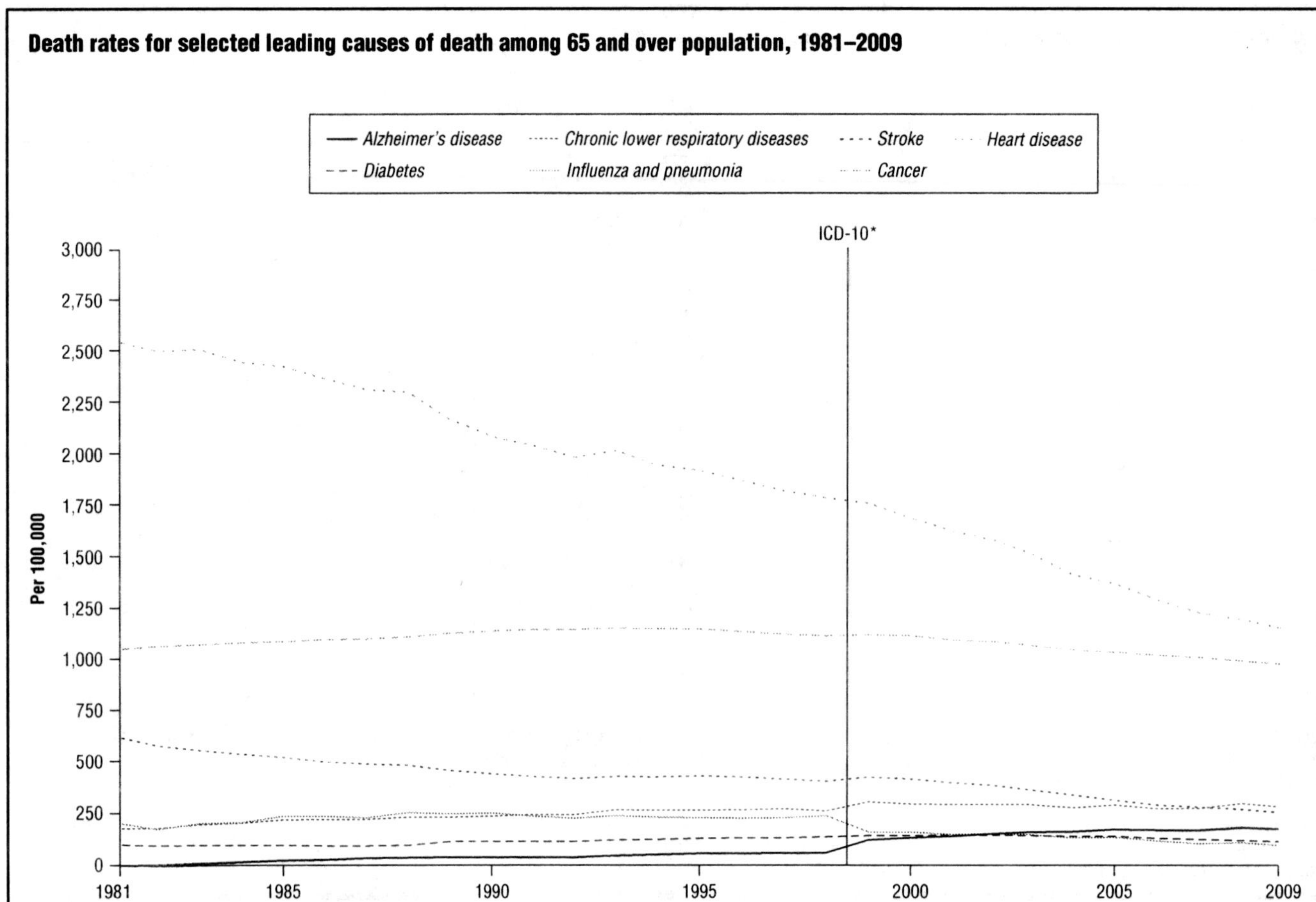

*Change calculated from 1999 when 10th revision of the International Classification of Diseases (ICD-10) was implemented.
Notes: Death rates for 1981–1998 are based on the 9th revision fo the International Classification of Diseases (ICD-9). Starting in 1999, death rates are based on ICD-10. For the period 1981–1998, causes were coded using ICD-9 codes that are nearly comparable with the 113 cause list for the ICD-10 and may differ from previously published estimates. Rates are age-adjusted using the 2000 standard population.
Reference population: These data refer to the resident population.

SOURCE: "Death Rates for Selected Leading Causes of Death among People Age 65 and over, 1981–2009," in *Older Americans 2012: Key Indicators of Well-Being*, Federal Interagency Forum on Aging Related Statistics, 2012, http://www.agingstats.gov/agingstatsdotnet/Main_Site/Data/2012_Documents/Docs/EntireChartbook.pdf (accessed February 7, 2014)

process. The Association of American Medical Colleges has responded to the need for geriatric care by developing minimum geriatrics-specific competencies. The competencies establish performance benchmarks for medical school graduates who will care for geriatric patients when they are first-year residents. The competencies are organized under eight general areas: medication management; cognitive and behavioral disorders; self-care capacity; falls, balance, and gait disorders; health care planning and promotion; atypical presentation of disease; palliative care (care that relieves the pain but does not cure the illness); and hospital care for elders.

Shortage of Geriatricians

According to the American Geriatrics Society (AGS), in the fact sheet "The Demand for Geriatric Care and the Evident Shortage of Geriatrics Healthcare Providers" (March 2013, http://www.americangeriatrics.org/files/documents/Adv_Resources/demand_for_geriatric_care.pdf), there are far fewer trained geriatricians than are necessary to meet the needs of a rapidly aging U.S. population. As of 2013, there were 7,500 geriatricians in the United States, each of which can care for approximately 700 elderly adults. This was enough geriatricians to serve approximately 5.3 million elderly patients, whereas there were closer to 12 million patients in need of geriatricians. As the elderly population continues to grow, the need for more geriatricians will only escalate. The AGS estimates that around 30,000 geriatricians will be needed by 2030, when the last of the Baby Boomers reach retirement age. To meet this demand, approximately 1,200 new geriatricians would have to be trained every year for the next 20 years.

This is unlikely to happen based on present medical school trends. The AGS reports that in 2010 only 75 residents in internal medicine or family medicine nationwide entered fellowship programs associated with geriatric medicine, down from 112 in 2005. Geriatric medicine, like the practice of internal and general medicine more generally,

FIGURE 5.8

Percentage of adults 65 and over who reported selected chronic health conditions, by sex, 2009–10

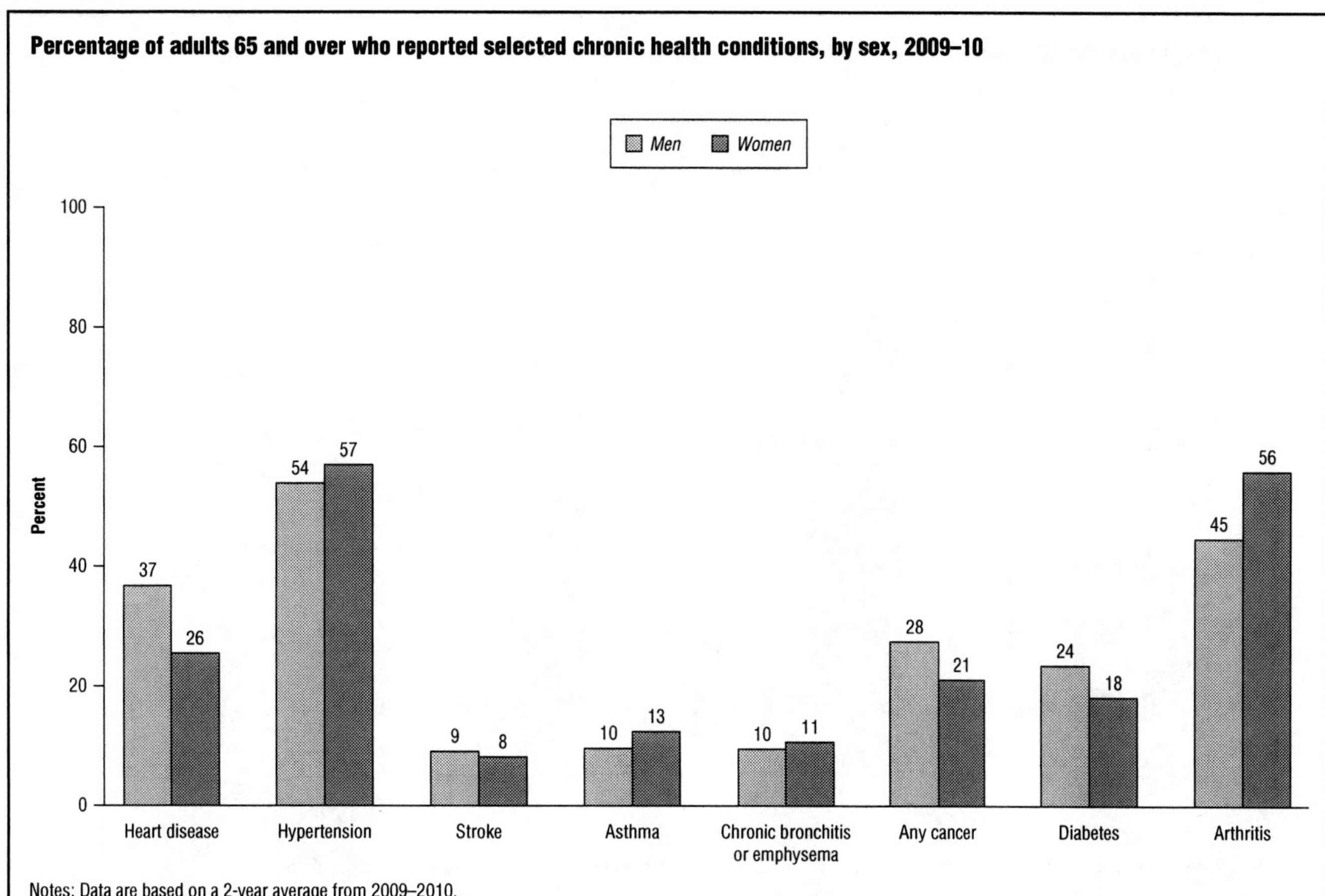

Notes: Data are based on a 2-year average from 2009–2010.
Reference population: These data refer to the civilian noninstitutionalized population.

SOURCE: "Percentage of People Age 65 and over Who Reported Having Selected Chronic Health Conditions, by Sex, 2009–2010," in *Older Americans 2012: Key Indicators of Well-Being*, Federal Interagency Forum on Aging Related Statistics, 2012, http://www.agingstats.gov/agingstatsdotnet/Main_Site/Data/2012_Documents/Docs/EntireChartbook.pdf (accessed February 7, 2014)

is one of the lowest paying of all medical and surgical specialties. The high cost of medical school and the large student loans that graduates must repay once they become licensed physicians are believed to be primary factors in steering medical students away from geriatrics and into more lucrative specialties.

The lack of geriatric expertise extends beyond the ranks of general physicians. According to the AGS, less than 1% of registered nurses, pharmacists, and physician assistants have geriatric training, and only 2.6% of advanced practice registered nurses (nurses with specialized postgraduate training) have geriatric training. Additionally, there are only around 1,600 geriatric psychiatrists in the United States, only 3% of psychologists have practices devoted primarily to older adults, and only 4% of social workers emphasize geriatric issues.

These shortages are expected to result in significant failures to deliver the health care that older Americans will need in the coming decades.

FIGURE 5.9

Percentage of adults 65 and over who reported good to excellent health status, by age, race, and Hispanic origin, 2008–10

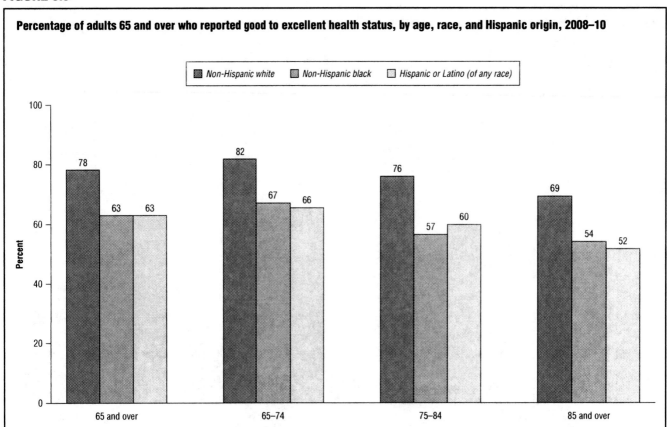

Non-Hispanic white | Non-Hispanic black | Hispanic or Latino (of any race)

Percent

	Non-Hispanic white	Non-Hispanic black	Hispanic or Latino (of any race)
65 and over	78	63	63
65–74	82	67	66
75–84	76	57	60
85 and over	69	54	52

Notes: Data are based on a 3-year average from 2008–2010. Reference population: These data refer to the civilian noninstitutionalized population.

SOURCE: "Percentage of People Age 65 and over with Respondent-Assessed Good to Excellent Health Status by Age Group and Race and Hispanic Origin, 2008–2010," in *Older Americans 2012: Key Indicators of Well-Being*, Federal Interagency Forum on Aging Related Statistics, 2012, http://www.agingstats.gov/agingstatsdotnet/Main_Site/Data/2012_Documents/Docs/EntireChartbook.pdf (accessed February 7, 2014)

FIGURE 5.10

Percentage of adults 65 and over with limitations on daily activities, by age group, 2010

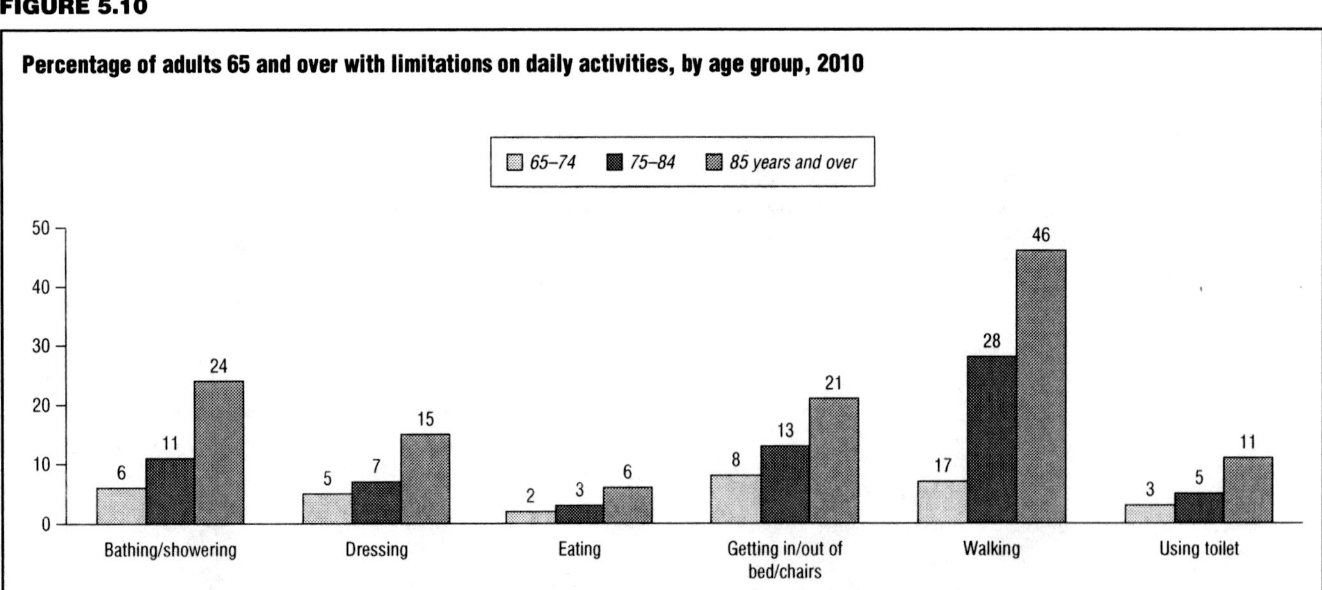

SOURCE: "Figure 9. Percent of Persons with Limitations in Activities of Daily Living by Age Group: 2010," in *A Profile of Older Americans: 2012*, U.S. Department of Health and Human Services, Administration on Aging, 2013, http://www.aoa.gov/AoARoot/(S(2ch3qw55k1qylo45dbihar2u))/Aging_Statistics/Profile/2012/docs/2012profile.pdf (accessed February 6, 2014)

TABLE 5.3

People without health insurance coverage, by selected characteristics, 2011 and 2012

[Numbers in thousands. People as of March of the following year.]

	2011			2012				
		Uninsured			Uninsured		Change in uninsured[a]	
Characteristic	Total	Number	Percent	Total	Number	Percent	Number	Percent
Total	**308,827**	**48,613**	**15.7**	**311,116**	**47,951**	**15.4**	**−663**	**−0.3**
Family status								
In families	252,316	36,749	14.6	252,863	35,830	14.2	−919	−0.4
Householder	80,529	11,870	14.7	80,944	11,921	14.7	52	Z
Related children under 18	72,568	6,647	9.2	72,545	6,348	8.8	−299	−0.4
Related children under 6	23,860	1,969	8.3	23,604	1,960	8.3	−8	0.1
In unrelated subfamilies	1,623	462	28.5	1,599	371	23.2	−91	−5.3
Unrelated individuals	54,888	11,402	20.8	56,654	11,749	20.7	347	Z
Race[b] and Hispanic origin								
White	241,586	35,991	14.9	242,469	35,625	14.7	−366	−0.2
White, not Hispanic	195,148	21,681	11.1	195,330	21,585	11.1	−96	−0.1
Black	39,696	7,722	19.5	40,208	7,629	19.0	−93	−0.5
Asian	16,094	2,696	16.8	16,433	2,477	15.1	−219	−1.7
Hispanic (any race)	52,358	15,776	30.1	53,230	15,500	29.1	−276	−1.0
Age								
Under age 65	267,320	47,923	17.9	267,829	47,312	17.7	−612	−0.3
Under age 18	74,108	6,964	9.4	74,187	6,586	8.9	−379	−0.5
Under age 19[c]	78,384	7,634	9.7	78,177	7,193	9.2	−441	−0.5
Aged 19 to 25[c]	29,909	8,272	27.7	30,207	8,205	27.2	−66	−0.5
Aged 26 to 34	37,174	10,237	27.5	37,631	10,228	27.2	−9	−0.4
Aged 35 to 44	39,927	8,399	21.0	39,877	8,428	21.1	29	0.1
Aged 45 to 64	81,926	13,382	16.3	81,937	13,257	16.2	−125	−0.2
Aged 65 and older	41,507	690	1.7	43,287	639	1.5	−51	−0.2
Nativity								
Native born	268,851	35,436	13.2	271,010	35,127	13.0	−309	−0.2
Foreign born	39,976	13,177	33.0	40,107	12,824	32.0	−353	−1.0
Naturalized citizen	17,934	3,431	19.1	18,200	3,322	18.3	−109	−0.9
Not a citizen	22,042	9,746	44.2	21,906	9,502	43.4	−244	−0.8
Region								
Northeast	55,035	6,061	11.0	55,135	5,939	10.8	−123	−0.2
Midwest	66,115	8,425	12.7	66,422	7,937	11.9	−489	−0.8
South	115,068	21,059	18.3	116,130	21,587	18.6	527	0.3
West	72,610	13,067	18.0	73,429	12,488	17.0	−579	−1.0
Residence								
Inside metropolitan statistical areas	261,455	41,299	15.8	263,328	40,694	15.5	−605	−0.3
Inside principal cities	100,302	19,045	19.0	101,363	18,836	18.6	−209	−0.4
Outside principal cities	161,153	22,255	13.8	161,965	21,859	13.5	−396	−0.3
Outside metropolitan statistical areas[d]	47,372	7,314	15.4	47,788	7,256	15.2	−58	−0.3
Work experience								
Total, aged 18 to 64	**193,213**	**40,959**	**21.2**	**193,642**	**40,726**	**21.0**	**−233**	**−0.2**
All workers	144,163	27,863	19.3	145,814	28,378	19.5	515	0.1
Worked full-time, year-round	97,443	14,926	15.3	98,715	15,309	15.5	383	0.2
Less than full-time, year-round	46,720	12,937	27.7	47,099	13,069	27.7	132	0.1
Did not work at least one week	49,049	13,096	26.7	47,828	12,348	25.8	−748	−0.9
Disability status[e]								
Total, aged 18 to 64	**193,213**	**40,959**	**21.2**	**193,642**	**40,726**	**21.0**	**−233**	**−0.2**
With a disability	14,968	2,484	16.6	14,996	2,493	16.6	8	Z
With no disability	177,309	38,473	21.7	177,727	38,233	21.5	−240	−0.2

TABLE 5.3

People without health insurance coverage, by selected characteristics, 2011 and 2012 [CONTINUED]

[Numbers in thousands. People as of March of the following year.]

Z Represents or rounds to zero.
[a]Details may not sum to totals because of rounding.
[b]Federal surveys give respondents the option of reporting more than one race. Therefore, two basic ways of defining a race group are possible. A group such as Asian may be defined as those who reported Asian and no other race (the race-alone or single-race concept) or as those who reported Asian regardless of whether they also reported another race (the race-alone-or-in-combination concept). This table shows data using the first approach (race alone). The use of the single-race population does not imply that it is the preferred method of presenting or analyzing data. The Census Bureau uses a variety of approaches. Information on people who reported more than one race, such as white ***and*** American Indian and Alaska Native or Asian ***and*** black or African American, is available from Census 2010 through American FactFinder. About 2.9 percent of people reported more than one race in Census 2010. Data for American Indians and Alaska Natives, Native Hawaiians and other Pacific Islanders, and those reporting two or more races are not shown separately.
[c]These age groups are of special interest because of the Affordable Care Act of 2010. Children under the age of 19 are eligible for Medicaid/CHIP, and individuals aged 19 to 25 may be a dependent on a parent's health plan.
[d]The "Outside metropolitan statistical areas" category includes both micropolitan statistical areas and territory outside of metropolitan and micropolitan statistical areas.
[e]The sum of those with and without a disability does not equal the total because disability status is not defined for individuals in the armed forces.

SOURCE: Carmen DeNavas-Walt, Bernadette D. Proctor, and Jessica C. Smith, "Table 7. People without Health Insurance Coverage by Selected Characteristics: 2011 and 2012," in *Income, Poverty, and Health Insurance Coverage in the United States: 2012*, U.S. Census Bureau, September 2013, http://www.census.gov/prod/2013pubs/p60-245.pdf (accessed February 10, 2014)

FIGURE 5.11

Percentage of adults 65 and over with health insurance coverage, 2011

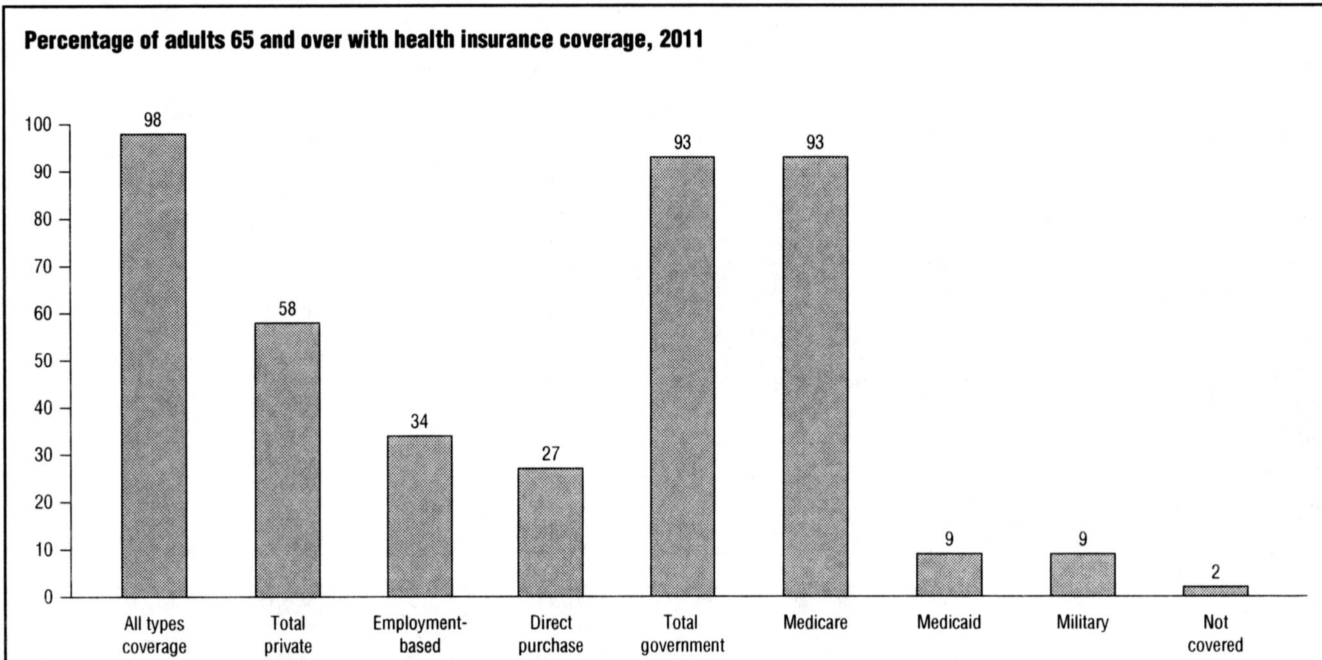

Note: Data are for the non-institutionalized elderly. A person can be represented in more than one category.

SOURCE: "Figure 8. Percentage of Persons 65+ with Health Insurance Coverage, 2011," in *A Profile of Older Americans: 2012*, U.S. Department of Health and Human Services, Administration on Aging, 2013, http://www.aoa.gov/AoARoot/(S(2ch3qw55k1qylo45dbihar2u))/Aging_Statistics/Profile/2012/docs/2012profile.pdf (accessed February 6, 2014)

FIGURE 5.12

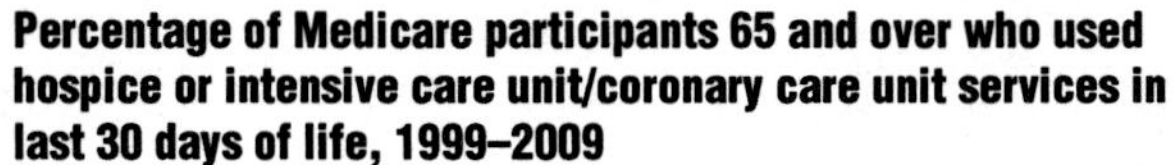

Percentage of Medicare participants 65 and over who used hospice or intensive care unit/coronary care unit services in last 30 days of life, 1999–2009

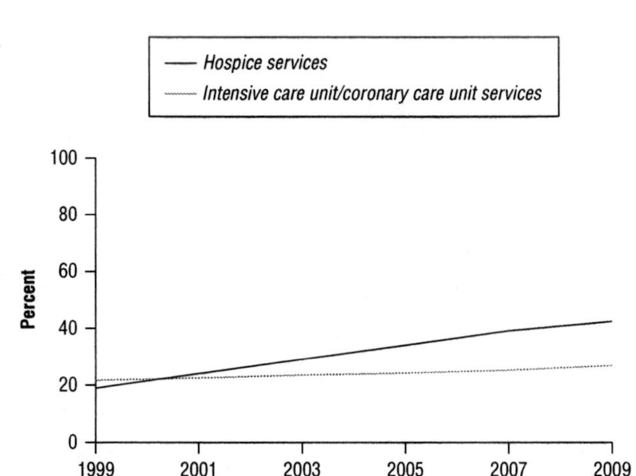

Notes: Chart is based on a 5 percent sample of deaths occurring between February and December of each year.
Reference population: These data refer to Medicare enrollees in fee-for-service.

SOURCE: "Percentage of Medicare Decedents Age 65 and over Who Used Hospice or Intensive Care Unit/Coronary Care Unit Services in Their Last 30 Days of Life, for Selected Years 1999–2009," in *Older Americans 2012: Key Indicators of Well-Being*, Federal Interagency Forum on Aging Related Statistics, 2012, http://www.agingstats.gov/agingstatsdotnet/Main_Site/Data/2012_Documents/Docs/EntireChartbook.pdf (accessed February 7, 2014)

FIGURE 5.13

Percentage distribution of deaths among adults 65 and over, by place of death, 1989–2009

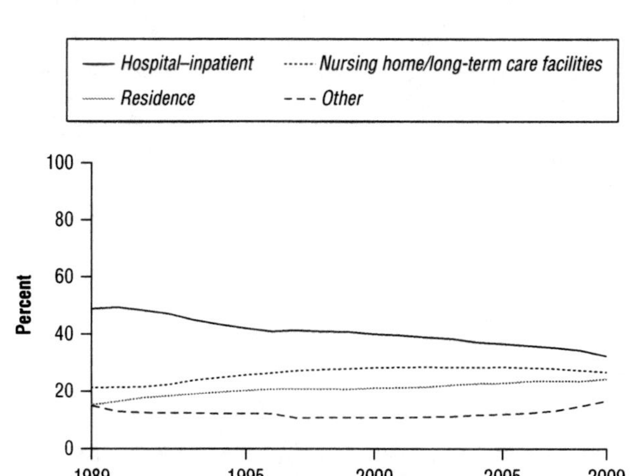

Notes: "Other" includes hospital outpatient or emergency department, including dead on arrival, inpatient hospice facilities, and all other places and unknown. Beginning in 2003, the term "long-term care facility" was added to the nursing home check box on the death certificate.
Reference population: These data refer to the resident population.

SOURCE: "Percent Distribution of Decedents Age 65 and over by Place of Death, 1989–2009," in *Older Americans 2012: Key Indicators of Well-Being*, Federal Interagency Forum on Aging Related Statistics, 2012, http://www.agingstats.gov/agingstatsdotnet/Main_Site/Data/2012_Documents/Docs/EntireChartbook.pdf (accessed February 7, 2014)

CHAPTER 6
INFANT AND CHILD DEATH

What greater pain could mortals have than this: To see their children dead before their eyes?

—Euripides

End-of-life issues are wrenching by definition, but those involving children have the potential to be particularly devastating. Parents who find themselves responsible for making decisions about how to handle their children's illnesses come into conflict with some of their most basic instincts, and unconditional love for a child can complicate rather than solve the dilemmas that arise in relation to the continuation of life support or other treatments. The parental need to protect one's child may be absolute, but what does protection mean in the case of a terminally ill child? Does protection translate into an infinite prolongation of life, even if this means exposing the child to unnecessary suffering? Or does protection translate into allowing the child to find relief from an agonizing existence even if the result is death?

Impossible as these decisions may seem, parents must regularly make them. In a best-case scenario, parents faced with such a terrible dilemma are aided by sensitive physicians and mental-health professionals, and they are able to make decisions with which they can eventually come to terms. Other cases present additional complications. What if the ailing child is an adolescent who refuses further treatment for a terminal illness? Whose wishes matter more: the suffering adolescent's, or the parent's?

This chapter focuses on infant and child death, the conditions that often cause mortality at young ages, and medical decision making for seriously ill children.

INFANT MORTALITY RATES AND CAUSES

Marian F. MacDorman and T. J. Mathews of the National Center for Health Statistics (NCHS) indicate in *Recent Trends in Infant Mortality in the United States* (October 2008, http://www.cdc.gov/nchs/data/databriefs/db09.pdf) that between 1900 and 2000 the U.S. infant mortality rate declined dramatically. In 1900 the infant mortality rate was approximately 100 deaths per 1,000 live births, whereas in 2000 it was 6.9 deaths per 1,000 live births. Between 2000 and 2007 the infant mortality rate appeared to have stopped decreasing, but between 2007 and 2011 it resumed a downward trend. (See Figure 6.1.)

This improvement in the prospects for newborn infants, which is common to all countries of the developed world, represents one of the most significant medical accomplishments in history. The same advances that prolonged life expectancies generally—especially those relating to sanitation, infectious diseases, antibiotics, and vaccination—played a major role in the early declines in infant mortality. Since 1960 advances in neonatology (the medical subspecialty that is concerned with the care of newborns) have been the primary drivers of the continued improvement in outcomes for newborn infants. Infants born prematurely or with low birth weights, who were once likely to die, now can survive life-threatening conditions because of the development of neonatal intensive care units, technologies, and treatments.

Babies of all races and ethnicities are more likely to die in the neonatal period (the first 28 days of life) than in the postneonatal period (28 days to 11 months of age). (See Table 6.1.) Of the 23,910 infant deaths in 2011, 15,954 (66.7%) occurred during the neonatal period, compared with 7,956 during the postneonatal period. Although the proportions of deaths that occurred during the neonatal versus postneonatal period differed slightly according to ethnic and racial identification, the general trend was consistent across groups.

U.S. Rates Compared with Those of Other Countries

Although infant mortality rates in the United States had reached historic lows by the early 21st century, they were considerably higher than rates in other wealthy countries.

FIGURE 6.1

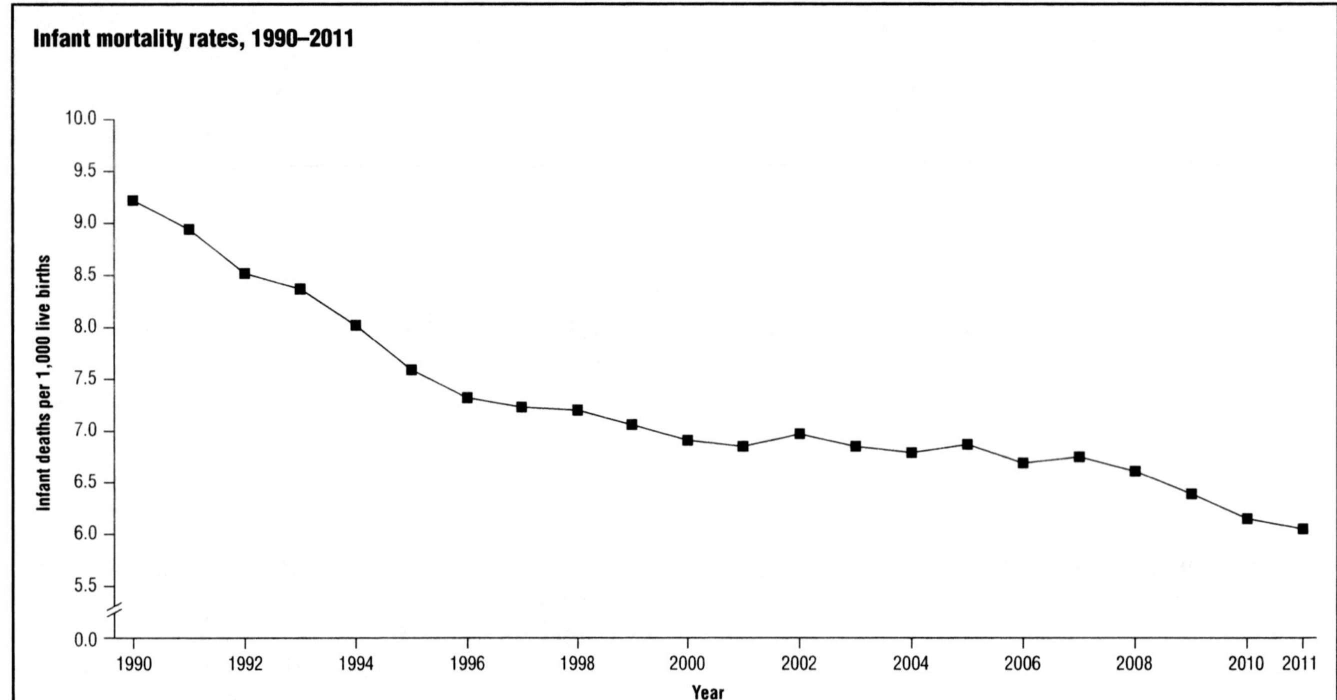

SOURCE: Arialdi M. Miniño, "Figure 5. Infant Mortality Rates: United States, 1990–2010 Final and Preliminary 2011," in "Death in the United States, 2011," *NCHS Data Brief*, no. 115, Centers for Disease Control and Prevention, National Center for Health Statistics, March 2013, http://www.cdc.gov/nchs/data/databriefs/db115.pdf (accessed December 27, 2013)

Table 6.2 shows the infant mortality rates for most of the current member countries of the Organisation for Economic Co-operation and Development (OECD), a group that promotes international economic and social well-being and that consists of most of the world's richest countries as well as a number of emerging countries. The United States has by far the largest economy of any OECD member country, but its 2009 infant mortality rate was surpassed by only those of Chile, Mexico, and Turkey, placing it 27th among the 31 countries for which data were available. (No 2009 data were available for Canada, so the numerical rankings in this table reach only 30. Canada's infant mortality rate was, however, known to be lower than that of the United States during this time.)

Moreover, between 1960 and 2009 the U.S. infant mortality rate fell more slowly than the rates of comparably developed countries: its 1960 rate of 26 infant deaths per 1,000 live births translated into a ranking of 12th among the 31 countries shown. Countries with comparable rates in 1960, such as Canada (27.3), France (27.7), the Slovak Republic (28.6), and Ireland (29.3), all reduced their infant mortality rates more quickly over the subsequent five decades. The U.S. rate was more than double that of all countries ranked one through nine in 2009 (because numerous countries had identical rates, there were 11 countries in this group), and it was more than triple that of Iceland, the country with the lowest infant mortality rate in the world (1.8 infant deaths per 1,000 births).

Some researchers have suggested that differences in the way countries classify live births explains some of the disparity between infant mortality rates in the United States and rates in the rest of the developed world. Specifically, some European countries use gestational weight, age, or both in their definition of what constitutes a live birth, classifying the deaths of babies who do not surpass these limits as stillbirths rather than as infant deaths. Because the United States considers all babies born alive to be live births, it would necessarily have a higher infant mortality rate than a country that does not consider all such deaths to be infant deaths.

However, since 1993 most developed countries have used the same definition as the United States, which is the definition recommended by the World Health Organization. The handful of countries that continue to classify some instances of infant mortality as stillbirths (the Czech Republic, France, Ireland, the Netherlands, and Poland) are not sufficient to skew the international data on their own. According to Elayne J. Heisler of the Congressional Research Service, in *The U.S. Infant Mortality Rate: International Comparisons, Underlying Factors, and Federal Programs* (April 4, 2012, https://www.fas.org/sgp/crs/misc/R41378.pdf), statisticians at the NCHS have concluded that, for the high U.S. rates to be explained by differences in the reporting of live births, all European countries "would have to misreport one-third of their infant deaths, which these researchers conclude is unlikely."

TABLE 6.1

Infant deaths and infant mortality rates, by age, race, and Hispanic origin, 2010–11

[Data are based on the continuous file of records received from the states. Rates per 1,000 live births. Figures for 2011 are based on weighted data rounded to the nearest individual, so categories may not add to totals. Race and Hispanic origin are reported separately on both the birth and death certificate. Rates for Hispanic origin should be interpreted with caution because of the inconsistencies between reporting Hispanic origin on birth and death certificates. Race categories are consistent with the 1977 Office of Management and Budget (OMB) standards. Multiple-race data were reported for deaths by 38 states and District of Columbia in 2011, and by 37 states and the District of Columbia in 2010, and were reported for births, by 40 states and District of Columbia in 2011, and by 38 states and the District of Columbia in 2010. The multiple-race data for these states were bridged to the single-race categories of the 1977 OMB standards for comparability with other states.]

Age, race, and Hispanic origin	2011		2010	
	Number	Rate	Number	Rate
All races[a]				
Under 1 year	23,910	6.05	24,586	6.15
Under 28 days	15,954	4.04	16,188	4.05
28 days–11 months	7,956	2.01	8,398	2.10
Total white				
Under 1 year	15,438	5.11	15,954	5.20
Under 28 days	10,422	3.45	10,612	3.46
28 days–11 months	5,016	1.66	5,342	1.74
Non-Hispanic white				
Under 1 year	10,872	5.05	11,025	5.10
Under 28 days	7,191	3.34	7,212	3.34
28 days–11 months	3,681	1.71	3,813	1.76
Total black				
Under 1 year	7,234	11.42	7,401	11.63
Under 28 days	4,719	7.45	4,769	7.49
28 days–11 months	2,515	3.97	2,632	4.14
Hispanic[b]				
Under 1 year	4,806	5.27	5,170	5.47
Under 28 days	3,353	3.68	3,524	3.73
28 days–11 months	1,453	1.59	1,646	1.74

[a]Includes races other than white and black.
[b]Includes all persons of Hispanic origin of any race.
Notes: Data are subject to sampling or random variation. Although the infant mortality rate is the preferred indicator of the risk of dying during the first year of life, another measure of infant mortality, the infant death rate, is shown elsewhere in this report. The two measures typically are similar, yet they can differ because the denominators used for these measures are different.

SOURCE: Donna L. Hoyert and Jiaquan Xu, "Table 4. Infant Deaths and Infant Mortality Rates, by Age, Race, and Hispanic Origin: United States, Final 2010 and Preliminary 2011," in "Deaths: Preliminary Data for 2011," *National Vital Statistics Reports*, vol. 61, no. 6, October 10, 2012, http://www.cdc.gov/nchs/data/nvsr/nvsr61/nvsr61_06.pdf (accessed December 23, 2013)

According to Heisler, NCHS researchers have shown that the high infant mortality rate in the United States is largely explained by its high rate of infant mortality due to short gestational age (prematurity) and low birth weight. The usual length of human pregnancy is 40 weeks, and infants born before 37 weeks of pregnancy are considered to be premature. A premature infant does not have fully formed organ systems. If the premature infant is born with a birth weight that is comparable to a full-term baby and has organ systems only slightly underdeveloped, the chances of survival are great. Conversely, premature infants of very low birth weight are susceptible to many risks and are less likely to survive. If they survive, they may suffer from intellectual disability and other abnormalities of the nervous system. A severe medical condition called respiratory distress syndrome (RDS) also commonly affects premature infants born before 35 weeks of pregnancy. In RDS immature lungs do not function properly and may cause infant death within hours after birth. Intensive care includes the use of a mechanical ventilator to facilitate breathing. Premature infants also commonly have immature gastrointestinal systems, which preclude them from taking in nourishment properly. Unable to suck and swallow, they must be fed through a stomach tube.

In the United States as in the rest of the developed world, birth defects—which are officially classified as congenital malformations, deformations, and chromosomal abnormalities—account for more cases of infant mortality than any other cause. In the United States, however, the number of infant deaths caused by disorders related to prematurity and low birth weight is nearly as high as the number due to birth defects. As Table 6.3 shows, birth defects accounted for 4,984 infant deaths in 2011, and short gestation and low birth weight led to death in 4,116 cases. Sudden infant death syndrome caused 1,711 infant deaths, maternal complications of pregnancy caused 1,578 infant deaths, and accidents caused 1,089 infant deaths. Although the United States' rate of infant mortality due to birth defects is similar to that of other developed countries, it has a far higher rate of low birth weight and short gestational age births. Heisler reports that "the U.S. [infant mortality rate] would be 3.9 if the United States had the same rate of low birthweight and short gestational age births as Sweden."

The prevalence of low birth weight and short gestational age births is, in turn, linked to disparities among different racial and ethnic groups in the United States. African American and Native American infants, exposed, in the aggregate, to inequalities in medical care and other social resources, have long been considerably more likely to die during the first year after birth than have babies of other races and ethnicities. As Table 6.4 shows, the infant mortality rate for African American mothers stood at 19.2 per 1,000 live births in 1983, and that of Native American mothers stood at 15.2. By comparison, the rate for Hispanic mothers was 9.5, the rate for white mothers was 9.3, and the rate for Asian or Pacific Islander mothers was 8.3. Since the 1980s, infant mortality rates have fallen faster for both African American and Native American mothers than for the other groups. By 1995 the African American infant mortality rate was 14.6, and the Native American rate was 9. Thereafter, the rate for Native American mothers fluctuated, remaining significantly higher than that for Hispanic, white, and Asian or Pacific Islander mothers. The rate for African American mothers continued to drop, but

TABLE 6.2

Infant mortality rates and rankings for Organisation for Economic Co-operation and Development (OECD) countries, selected years 1960–2009

[Data are based on reporting by OECD countries]

Country[b]	1960	1970	1980	1990	2000	2007	2008	2009	International rankings[a] 1960	International rankings[a] 2009
	Infant[c] deaths per 1,000 live births									
Australia	20,2	17.9	10.7	8.2	5.2	4.2	4.1	4.3	6	20
Austria	37.5	25.9	14.3	7.8	4.8	3.7	3.7	3.8	20	15
Belgium	31.4	21.1	12.1	8.0	4.8	3.9	3.7	3.4	18	12
Canada	27.3	18.8	10.4	6.8	5.3	5.1	5.1	—	13	—
Chile	120.3	79.3	33.0	16.0	8.9	8.3	7.8	7.9	28	28
Czech Republic	20.0	20.2	16.9	10.8	4.1	3.1	2.8	2.9	5	5
Denmark	21.5	14.2	8.4	7.5	5.3	4.0	4.0	3.1	9	6
Finland	21.0	13.2	7.6	5.6	3.8	2.7	2.6	2.6	7	4
France	27.7	18.2	10.0	7.3	4.5	3.8	3.8	3.9†	14	18
Germany	35.0	22.5	12.4	7.0	4.4	3.9	3.5	3.5	19	13
Greece	40.1	29.6	17.9	9.7	5.9	3.5	2.7	3.1	21	6
Hungary	47.6	35.9	23.2	14.8	9.2	5.9	5.6	5.1	24	23
Iceland	13.0	13.2	7.7	5.9	3.0	2.0	2.5	1.8	1	1
Ireland	29.3	19.5	11.1	8.2	6.2	3.1	3.8	3.2	16	9
Israel[d]	—	24.2	15.6	9.9	5.5	3.9	3.8	3.8	—	15
Italy	43.9	29.6	14.6	8.1	4.3	3.5	3.3	3.9	23	18
Japan	30.7	13.1	7.5	4.6	3.2	2.6	2.6	2.4	17	2
Korea	—	45.0	—	—	—	3.6	3.5	3.2	—	9
Mexico	92.3	—	52.6	—	19.4	15.7	15.2	14.7	27	30
Netherlands	16.5	12.7	8.6	7.1	5.1	4.1	3.8	3.8	3	15
New Zealand	22.6	16.7	13.0	8.4	6.3	4.8	5.0	5.2	11	24
Norway	16.0	11.3	8.1	6.9	3.8	3.1	2.7	3.1	2	6
Poland	56.1	36.4	25.4	19.4	8.1	6.0	5.6	5.6	25	25
Portugal	77.5	55.5	24.3	10.9	5.5	3.4	3.3	3.6	26	14
Slovak Republic	28.6	25.7	20.9	12.0	8.6	6.1	5.9	5.7	15	26
Spain	43.7	28.1	12.3††	7.6	4.3	3.4	3.3	3.2	22	9
Sweden	16.6	11.0	6.9	6.0	3.4	2.5	2.5	2.5	4	3
Switzerland	21.1	15.1	9.1	6.8	4.9	3.9	4.0	4.3	8	20
Turkey	189.5	145.0	117.5	51.5††	31.6	15.9	14.9	13.1	29	29
United Kingdom	22.5	18.5	12.1	7.9	5.6	4.8	4.7	4.6	10	22
United States	26.0	20.0	12.6	9.2	6.9	6.8	6.6	6.4	12	27

—Data not available.
†Data are estimated.
††Break in series.
[a]Rankings are from lowest to highest infant mortality rates (IMR). Countries with the same IMR receive the same rank. The country with the next highest IMR is assigned the rank it would have received had the lower-ranked countries not been tied, i.e., skip a rank. The latest year's international rankings are based on 2009 data because that is the most current data year for which most countries have reported their final data to OECD. Countries without an estimate in the OECD database are omitted from this table. Relative rankings for individual countries may be affected if not all countries have reported data to OECD.
[b]Refers to countries, territories, cities, or geographic areas with at least 2.5 million population and with complete counts of live births and infant deaths according to the United Nations Demographic Yearbook.
[c]Under 1 year of age.
[d]The statistical data for Israel are supplied by, and under the responsibility of, the relevant Israeli authorities. The use of such data by the OECD is without prejudice to the status of the Golan Heights, East Jerusalem, and Israeli settlements in the West Bank under the terms of international law.
Notes: Some rates for selected countries and selected years were revised and differ from previous editions of *Health, United States*.

SOURCE: "Table 16. Infant Mortality Rates and International Rankings: Organisation for Economic Co-operation and Development (OECD) Countries, Selected Years 1960–2009," in *Health, United States, 2012: With Special Feature on Emergency Care*, Centers for Disease Control and Prevention, National Center for Health Statistics, 2013, http://www.cdc.gov/nchs/data/hus/hus12.pdf (accessed December 27, 2013). Data from the Organisation for Economic Co-operation and Development (OECD) Health Data 2012.

throughout the early years of the new century, it remained more than double that of Hispanic, white, and Asian mothers. As of 2011, the total infant mortality rate was 6.1 per 1,000 live births, the non-Hispanic white rate was 5, the Hispanic rate was 5.3, and the African American rate was 11.4. (See Table 6.1.)

As Table 6.3 shows, whereas birth defects were the leading cause of infant death among whites and Hispanics in 2011, disorders related to short gestation and low birth weight were the leading cause of infant death among African Americans. Short gestation and low birth weight caused the deaths of 1,576 African American babies, whereas birth defects led to death in 994 cases. The African American infant mortality rate associated with short gestation and low birth weight, at 248.8 per 100,000 live births, was more than three times greater than that for non-Hispanic whites (73.3) and nearly three times greater than that for Hispanics (85.9).

These infant deaths are to a substantial degree preventable, given access to high-quality prenatal care. According to the U.S. Department of Health and Human Services' Office of Minority Health, in "Infant

TABLE 6.3

Infant deaths and infant mortality rates for the 10 leading causes of infant death, by race and Hispanic origin, 2011

[Data are based on a continuous file of records received from the states. Rates are per 100,000 live births. Figures are based on weighted data rounded to the nearest individual, so categories may not add to totals or subtotals. Race and Hispanic origin are reported separately on both the birth and death certificate. Rates for Hispanic origin should be interpreted with caution because of inconsistencies between reporting Hispanic origin on birth and death certificates. Race categories are consistent with the 1977 Office of Management and Budget (OMB) standards. Multiple-race data were reported for deaths by 38 states and District of Columbia and for births by 40 states and District of Columbia. The multiple-race data for these states were bridged to the single-race categories of the 1977 OMB standards for comparability with other states. Data for persons of Hispanic origin are included in the data for each race group, according to the decedent's reported race.]

Rank[a]	Cause of death, race, and Hispanic origin	Number	Rate
	All races[b]		
...	All causes	23,907	604.7
1	Congenital malformations, deformations and chromosomal abnormalities	4,984	126.1
2	Disorders related to short gestation and low birth weight, not elsewhere classified	4,116	104.1
3	Sudden infant death syndrome	1,711	43.3
4	Newborn affected by maternal complications of pregnancy	1,578	39.9
5	Accidents (unintentional injuries)	1,089	27.5
6	Newborn affected by complications of placenta, cord and membranes	992	25.1
7	Bacterial sepsis of newborn	526	13.3
8	Respiratory distress of newborn	514	13.0
9	Diseases of the circulatory system	496	12.5
10	Neonatal hemorrhage	444	11.2
...	All other causes	7,457	188.6
	Total white		
...	All causes	15,451	511.7
1	Congenital malformations, deformations and chromosomal abnormalities	3,732	123.6
2	Disorders related to short gestation and low birth weight, not elsewhere classified	2,330	77.2
3	Sudden infant death syndrome	1,126	37.3
4	Newborn affected by maternal complications of pregnancy	962	31.9
5	Accidents (unintentional injuries)	678	22.5
6	Newborn affected by complications of placenta, cord and membranes	642	21.3
7	Respiratory distress of newborn	341	11.3
8	Bacterial sepsis of newborn	326	10.8
9	Diseases of the circulatory system	317	10.5
10	Neonatal hemorrhage	315	10.4
...	All other causes	4,682	155.0
	Non-Hispanic white		
...	All causes	10,883	506.0
1	Congenital malformations, deformations and chromosomal abnormalities	2,496	116.0
2	Disorders related to short gestation and low birth weight, not elsewhere classified	1,577	73.3
3	Sudden infant death syndrome	904	42.0
4	Newborn affected by maternal complications of pregnancy	645	30.0
5	Accidents (unintentional injuries)	550	25.6
6	Newborn affected by complications of placenta, cord and membranes	456	21.2
7	Respiratory distress of newborn	243	11.3
8	Neonatal hemorrhage	227	10.6
8	Bacterial sepsis of newborn	227	10.6
10	Diseases of the circulatory system	220	10.2
...	All other causes	3,338	155.2
	Total black		
...	All causes	7,221	1,139.8
1	Disorders related to short gestation and low birth weight, not elsewhere classified	1,576	248.8
2	Congenital malformations, deformations and chromosomal abnormalities	994	156.9
3	Newborn affected by maternal complications of pregnancy	535	84.4
4	Sudden infant death syndrome	517	81.6
5	Accidents (unintentional injuries)	355	56.0
6	Newborn affected by complications of placenta, cord and membranes	314	49.6
7	Bacterial sepsis of newborn	178	28.1
8	Diseases of the circulatory system	152	24.0
9	Necrotizing enterocolitis of newborn	150	23.7
10	Respiratory distress of newborn	148	23.4
...	All other causes	2,302	363.4

Mortality and African Americans" (July 29, 2013, http://minorityhealth.hhs.gov/templates/content.aspx?ID=3021), non-Hispanic African American mothers were almost as likely as non-Hispanic white mothers to receive prenatal care of some sort as of 2011: 80.9% of African American mothers received prenatal care that year, compared with 85.7% of white mothers. Nevertheless, there can be wide variations in the quality and consistency of prenatal care. Adequate care should start during the first trimester of pregnancy, and the Office of Minority Health notes that as of 2008 (the most recent year for which data were available as of April 2014), African American mothers were more than twice as likely as non-Hispanic whites to receive prenatal care either not at all or beginning in the third trimester of pregnancy.

TABLE 6.3

Infant deaths and infant mortality rates for the 10 leading causes of infant death, by race and Hispanic origin, 2011 [CONTINUED]

[Data are based on a continuous file of records received from the states. Rates are per 100,000 live births. Figures are based on weighted data rounded to the nearest individual, so categories may not add to totals or subtotals. Race and Hispanic origin are reported separately on both the birth and death certificate. Rates for Hispanic origin should be interpreted with caution because of inconsistencies between reporting Hispanic origin on birth and death certificates. Race categories are consistent with the 1977 Office of Management and Budget (OMB) standards. Multiple-race data were reported for deaths by 38 states and District of Columbia and for births by 40 states and District of Columbia. The multiple-race data for these states were bridged to the single-race categories of the 1977 OMB standards for comparability with other states. Data for persons of Hispanic origin are included in the data for each race group, according to the decedent's reported race.]

Rank[a]	Cause of death, race, and Hispanic origin	Number	Rate
	Hispanic[c]		
...	All causes	4,804	526.6
1	Congenital malformations, deformations and chromosomal abnormalities	1,282	140.5
2	Disorders related to short gestation and low birth weight, not elsewhere classified	784	85.9
3	Newborn affected by maternal complications of pregnancy	330	36.2
4	Sudden infant death syndrome	239	26.2
5	Newborn affected by complications of placenta, cord and membranes	193	21.2
6	Accidents (unintentional injuries)	142	15.6
7	Bacterial sepsis of newborn	106	11.6
8	Diseases of the circulatory system	105	11.5
9	Respiratory distress of newborn	99	10.9
10	Neonatal hemorrhage	94	10.3
...	All other causes	1,430	156.7

. . .Category not applicable.
[a]Rank based on number of deaths.
[b]Includes races other than white and black.
[c]Includes all persons of Hispanic origin of any race.
Note: For certain causes of death such as unintentional injuries, homicides, sudden infant death syndrome, and respiratory diseases, preliminary and final data differ because of the truncated nature of the preliminary file. Data are subject to sampling or random variation. Although the infant mortality rate is the preferred indicator of the risk of dying during the first year of life, another measure of infant mortality, the infant death rate, is shown elsewhere in the report. The two measures typically are similar, yet they can differ because the denominators used for these measures are different.

SOURCE: Donna L. Hoyert and Jiaquan Xu, "Table 8. Infant Deaths and Infant Mortality Rates for the 10 Leading Causes of Infant Death, by Race and Hispanic Origin: United States, Preliminary 2011," in "Deaths: Preliminary Data for 2011," *National Vital Statistics Reports*, vol. 61, no. 6, October 10, 2012, http://www.cdc.gov/nchs/data/nvsr/nvsr61/nvsr61_06.pdf (accessed December 23, 2013)

The Causes of Low Birth Weight and Prematurity

As Figure 6.2 shows, the prevalence of preterm births in the United States (births that occurred earlier than week 39 of pregnancy) increased markedly between 1990 and 2006. This was true among both subgroups of premature births: births occurring in the early preterm period (at less than 34 weeks of gestation) and births occurring in the late preterm period (34 to 36 weeks). During this same period the number of births occurring in the early term period (37 to 38 weeks), a time when babies can usually be delivered without complication—although the risks are still greater than at full term (39 to 40 weeks)—also increased significantly. Since 2006 the prevalence of preterm and early term births has declined, although it remains elevated relative to rates during the 1980s and 1990s. Low birth weight rates have followed a similar pattern, which is understandable given that premature babies typically weigh less than full-term babies. Among all races, the low birth weight (less than 5 pounds, 8 ounces [2,500 g]) and very low birth weight (less than 3 pounds, 4 ounces [1,500 g]) rates both rose steadily from 1990 and peaked in 2006 before beginning to decline gradually. (See Table 6.5.) The same was true of both preterm (less than 37 weeks of gestation) and very preterm (less than 32 weeks) rates.

According to Joyce A. Martin et al. of the NCHS, in "Births: Final Data for 2011" (*National Vital Statistics Reports*, vol. 61, no. 1, June 28, 2013), one reason for the rise in births prior to 39 weeks may have been an increase in the rates of delivery via cesarean section (delivery of a fetus by surgical incision through the abdominal wall and uterus) between 1996 and 2009. The subsequent declines, from 2009 to 2011, may also be partly linked to efforts on behalf of medical professionals and other experts to dissuade people from delivering via cesarean section except in cases when it is medically necessary.

Another reason for the rise in low birth weight and preterm babies may be the dramatic rise in the multiple-birth rate between the 1980s and 2005. Twins, triplets, and higher-order multiple births are more likely to be born prematurely than are single infants; and even when they are born closer to full term, they are more likely to weigh less than single infants. Between 1980 and 2011 the multiple-birth rate for all races and ethnicities rose dramatically, from 19.3 per 1,000 live births to 34.6 per 1,000. (See Table 6.6.) The 2011 multiple-birth rate was identical for both non-Hispanic white mothers and non-Hispanic African American mothers, at 38.3 per 1,000. The multiple-birth rate for Hispanic mothers was much lower throughout this period, although it rose, as well, from 18.4 in 1990 to 23.9 in 2011.

Preterm delivery and low birth weight rates are clearly correlated with maternal age. As Table 6.7 shows,

TABLE 6.4

Infant, neonatal, and postneonatal mortality rates, by race and Hispanic origin of mother, selected years 1983–2008

[Data are based on linked birth and death certificates for infants]

Maternal race and Hispanic origin	1983[a]	1985[a]	1990[a]	1995[b]	2000[b]	2005[b]	2007[b]	2008[b]
				Infant[c] deaths per 1,000 live births				
All mothers	**10.9**	**10.4**	**8.9**	**7.6**	**6.9**	**6.9**	**6.8**	**6.6**
White	9.3	8.9	7.3	6.3	5.7	5.7	5.6	5.6
Black or African American	19.2	18.6	16.9	14.6	13.5	13.3	12.9	12.4
American Indian or Alaska Native	15.2	13.1	13.1	9.0	8.3	8.1	9.2	8.4
Asian or Pacific Islander[d]	8.3	7.8	6.6	5.3	4.9	4.9	4.8	4.5
Hispanic or Latina[e, f]	9.5	8.8	7.5	6.3	5.6	5.6	5.5	5.6
Mexican	9.1	8.5	7.2	6.0	5.4	5.5	5.4	5.6
Puerto Rican	12.9	11.2	9.9	8.9	8.2	8.3	7.7	7.3
Cuban	7.5	8.5	7.2	5.3	4.6	4.4	5.2	4.9
Central and South American	8.5	8.0	6.8	5.5	4.6	4.7	4.6	4.8
Other and unknown Hispanic or Latina	10.6	9.5	8.0	7.4	6.9	6.4	6.4	5.9
Not Hispanic or Latina[f]:								
White	9.2	8.6	7.2	6.3	5.7	5.8	5.6	5.5
Black or African American	19.1	18.3	16.9	14.7	13.6	13.6	13.3	12.7
				Neonatal[c] deaths per 1,000 live births				
All mothers	**7.1**	**6.8**	**5.7**	**4.9**	**4.6**	**4.5**	**4.4**	**4.3**
White	6.1	5.8	4.6	4.1	3.8	3.8	3.7	3.6
Black or African American	12.5	12.3	11.1	9.6	9.1	8.9	8.5	8.1
American Indian or Alaska Native	7.5	6.1	6.1	4.0	4.4	4.0	4.6	4.2
Asian or Pacific Islander[d]	5.2	4.8	3.9	3.4	3.4	3.4	3.4	3.1
Hispanic or Latina[e, f]	6.2	5.7	4.8	4.1	3.8	3.9	3.7	3.8
Mexican	5.9	5.4	4.5	3.9	3.6	3.8	3.7	3.8
Puerto Rican	8.7	7.6	6.9	6.1	5.8	5.9	5.1	5.0
Cuban	5.0*	6.2	5.3	3.6*	3.2*	3.1*	3.7	3.3
Central and South American	5.8	5.6	4.4	3.7	3.3	3.2	3.1	3.2
Other and unknown Hispanic or Latina	6.4	5.6	5.0	4.8	4.6	4.3	4.1	3.8
Not Hispanic or Latina[f]:								
White	5.9	5.6	4.5	4.0	3.8	3.7	3.6	3.5
Black or African American	12.0	11.9	11.0	9.6	9.2	9.1	8.7	8.3
				Postneonatal[c] deaths per 1,000 live births				
All mothers	**3.8**	**3.6**	**3.2**	**2.6**	**2.3**	**2.3**	**2.3**	**2.3**
White	3.2	3.1	2.7	2.2	1.9	2.0	1.9	2.0
Black or African American	6.7	6.3	5.9	5.0	4.3	4.3	4.4	4.3
American Indian or Alaska Native	7.7	7.0	7.0	5.1	3.9	4.0	4.7	4.2
Asian or Pacific Islander[d]	3.1	2.9	2.7	1.9	1.4	1.5	1.4	1.4
Hispanic or Latina[e, f]	3.3	3.2	2.7	2.1	1.8	1.8	1.8	1.8
Mexican	3.2	3.2	2.7	2.1	1.8	1.7	1.7	1.8
Puerto Rican	4.2	3.5	3.0	2.8	2.4	2.4	2.6	2.3
Cuban	2.5*	2.3*	1.9*	1.7*	*	1.4*	1.5*	1.6*
Central and South American	2.6	2.4	2.4	1.9	1.4	1.5	1.4	1.6
Other and unknown Hispanic or Latina	4.2	3.9	3.0	2.6	2.3	2.1	2.3	2.1
Not Hispanic or Latina[f]:								
White	3.2	3.0	2.7	2.2	1.9	2.1	2.0	2.0
Black or African American	7.0	6.4	5.9	5.0	4.4	4.5	4.6	4.4

*Estimates are considered unreliable. Rates preceded by an asterisk are based on fewer than 50 deaths in the numerator. Rates not shown are based on fewer than 20 deaths in the numerator.
[a]Rates based on unweighted birth cohort data.
[b]Rates based on a period file using weighted data.
[c]Infant (under 1 year of age), neonatal (under 28 days), and postneonatal (28 days–11 months).
[d]Estimates are not available for Asian or Pacific Islander subgroups because not all states have adopted the 2003 revision of the U.S. Standard Certificate of Live Birth.
[e]Persons of Hispanic origin may be of any race.
[f]Prior to 1995, data are shown only for states with an Hispanic-origin item on their birth certificates.
Notes: The race groups white, black, American Indian or Alaska Native, and Asian or Pacific Islander include persons of Hispanic and non-Hispanic origin. Starting with 2003 data, some states reported multiple-race data. The multiple-race data for these states were bridged to the single-race categories of the 1977 Office of Management and Budget standards, for comparability with other states. National linked files do not exist for 1992–1994. Data for additional years are available.

SOURCE: "Table 11. Infant, Neonatal, and Postneonatal Mortality Rates, by Detailed Race and Hispanic Origin of Mother: United States, Selected Years 1983–2008," in *Health, United States, 2012: With Special Feature on Emergency Care*, Centers for Disease Control and Prevention, National Center for Health Statistics, 2013, http://www.cdc.gov/nchs/data/hus/hus12.pdf (accessed December 27, 2013)

both teen mothers and mothers over the age of 40 years were significantly more likely to have preterm and low birth weight babies in 2011. This was true of mothers across racial and ethnic categories. The average age at which women begin to have children has significantly increased since the late 20th century, and it has become much more common for women over the age of 40 years to give birth, thanks to advancements in fertility treatments. Additionally, some fertility treatments increase rates of prematurity and low birth weight because they

FIGURE 6.2

Preterm births, 1990 and 2006–11

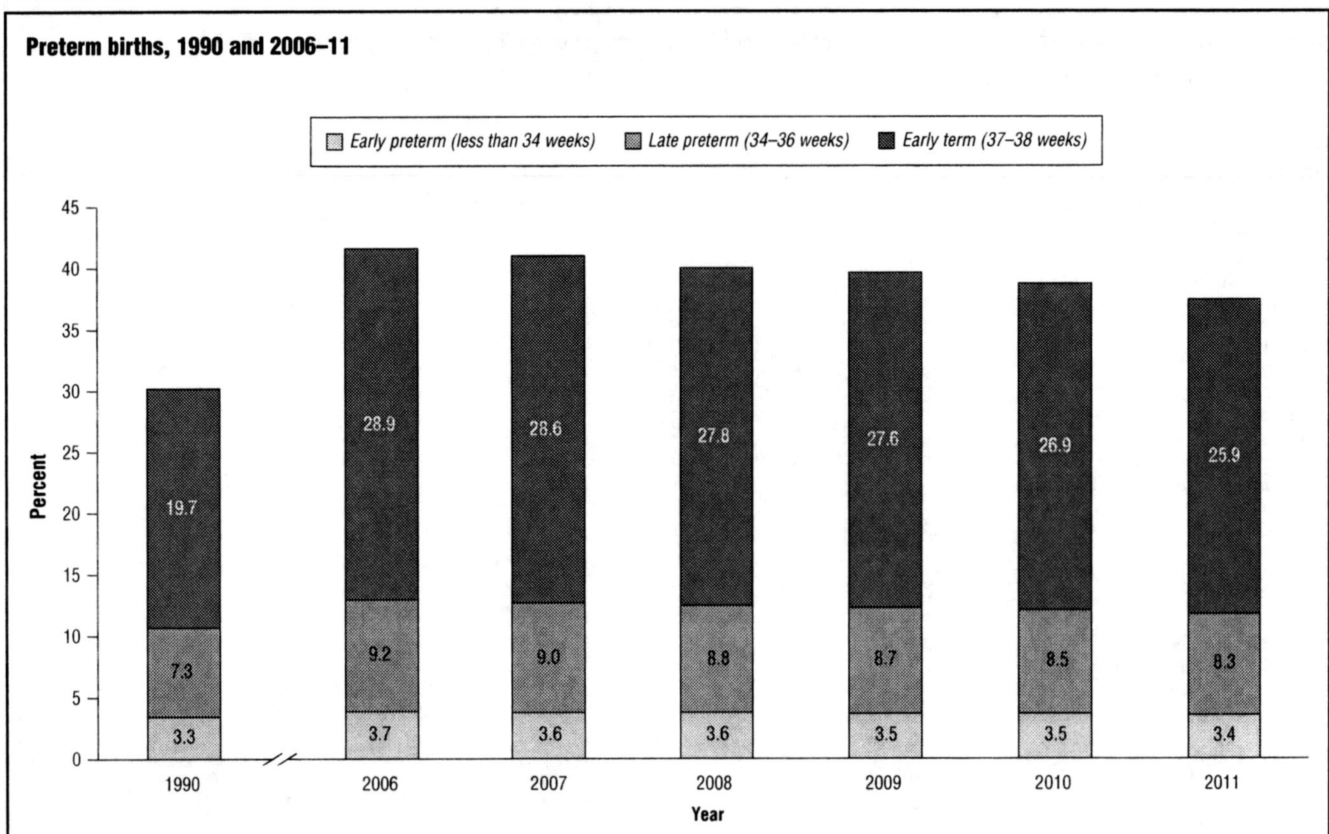

SOURCE: Joyce A. Martin et al., "Figure 1. Births at Less Than 39 Weeks of Gestation: United States, 1990 and 2006–2011," in "Births: Final Data for 2011," *National Vital Statistics Reports*, vol. 62, no. 1, June 28, 2013, http://www.cdc.gov/nchs/data/nvsr/nvsr62/nvsr62_01.pdf#table01 (accessed December 27, 2013)

are more likely to result in multiple births. However, women between the ages of 20 and 34 years accounted for the overwhelming majority of both preterm and low birth weight babies in 2011. Thus, the prevalence of prematurity and low birth weight in the United States cannot be fully explained by trends in maternal age.

Other factors that commonly result in prematurity and low birth weight include poor maternal nutrition, drug and alcohol use, smoking, and sexually transmitted infections.

Birth Defects and End-of-Life Issues

According to the Centers for Disease Control and Prevention (CDC), in "Birth Defects: Data and Statistics" (July 15, 2013, http://www.cdc.gov/ncbddd/birthdefects/data.html), one out of every 33 babies born in the United States each year has a birth defect. The CDC notes that babies born with birth defects are more likely to have poor health and long-term disabilities than babies born without birth defects. Babies born with birth defects typically account for around 20% of total infant mortality.

Some of the more serious birth defects are anencephaly (absence of the majority of the brain) and spina bifida (incomplete development of the back and spine), both of which are classified as neural tube defects (NTDs), because they result from the failure of the neural tube (the embryo's precursor to the central nervous system) to develop properly during early pregnancy. Down syndrome, a condition in which babies are born with an extra copy of chromosome 21 in their cells, results in anatomical and developmental problems along with cognitive deficits. Down syndrome children may be born with birth defects that are fatal, including defects of the heart, lungs, and gastrointestinal tract. Many Down syndrome children, however, live well into their 50s and beyond.

Some birth defects are genetic in nature. For example, Tay-Sachs disease, a fatal condition, primarily affects children of east European Jewish ancestry as a result of inherited genetic irregularities. Down syndrome is also genetically transmitted, although it is not specific to any particular genetic subgroup. Other birth defects result from environmental factors such as maternal drug use or infections during pregnancy. The specific causes of many birth defects are unknown, but scientists theorize that a combination of genetic and environmental factors may explain numerous conditions. Most birth defects cannot be prevented. Exceptions include those caused by maternal alcohol and drug consumption during pregnancy.

TABLE 6.5

Very preterm and preterm births, and very low birthweight and low birthweight births, by race and Hispanic origin of mother, 1981–2011

Year	Very preterm[a] All races[c]	Very preterm Non-Hispanic White[d]	Very preterm Non-Hispanic Black[d]	Very preterm Hispanic[e]	Preterm[b] All races[c]	Preterm Non-Hispanic White[d]	Preterm Non-Hispanic Black[d]	Preterm Hispanic[e]
	Percent							
2011	1.93	1.54	3.76	1.76	11.73	10.50	16.77	11.65
2010	1.96	1.58	3.79	1.78	11.99	10.77	17.12	11.79
2009	1.97	1.57	3.87	1.77	12.18	10.92	17.47	11.97
2008	1.99	1.60	3.84	1.80	12.33	11.14	17.54	12.10
2007	2.04	1.64	4.08	1.82	12.68	11.50	18.29	12.29
2006	2.04	1.66	4.08	1.80	12.80	11.70	18.46	12.25
2005	2.03	1.64	4.17	1.79	12.73	11.69	18.43	12.13
2004	2.01	1.63	4.05	1.77	12.49	11.50	17.91	12.00
2003	1.97	1.60	3.99	1.73	12.33	11.30	17.83	11.87
2002	1.96	1.56	4.04	1.72	12.08	10.98	17.66	11.61
2001	1.95	1.55	4.05	1.69	11.95	10.81	17.63	11.45
2000	1.93	1.51	4.09	1.69	11.64	10.43	17.41	11.24
1999	1.96	1.54	4.18	1.68	11.77	10.52	17.63	11.43
1998	1.96	1.52	4.15	1.72	11.69	10.24	17.60	11.43
1997	1.94	1.49	4.19	1.68	11.36	9.94	17.61	11.20
1996	1.89	1.43	4.17	1.66	10.99	9.50	17.51	10.89
1995	1.89	1.41	4.29	1.66	10.99	9.40	17.77	10.91
1994	1.91	1.39	4.36	1.67	11.02	9.27	18.18	10.94
1993	1.93	1.39	4.45	1.67	10.99	9.08	18.58	10.98
1992[f]	1.91	1.33	4.50	1.64	10.69	8.72	18.49	10.75
1991[f]	1.94	1.35	4.65	1.65	10.82	8.73	19.00	10.96
1990[g]	1.92	1.33	4.63	1.69	10.62	8.50	18.89	10.96
1989[h]	1.95	1.34	4.68	1.76	10.58	8.40	19.05	11.10
1988	1.96	—	—	—	10.22	—	—	—
1987	1.96	—	—	—	10.20	—	—	—
1986	1.90	—	—	—	9.97	—	—	—
1985	1.88	—	—	—	9.76	—	—	—
1984	1.83	—	—	—	9.40	—	—	—
1983	1.86	—	—	—	9.61	—	—	—
1982	1.84	—	—	—	9.50	—	—	—
1981	1.81	—	—	—	9.44	—	—	—

Year	Very low birth weight[i] All races[c]	Very low birth weight Non-Hispanic White[d]	Very low birth weight Non-Hispanic Black[d]	Very low birth weight Hispanic[e]	Low birth weight[j] All races[c]	Low birth weight Non-Hispanic White[d]	Low birth weight Non-Hispanic Black[d]	Low birth weight Hispanic[e]
	Percent							
2011	1.44	1.14	2.99	1.20	8.10	7.09	13.33	7.02
2010	1.45	1.16	2.98	1.20	8.15	7.14	13.53	6.97
2009	1.45	1.16	3.06	1.19	8.16	7.19	13.61	6.94
2008	1.46	1.18	3.01	1.20	8.18	7.22	13.71	6.96
2007	1.49	1.19	3.20	1.21	8.22	7.28	13.90	6.93
2006	1.49	1.20	3.15	1.19	8.26	7.32	13.97	6.99
2005	1.49	1.21	3.27	1.20	8.19	7.29	14.02	6.88
2004	1.48	1.20	3.15	1.20	8.08	7.20	13.74	6.79
2003	1.45	1.18	3.12	1.16	7.93	7.04	13.55	6.69
2002	1.46	1.17	3.15	1.17	7.82	6.91	13.39	6.55
2001	1.44	1.17	3.08	1.14	7.68	6.76	13.07	6.47
2000	1.43	1.14	3.10	1.14	7.57	6.60	13.13	6.41
1999	1.45	1.15	3.18	1.14	7.62	6.64	13.23	6.38
1998	1.45	1.15	3.11	1.15	7.57	6.55	13.17	6.44
1997	1.42	1.12	3.05	1.13	7.51	6.47	13.11	6.42
1996	1.37	1.08	3.02	1.12	7.39	6.36	13.12	6.28
1995	1.35	1.04	2.98	1.11	7.32	6.20	13.21	6.29
1994	1.33	1.01	2.99	1.08	7.28	6.06	13.34	6.25
1993	1.33	1.00	2.99	1.06	7.22	5.92	13.43	6.24
1992[f]	1.29	0.94	2.97	1.04	7.08	5.73	13.40	6.10
1991[f]	1.29	0.94	2.97	1.02	7.12	5.72	13.62	6.15
1990[g]	1.27	0.93	2.93	1.03	6.97	5.61	13.32	6.06
1989[h]	1.28	0.93	2.97	1.05	7.05	5.62	13.61	6.18
1988	1.24	—	—	—	6.93	—	—	—
1987	1.24	—	—	—	6.90	—	—	—
1986	1.21	—	—	—	6.81	—	—	—
1985	1.21	—	—	—	6.75	—	—	—
1984	1.19	—	—	—	6.72	—	—	—
1983	1.19	—	—	—	6.82	—	—	—
1982	1.18	—	—	—	6.75	—	—	—
1981	1.16	—	—	—	6.81	—	—	—

TABLE 6.5

Very preterm and preterm births, and very low birthweight and low birthweight births, by race and Hispanic origin of mother, 1981–2011
[CONTINUED]

—Data not available.
[a]Births of less than 32 completed weeks of gestation.
[b]Births of less than 37 completed weeks of gestation.
[c]Includes races other than white and black and origin not stated.
[d]Race and Hispanic origin are reported separately on birth certificates. Persons of Hispanic origin may be of any race. Race categories are consistent with the 1977 Office of Management and Budget standards. Forty states and the District of Columbia reported multiple-race data for 2011 that were bridged to single-race categories for comparability with other states. Multiple-race reporting areas vary for 2003–2011.
[e]Includes all persons of Hispanic origin of any race.
[f]Data by Hispanic origin exclude New Hampshire, which did not report Hispanic origin.
[g]Data by Hispanic origin exclude New Hampshire and Oklahoma, which did not report Hispanic origin.
[h]Data by Hispanic origin exclude New Hampshire, Oklahoma, and Louisiana, which did not report Hispanic origin.
[i]Less than 1,500 grams (3 pounds, 4 ounces).
[j]Less than 2,500 grams (5 pounds, 8 ounces).

SOURCE: Joyce A. Martin et al., "Table 24. Very Preterm and Preterm Births, and Very Low Birthweight and Low Birthweight Births, by Race and Hispanic Origin of Mother: United States, 1981–2011," in "Births: Final Data for 2011," *National Vital Statistics Reports*, vol. 62, no. 1, June 28, 2013, http://www.cdc.gov/nchs/data/nvsr/nvsr62/nvsr62_01.pdf#table01 (accessed December 27, 2013)

Additionally, prenatal consumption of folic acid, a B vitamin, can help prevent NTDs such as anencephaly and spina bifida.

Racial and ethnic variations in birth defects are not well understood, although differences in the prevalence of individual conditions have been observed. As Table 6.8 shows, non-Hispanic African American mothers are more likely than non-Hispanic white mothers to have babies with tetralogy of Fallot (malformations of the heart that affect blood flow), lower limb reduction defects (incomplete development of one or both legs), and trisomy 18 (a chromosomal defect that is frequently fatal). Hispanic mothers are more likely than non-Hispanic white mothers to have babies with anencephaly, spina bifida, encephalocele (an NTD involving a protrusion of the brain through a hole in the skull), and gastroschisis (a malformation of the abdominal wall resulting in the protrusion of the intestines outside of the body).

NEURAL TUBE DEFECTS: ANENCEPHALY AND SPINA BIFIDA. The two most common NTDs, and therefore the ones that raise the most questions regarding end-of-life care, are anencephaly and spina bifida. Anencephalic infants die before birth (in utero or stillborn) or shortly thereafter. Medical advances have not meaningfully increased the chances for survival of these infants. Spina bifida was once a death sentence for most babies. However, with the advent of antibiotics and advanced surgical techniques, some newborns with spina bifida can now be saved.

According to T. J. Mathews in *Trends in Spina Bifida and Anencephalus in the United States, 1991–2006* (April 2009, http://www.cdc.gov/nchs/data/hestat/spine_anen/spine_anen.pdf), the most recent comprehensive report on this topic as of April 2014, the incidence of anencephaly decreased significantly from 18.4 cases per 100,000 live births in 1991 to 9.4 cases per 100,000 live births in 2001. (See Figure 6.3 and Table 6.9.) The largest drop during this period was between 1991 and 1992. Between 1993 and 2001 the general trend was downward. Between 2002 and 2003 the rates increased from 9.6 cases per 100,000 live births to 11.1 cases per 100,000 live births. Since 2003 rates have stabilized somewhat, standing at 11.2 cases per 100,000 live births in 2006.

Mathews notes that spina bifida rates increased from 22.8 cases per 100,000 live births in 1992 to 28 cases per 100,000 live births in 1995, and that after 1995 the rates declined to 18 cases per 100,000 live births in 2005 and 2006—the lowest spina bifida rates ever reported. (See Figure 6.4 and Table 6.10.) The CDC attributes some of the success in reducing spina bifida rates to the preventive use of folic acid during pregnancy. Women who receive adequate prenatal care are generally directed to ingest prenatal vitamins that contain folic acid. Additionally, in 1992 the U.S. Food and Drug Administration issued a directive mandating that, by 1998, cereal manufacturers add folic acid to their enriched cereal grain products.

Issues related to brain death and organ donation sometimes arise in cases of anencephaly. One case that gained national attention was that of Theresa Ann Campo in 1992. Before their daughter's birth, Theresa's parents discovered through prenatal testing that their baby would be born without a fully developed brain. They decided to carry the fetus to term and donate her organs for transplantation. When baby Theresa was born, her parents asked for her to be declared brain dead. However, Theresa's brain stem was still functioning, so the court ruled against the parents' request. Baby Theresa died 10 days later and her organs were not usable for transplant because they had deteriorated as a result of oxygen deprivation.

Some physicians and ethicists argue that even if anencephalic babies have a brain stem, they should be considered brain dead. Lacking a functioning higher brain, these babies can feel nothing and have no consciousness.

TABLE 6.6

Twin, triplet, and higher-order multiple births, by race and Hispanic origin of mother, 1980–2011

Year and race and Hispanic origin of mother	Total births	Twin births	Triplet or higher-order births	Multiple birth rate[a]	Twin birth rate[b]	Triplet or higher-order birthrate[c]
All races[d]						
2011	3,953,590	131,269	5,417	34.6	33.2	137.0
2010	3,999,386	132,562	5,503	34.5	33.1	137.6
2009	4,130,665	137,217	6,340	34.8	33.2	153.5
2008	4,247,694	138,660	6,268	34.1	32.6	147.6
2007	4,316,233	138,961	6,427	33.7	32.2	148.9
2006	4,265,555	137,085	6,540	33.7	32.1	153.3
2005	4,138,349	133,122	6,694	33.8	32.2	161.8
2004	4,112,052	132,219	7,275	33.9	32.2	176.9
2003	4,089,950	128,665	7,663	33.3	31.5	187.4
2002	4,021,726	125,134	7,401	33.0	31.1	184.0
2001	4,025,933	121,246	7,471	32.0	30.1	185.6
2000	4,058,814	118,916	7,325	31.1	29.3	180.5
1999	3,959,417	114,307	7,321	30.7	28.9	184.9
1998	3,941,553	110,670	7,625	30.0	28.1	193.5
1997	3,880,894	104,137	6,737	28.6	26.8	173.6
1996	3,891,494	100,750	5,939	27.4	25.9	152.6
1995	3,899,589	96,736	4,973	26.1	24.8	127.5
1994	3,952,767	97,064	4,594	25.7	24.6	116.2
1993	4,000,240	96,445	4,168	25.2	24.1	104.2
1992	4,065,014	95,372	3,883	24.4	23.5	95.5
1991	4,110,907	94,779	3,346	23.9	23.1	81.4
1990	4,158,212	93,865	3,028	23.3	22.6	72.8
1989	4,040,958	90,118	2,798	23.0	22.3	69.2
1988	3,909,510	85,315	2,385	22.4	21.8	61.0
1987	3,809,394	81,778	2,139	22.0	21.5	56.2
1986	3,756,547	79,485	1,814	21.6	21.2	48.3
1985	3,760,561	77,102	1,925	21.0	20.5	51.2
1984	3,669,141	72,949	1,653	20.3	19.9	45.1
1983	3,638,933	72,287	1,575	20.3	19.9	43.3
1982	3,680,537	71,631	1,484	19.9	19.5	40.3
1981	3,629,238	70,049	1,385	19.7	19.3	38.2
1980	3,612,258	68,339	1,337	19.3	18.9	37.0
Non-Hispanic white[e]						
2011	2,146,566	78,638	3,670	38.3	36.6	171.0
2010	2,162,406	79,728	3,842	38.6	36.9	177.7
2009	2,212,552	81,954	4,457	39.1	37.0	201.4
2008	2,267,817	82,903	4,493	38.5	36.6	198.1
2007	2,310,333	83,632	4,559	38.2	36.2	197.3
2006	2,308,640	83,108	4,805	38.1	36.0	208.1
2005	2,279,768	82,223	4,966	38.2	36.1	217.8
2004	2,296,683	83,346	5,590	38.7	36.3	243.4
2003	2,321,904	81,691	5,922	37.7	35.2	255.0
2002	2,298,156	79,949	5,754	37.3	34.8	250.4
2001	2,326,578	77,882	5,894	36.0	33.5	253.3
2000	2,362,968	76,018	5,821	34.6	32.2	246.3
1999	2,346,450	73,964	5,909	34.0	31.5	251.8
1998	2,362,462	71,270	6,206	32.8	30.2	262.8
1997	2,333,363	67,191	5,386	31.1	28.8	230.8
1996	2,358,989	65,523	4,885	29.8	27.8	207.1
1995	2,382,638	62,370	4,050	27.9	26.2	170.0
1994	2,438,855	62,476	3,721	27.1	25.6	152.6
1993	2,472,031	61,525	3,360	26.2	24.9	135.9
1992[f]	2,527,207	60,640	3,115	25.2	24.0	123.3
1991[f]	2,589,878	60,904	2,612	24.5	23.5	100.9
1990[g]	2,626,500	60,210	2,358	23.8	22.9	89.8
Non-Hispanic black[e]						
2011	582,345	21,681	634	38.3	37.2	108.9
2010	589,808	21,804	574	37.9	37.0	97.3
2009	609,584	23,159	644	39.0	38.0	105.6
2008	623,029	22,924	569	37.7	36.8	91.3
2007	627,191	23,101	612	37.8	36.8	97.6
2006	617,247	22,702	580	37.7	36.8	94.0
2005	583,759	21,254	616	37.5	36.4	105.5

Others fear that declaring anencephalic babies dead could be the start of a slippery slope that might eventually include babies with other birth defects in the same category. Other people are concerned that anencephalic babies may be kept alive for the purpose of harvesting their organs for transplant at a later date.

TABLE 6.6

Twin, triplet, and higher-order multiple births, by race and Hispanic origin of mother, 1980–2011 [CONTINUED]

Year and race and Hispanic origin of mother	Total births	Twin births	Triplet or higher-order births	Multiple birth rate[a]	Twin birth rate[b]	Triplet or higher-order birthrate[c]
2004	578,772	20,605	577	36.6	35.6	99.7
2003	576,033	20,010	631	35.8	34.7	109.5
2002	578,335	20,064	591	35.7	34.7	102.2
2001	589,917	19,974	531	34.8	33.9	90.0
2000	604,346	20,173	506	34.2	33.4	83.7
1999	588,981	18,920	561	33.1	32.1	95.2
1998	593,127	18,589	518	32.2	31.3	87.3
1997	581,431	17,472	523	30.9	30.0	90.0
1996	578,099	16,873	425	29.9	29.2	73.5
1995	587,781	16,622	340	28.9	28.3	57.8
1994	619,198	17,934	357	29.5	29.0	57.7
1993	641,273	18,115	314	28.7	28.2	49.0
1992[f]	657,450	18,294	346	28.4	27.8	52.6
1991[f]	666,758	18,243	367	27.9	27.4	55.0
1990[g]	661,701	17,646	306	27.1	26.7	46.2
Hispanic[h]						
2011	918,129	21,236	723	23.9	23.1	78.7
2010	945,180	21,359	721	23.4	22.6	76.3
2009	999,548	22,481	835	23.3	22.5	83.5
2008	1,041,239	23,266	834	23.1	22.3	80.1
2007	1,062,779	23,405	857	22.8	22.0	80.6
2006	1,039,077	22,698	787	22.6	21.8	75.7
2005	985,505	21,723	761	22.8	22.0	77.2
2004	946,349	20,351	723	22.3	21.5	76.4
2003	912,329	19,472	784	22.2	21.3	85.9
2002	876,642	18,128	737	21.5	20.7	84.1
2001	851,851	17,257	710	21.1	20.3	83.3
2000	815,868	16,470	659	21.0	20.2	80.8
1999	764,339	15,388	583	20.9	20.1	76.3
1998	734,661	15,015	553	21.2	20.4	75.3
1997	709,767	13,821	516	20.2	19.5	72.7
1996	701,339	13,014	409	19.1	18.6	58.3
1995	679,768	12,685	355	19.2	18.7	52.2
1994	665,026	12,206	348	18.9	18.4	52.3
1993	654,418	12,294	321	19.3	18.8	49.1
1992[f]	643,271	11,932	239	18.9	18.5	37.2
1991[f]	623,085	11,356	235	18.6	18.2	37.7
1990[g]	595,073	10,713	235	18.4	18.0	39.5

[a]The number of live births in all multiple deliveries per 1,000 live births.
[b]The number of live births in twin deliveries per 1,000 live births.
[c]The number of live births in triplet and other higher-order deliveries per 100,000 live births.
[d]Includes races other than white and black and origin not stated.
[e]Race and Hispanic origin are reported separately on birth certificates. Persons of Hispanic origin may be of any race. Race categories are consistent with the 1977 Office of Management and Budget standards. Forty states and the District of Columbia reported multiple-race data for 2011 that were bridged to single-race categories for comparability with other states. Multiple-race reporting areas vary for 2003–2011.
[f]Excludes data for New Hampshire, which did not report Hispanic origin.
[g]Excludes data for New Hampshire and Oklahoma, which did not report Hispanic origin.
[h]Includes all persons of Hispanic origin of any race.

SOURCE: Joyce A. Martin et al., "Table 27. Twin and Triplet or Higher-Order Multiple Births, by Race and Hispanic Origin of Mother, United States: 1980–2011," in "Births: Final Data for 2011," *National Vital Statistics Reports*, vol. 62, no. 1, June 28, 2013, http://www.cdc.gov/nchs/data/nvsr/nvsr62/nvsr62_01.pdf#table01 (accessed December 27, 2013)

The treatment of newborns with spina bifida can also pose serious ethical dilemmas. Should an infant with a milder form of the disease be treated actively and another with severe defects be left untreated? In severe cases, should the newborn be sedated and not be given nutrition and hydration until death occurs? Or should this seriously disabled infant be cared for while suffering from bladder and bowel malfunctions, infections, and paralysis? What if infants who have been left to die unexpectedly survive? Would they be more disabled than if they had been treated right away?

The development of fetal surgery to correct spina bifida before birth added another dimension to the debate. There are risks for both the mother and the fetus during and after fetal surgery, but techniques have improved since the first successful surgery of this type in 1997.

CHILD MORTALITY

Once a U.S. child reaches the age of one, his or her statistical chances of survival improve dramatically. As Table 6.11 shows, the 2011 death rate for infants in the United States was 598.3 deaths per 100,000 people. The death rate for children aged one to four years, 26.2 deaths per 100,000, was nearly 23 times less than that of infants;

TABLE 6.7

Preterm and low birthweight births, by age and race and Hispanic origin of mother, 2011

Age and race and Hispanic origin of mother	Preterm[a]							Low birthweight[b]						
	Percent			Number				Percent			Number			
	Total	Early[c]	Late[d]	Total	Early[c]	Late[d]	Unknown	Total	Very[e]	Moderately[f]	Total	Very[e]	Moderately[f]	Unknown
All races[g]														
All ages	11.73	3.44	8.28	463,163	136,030	327,133	4,846	8.10	1.44	6.66	319,711	56,754	262,957	4,549
Under 15 years	21.12	7.94	13.18	835	314	521	21	11.68	2.72	8.95	463	108	355	9
15–19 years	13.51	4.40	9.11	44,507	14,496	30,011	438	9.59	1.70	7.88	31,584	5,615	25,969	325
15 years	16.52	5.95	10.57	1,933	696	1,237	39	10.47	2.18	8.29	1,228	256	972	13
16 years	15.39	5.42	9.97	4,468	1,574	2,894	47	9.82	1.94	7.88	2,853	564	2,289	26
17 years	14.23	4.75	9.49	7,779	2,595	5,184	75	9.90	1.72	8.18	5,411	941	4,470	55
18 years	13.49	4.39	9.10	12,480	4,059	8,421	113	9.66	1.69	7.97	8,941	1,564	7,377	95
19 years	12.62	3.94	8.68	17,847	5,572	12,275	164	9.30	1.62	7.68	13,151	2,290	10,861	136
20–24 years	11.67	3.45	8.22	107,858	31,916	75,942	1,127	8.31	1.43	6.88	76,840	13,255	63,585	986
25–29 years	10.70	3.04	7.66	120,486	34,218	86,268	1,449	7.31	1.26	6.05	82,356	14,241	68,115	1,331
30–34 years	11.11	3.18	7.94	109,509	31,303	78,206	1,108	7.53	1.36	6.18	74,256	13,387	60,869	1,131
35–39 years	13.16	3.86	9.30	60,980	17,894	43,086	539	8.81	1.64	7.17	40,821	7,590	33,231	602
40–44 years	15.55	4.75	10.80	16,913	5,167	11,746	153	10.82	2.06	8.75	11,764	2,242	9,522	152
45 years and over	27.31	9.50	17.80	2,075	722	1,353	11	21.42	4.16	17.26	1,627	316	1,311	13
Non-Hispanic white[h]														
All ages	10.50	2.88	7.62	225,150	61,754	163,396	2,380	7.09	1.14	5.95	152,047	24,461	127,586	2,344
Under 15 years	17.80	5.78	12.02	154	50	104	4	10.06	2.54	7.51	87	22	65	4
15–19 years	11.90	3.70	8.20	15,371	4,773	10,598	162	8.39	1.43	6.96	10,845	1,850	8,995	116
15 years	14.71	4.89	9.82	481	160	321	8	9.39	1.80	7.58	307	59	248	6
16 years	13.80	5.06	8.74	1,246	457	789	17	9.09	1.91	7.17	821	173	648	15
17 years	12.50	4.12	8.37	2,388	788	1,600	24	8.68	1.67	7.01	1,659	319	1,340	18
18 years	11.86	3.66	8.20	4,336	1,337	2,999	45	8.50	1.38	7.12	3,109	505	2,604	28
19 years	11.31	3.32	7.99	6,920	2,031	4,889	68	8.09	1.30	6.79	4,949	794	4,155	49
20–24 years	10.34	2.86	7.48	46,696	12,932	33,764	489	7.22	1.14	6.09	32,613	5,139	27,474	452
25–29 years	9.69	2.61	7.08	62,688	16,869	45,819	730	6.48	1.03	5.45	41,943	6,676	35,267	686
30–34 years	10.06	2.69	7.37	59,393	15,863	43,530	602	6.64	1.07	5.57	39,229	6,306	32,923	657
35–39 years	12.00	3.24	8.76	31,229	8,441	22,788	311	7.88	1.27	6.61	20,508	3,297	17,211	340
40–44 years	14.04	4.05	9.99	8,514	2,457	6,057	76	9.86	1.70	8.17	5,980	1,028	4,952	81
45 years and over	25.60	8.55	17.05	1,105	369	736	6	19.51	3.31	16.20	842	143	699	8
Non-Hispanic black[h]														
All ages	16.77	6.03	10.74	97,543	35,090	62,453	828	13.33	2.99	10.35	77,518	17,361	60,157	877
Under 15 years	25.47	11.02	14.45	349	151	198	8	14.55	3.35	11.20	200	46	154	3
15–19 years	17.26	6.42	10.84	13,536	5,032	8,504	137	13.73	2.76	10.98	10,775	2,162	8,613	103
15 years	20.87	8.03	12.84	681	262	419	18	14.04	3.30	10.74	460	108	352	5
16 years	18.78	7.35	11.43	1,354	530	824	7	13.39	2.93	10.47	966	211	755	3
17 years	18.37	6.86	11.51	2,413	901	1,512	29	13.93	2.60	11.33	1,831	342	1,489	20
18 years	17.25	6.40	10.85	3,778	1,401	2,377	26	13.73	2.68	11.05	3,007	587	2,420	27
19 years	16.13	5.89	10.24	5,310	1,938	3,372	57	13.70	2.78	10.93	4,511	914	3,597	48
20–24 years	15.97	5.57	10.40	29,692	10,359	19,333	271	13.17	2.70	10.47	24,497	5,024	19,473	275
25–29 years	15.86	5.58	10.27	23,391	8,234	15,157	193	12.57	2.81	9.77	18,545	4,138	14,407	215
30–34 years	17.12	6.22	10.90	17,826	6,477	11,349	147	13.25	3.33	9.91	13,789	3,470	10,319	169
35–39 years	19.24	7.30	11.94	9,655	3,664	5,991	57	14.65	3.81	10.84	7,348	1,913	5,435	92
40–44 years	21.56	8.05	13.51	2,790	1,042	1,748	14	16.32	4.21	12.11	2,111	545	1,566	19
45 years and over	30.40	13.10	17.30	304	131	173	1	25.30	6.30	19.00	253	63	190	1

TABLE 6.7

Preterm and low birthweight births, by age and race and Hispanic origin of mother, 2011 [CONTINUED]

Age and race and Hispanic origin of mother	Preterm[a]							Low birthweight[b]						
	Percent			Number				Percent			Number			
	Total	Early[c]	Late[d]	Total	Early[c]	Late[d]	Unknown	Total	Very[e]	Moderately[f]	Total	Very[e]	Moderately[f]	Unknown
Hispanic[i]														
All ages	11.65	3.25	8.40	106,884	29,859	77,025	780	7.02	1.20	5.82	64,449	11,022	53,427	600
Under 15 years	18.56	6.19	12.37	291	97	194	8	10.16	2.29	7.87	160	36	124	1
15–19 years	12.65	3.76	8.89	13,860	4,117	9,743	101	8.06	1.29	6.77	8,832	1,410	7,422	82
15 years	14.88	5.25	9.63	706	249	457	12	8.87	1.77	7.11	422	84	338	1
16 years	14.40	4.45	9.95	1,694	523	1,171	15	8.11	1.26	6.86	955	148	807	7
17 years	13.07	3.93	9.14	2,669	802	1,867	16	8.42	1.23	7.20	1,721	251	1,470	12
18 years	12.67	3.85	8.82	3,883	1,180	2,703	31	8.27	1.39	6.88	2,533	425	2,108	34
19 years	11.69	3.25	8.44	4,908	1,363	3,545	27	7.62	1.20	6.43	3,201	502	2,699	28
20–24 years	10.83	2.96	7.87	26,365	7,212	19,153	217	6.66	1.05	5.61	16,224	2,568	13,656	142
25–29 years	10.54	2.78	7.76	26,150	6,908	19,242	216	6.24	1.02	5.22	15,470	2,523	12,947	180
30–34 years	11.76	3.33	8.44	22,631	6,404	16,227	154	6.94	1.27	5.67	13,360	2,449	10,911	118
35–39 years	13.83	3.99	9.84	13,593	3,926	9,667	60	8.05	1.55	6.49	7,909	1,528	6,381	57
40–44 years	16.10	4.80	11.30	3,668	1,093	2,575	24	9.86	2.01	7.85	2,246	458	1,788	18
45 years and over	26.38	8.25	18.12	326	102	224	0	20.10	4.05	16.05	248	50	198	2

[a]Less than 37 completed weeks of gestation.
[b]Less than 2,500 grams.
[c]Less than 34 completed weeks of gestation.
[d]34–36 completed weeks of gestation.
[e]Less than 1,500 grams.
[f]1,500–2,499 grams.
[g]Includes races other than white and black and origin not stated.
[h]Race and Hispanic origin are reported separately on birth certificates. Persons of Hispanic origin may be of any race. Race categories are consistent with the 1977 Office of Management and Budget standards. Forty states and the District of Columbia reported multiple-race data for 2011 that were bridged to single-race categories for comparability with other states.
[i]Includes all persons of Hispanic origin of any race.

SOURCE: Joyce A. Martin et al., "Table 25. Preterm and Low Birthweight Births, by Age and Race and Hispanic Origin of Mother: United States, 2011," in "Births: Final Data for 2011," *National Vital Statistics Reports*, vol. 62, no. 1, June 28, 2013, http://www.cdc.gov/nchs/data/nvsr/nvsr62/nvsr62_01.pdf#table01 (accessed December 27, 2013)

TABLE 6.8

The prevalence of birth defects by race and ethnicity

[Compared with infants of non-Hispanic white mothers]

Infants of non-Hispanic black or African-American mothers had		Infants of Hispanic mothers had	
Higher birth prevalence of these birth defects:	**Lower birth prevalence of these birth defects**	**Higher birth prevalence of these birth defects:**	**Lower birth prevalence of these birth defects**
Tetralogy of Fallot	Cleft palate	Anencephaly	Tetralogy of Fallot
Lower limb reduction defects	Cleft lip with or without cleft palate	Spina bifida	Hypoplastic left heart syndrome
Trisomy 18	Esophageal atresia or tracheoesophageal fistula	Encephalocele	Cleft palate
	Gastroschisis	Gastroschisis	Esophageal atresia or tracheoesophageal fistula
	Down syndrome	Down syndrome	

SOURCE: "Race/Ethnicity," in *Birth Defects: Data and Statistics*, Centers for Disease Control and Prevention, July 15, 2013, http://www.cdc.gov/ncbddd/birthdefects/data.html (accessed January 21, 2014)

FIGURE 6.3

Anencephalus rates, 1991–2006

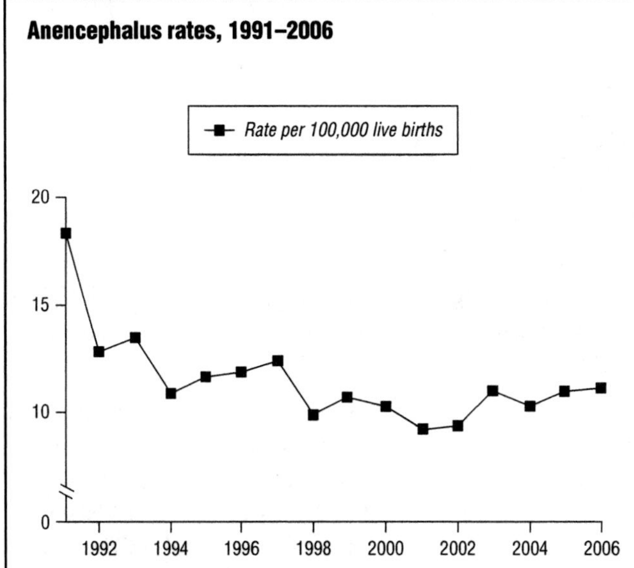

Note: Excludes data for Maryland, New Mexico, and New York, which did not require reporting for anencephalus for some years.

SOURCE: Adapted from T. J. Mathews, "Figure 2. Anencephalus Rates, 1991–2006," in *Trends in Spina Bifida and Anencephalus in the United States, 1991–2006*, Health E-Stats, Centers for Disease Control and Prevention, National Center for Health Statistics, April 2009, http://www.cdc.gov/nchs/data/hestat/spine_anen/spine_anen.pdf (accessed December 27, 2013)

TABLE 6.9

Number of live births, anencephalus cases, and anencephalus rates, 1991–2006

	Anencephalus cases	Total live births	Rate
2006	436	3,890,949	11.21
2005	432	3,887,109	11.11
2004	401	3,860,720	10.39
2003	441	3,715,577	11.14
2002	348	3,645,770	9.55
2001	343	3,640,555	9.42
2000	376	3,640,376	10.33
1999	382	3,533,565	10.81
1998	349	3,519,240	9.92
1997	434	3,469,667	12.51
1996	416	3,478,723	11.96
1995	408	3,484,539	11.71
1994	387	3,527,482	10.97
1993	481	3,562,723	13.50
1992	457	3,572,890	12.79
1991	655	3,564,453	18.38

Note: Excludes data for Maryland, New Mexico, and New York, which did not require reporting for anencephalus for some years.

SOURCE: Adapted from T. J. Mathews, "Table 2. Number of Live Births with Anencephalus and Rates per 100,000 Live Births: United States, 1991–2006," in *Trends in Spina Bifida and Anencephalus in the United States, 1991–2006*, Health E-Stats, Centers for Disease Control and Prevention, National Center for Health Statistics, April 2009, http://www.cdc.gov/nchs/data/hestat/spine_anen/spine_anen.pdf (accessed December 27, 2013)

and the death rate of children aged five to 14 years, 13.1 deaths per 100,000, was nearly 46 times less than that of infants. Only past age 55 did the average U.S. resident have a greater statistical probability of dying than the average infant.

Child mortality is thus much rarer in developed countries such as the United States than infant mortality. This is a historically unique phenomenon: researchers believe that for most of human history, people were more likely to die as children than as infants, and they were roughly as likely to die between the age of one and the onset of adolescence as they were to survive to adolescence. In a paper considering the role that child mortality played in human evolution, "Is Child Death the Crucible of Human Evolution?" (*Journal of Social, Evolutionary, and Cultural Psychology*, vol. 2, no. 4, December 2008), Tony Volk and Jeremy Atkinson provide a survey of scholarly estimates of the child mortality rates in various ancient and medieval societies. Evidence suggests, for example, that in ancient Rome (200 BC–AD 200) the infant mortality rate was approximately 30% (i.e., 30% of children did not survive their first year of life), while the child mortality rate was 50% (only half of children made it to adolescence). Volk and Atkinson find that evidence points to similar rates of infant and child

FIGURE 6.4

Spina bifida rates, 1991–2006

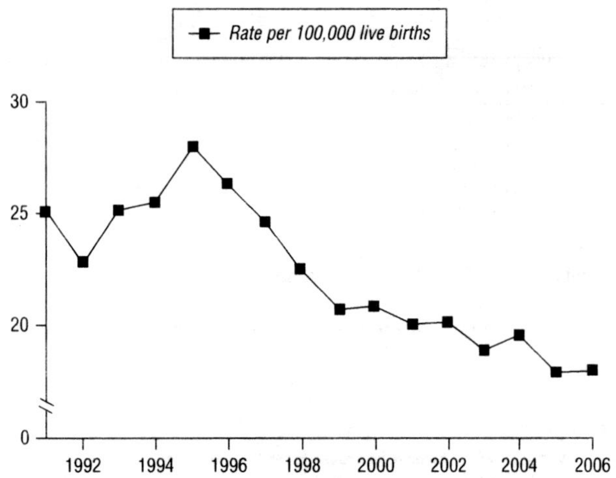

Note: Excludes data for Maryland, New Mexico, and New York, which did not require reporting for spina bifida for some years.

SOURCE: Adapted from T. J. Mathews, "Figure 1. Spina Bifida Rates, 1991–2006," in *Trends in Spina Bifida and Anencephalus in the United States, 1991–2006*, Health E-Stats, Centers for Disease Control and Prevention, National Center for Health Statistics, April 2009, http://www.cdc.gov/nchs/data/hestat/spine_anen/spine_anen.pdf (accessed December 27, 2013)

TABLE 6.10

Number of live births, spina bifida cases, and spina bifida rates, 1991–2006

	Spina bifida cases	Total live births	Rate
2006	700	3,890,949	17.99
2005	698	3,887,109	17.96
2004	755	3,860,720	19.56
2003	702	3,715,577	18.89
2002	734	3,645,770	20.13
2001	730	3,640,555	20.05
2000	759	3,640,376	20.85
1999	732	3,533,565	20.72
1998	790	3,519,240	22.45
1997	857	3,469,667	24.70
1996	917	3,478,723	26.36
1995	975	3,484,539	27.98
1994	900	3,527,482	25.51
1993	896	3,562,723	25.15
1992	816	3,572,890	22.84
1991	887	3,564,453	24.88

Note: Excludes data for Maryland, New Mexico, and New York, which did not require reporting for spina bifida for some years.

SOURCE: Adapted from T. J. Mathews, "Table 1. Number of Live Births with Spina Bifida and Rates per 100,000 Live Births: United States, 1991–2006," in *Trends in Spina Bifida and Anencephalus in the United States, 1991–2006*, Health E-Stats, Centers for Disease Control and Prevention, National Center for Health Statistics, April 2009, http://www.cdc.gov/nchs/data/hestat/spine_anen/spine_anen.pdf (accessed December 27, 2013)

mortality in 14th-century Japan, 17th-century France and Sweden, and 17th- and 18th-century China. They also find similar rates of infant (23%) and child (46%) mortality among hunter-gatherers in the modern age, who live without access to advanced medicine or sanitation.

Infant and child mortality rates began to decline during the mid-19th century, with improvements in sanitation, nutrition, and medical practices. Through the early 20th century, the death of children, although much rarer in the developed world than in ancient and medieval times, remained tragically commonplace. According to Gopal K. Singh of the U.S. Department of Health and Human Services, in *Child Mortality in the United States, 1935–2007: Large Racial and Socioeconomic Disparities Have Persisted over Time* (2010, http://www.hrsa.gov/healthit/images/mchb_child_mortality_pub.pdf), between 1900 and 1902, 90.2% of U.S. children who made it to their first birthday survived to age 15. The mortality rate for U.S. children aged one to four years was 1,418.8 deaths per 100,000 people in 1907, and the rate for children aged five to 14 years was 307.5. Figure 6.5 and Figure 6.6 show the precipitous declines in the rates of death for both groups of children between 1935 and 2007. Although declines were comparably dramatic for both white and African American children, African American children had a substantially higher likelihood of dying at all points throughout this period. By 2007, 99.7% of U.S. children who reached their first birthday survived to age 15.

Because childhood mortality from infectious diseases and other illnesses has been drastically reduced, accidents have consistently been the leading cause of death for children. Among the 39,213 deaths of U.S. residents aged one to 24 years in 2011, 38% were the result of accidents. (See Figure 6.7.) Homicide and suicide each accounted for an additional 13% of deaths. Cancer (7%) and heart disease (3%) were the next most-common causes of death for children and young adults in 2011.

CARING FOR TERMINALLY ILL INFANTS AND CHILDREN

According to Kelly Nicole Michelson and David M. Steinhorn, in "Pediatric End-of-Life Issues and Palliative Care" (*Clinical Pediatric Emergency Medicine*, vol. 8, no. 3, September 2007), since 2005 more than 56% of the annual average of 55,000 pediatric deaths (including both infant deaths and the deaths of children and young people up to the age of 19 years) occur in hospitals. Almost all of these hospital deaths occur in pediatric or neonatal intensive care units; a small minority occur in emergency departments. Whereas end-of-life care for adults is often focused on chronic conditions, especially heart disease and cancer, palliative care for children must address a wider array of concerns, on average. Michelson and Steinhorn note that this is evident in the statistics for one hospital, where

TABLE 6.11

Deaths and death rates, by age, 2010 and 2011

[Data are based on a continuous file of records received from the states. Age-specific rates are per 100,000 population in specified group. Age-adjusted rates are per 100,000 U.S. standard population. Figures for 2011 are based on weighted data rounded to the nearest individual, so categories may not add to totals. Race and Hispanic origin are reported separately on the death certificate. Data for Hispanic origin and specified races other than white and black should be interpreted with caution because of inconsistencies between reporting Hispanic origin and race on death certificates and on censuses and surveys. Race categories are consistent with the 1977 Office of Management and Budget (OMB) standards. Multiple-race data were reported by 38 states and the District of Columbia in 2011 and by 37 states and the District of Columbia in 2010. The multiple-race data for these states were bridged to the single-race categories of the 1977 OMB standards for comparability with other states. Data for persons of Hispanic origin are included in the data for each race group, according to the decedent's reported race.]

	2011		2010	
Age, sex, race, and Hispanic origin	**Number**	**Rate**	**Number**	**Rate**
Both sexes				
All ages	2,513,171	806.6	2,468,435	799.5
Under 1 year*	23,910	598.3	24,586	623.4
1–4 years	4,236	26.2	4,316	26.5
5–14 years	5,377	13.1	5,279	12.9
15–24 years	29,624	67.6	29,551	67.7
25–34 years	43,631	104.4	42,259	102.9
35–44 years	69,746	171.7	70,033	170.5
45–54 years	182,994	409.2	183,207	407.1
55–64 years	323,015	848.7	310,802	851.9
65–74 years	414,792	1,845.0	407,151	1,875.1
75–84 years	625,860	4,750.3	625,651	4,790.2
85 years and over	789,854	13,767.3	765,474	13,934.3
Not stated	132	—	126	—
Age-adjusted rate	—	740.6	—	747.0
Male				
All ages	1,253,716	817.9	1,232,432	812.0
Under 1 year*	13,259	648.8	13,702	680.2
1–4 years	2,393	29.0	2,460	29.6
5–14 years	3,163	15.1	3,054	14.6
15–24 years	21,894	97.6	21,790	97.6
25–34 years	30,003	142.6	29,192	141.5
35–44 years	43,152	213.4	43,434	212.5
45–54 years	111,552	506.6	112,018	505.9
55–64 years	196,424	1,070.0	189,295	1,075.5
65–74 years	234,102	2,234.6	229,704	2,275.1
75–84 years	312,543	5,608.1	311,830	5,693.7
85 years and over	285,134	15,054.4	275,866	15,414.3
Not stated	96	—	87	—
Age-adjusted rate	—	874.5	—	887.1
Female				
All ages	1,259,456	795.6	1,236,003	787.4
Under 1 year*	10,651	545.4	10,884	564.0
1–4 years	1,843	23.3	1,856	23.3
5–14 years	2,214	11.0	2,225	11.1
15–24 years	7,730	36.2	7,761	36.4
25–34 years	13,628	65.7	13,067	64.0
35–44 years	26,594	130.3	26,599	128.9
45–54 years	71,442	314.7	71,189	311.4
55–64 years	126,591	642.5	121,507	643.5
65–74 years	180,690	1,505.1	177,447	1,527.5
75–84 years	313,317	4,121.4	313,821	4,137.7
85 years and over	504,720	13,133.0	489,608	13,219.2
Not stated	36	—	39	—
Age-adjusted rate	—	631.9	—	634.9

—Category not applicable.
*Death rates for "Under 1 year" (based on population estimates) differ from infant mortality rates (based on live births).
Note: Data are subject to sampling or random variation.

SOURCE: Adapted from Donna L. Hoyert and Jiaquan Xu, "Table 1. Deaths and Death Rates, by Age, Sex, Race, and Hispanic Origin, and Age-Adjusted Death Rates, by Sex, Race, and Hispanic Origin: United States, Final 2010 and Preliminary 2011," in "Deaths: Preliminary Data for 2011," *National Vital Statistics Reports*, vol. 61, no. 6, October 10, 2012, http://www.cdc.gov/nchs/data/nvsr/nvsr61/nvsr61_06.pdf (accessed December 23, 2013)

approximately one-third of pediatric deaths were associated with cardiac events or conditions; around 40% were split roughly evenly between the diagnostic categories of neonatal-specific diagnoses, birth defects, and infectious conditions; 10% were due to cancer; and 6% were due to trauma (major injuries caused by an external source).

In spite of the significant differences in the distribution of conditions, palliative care for children follows much the same template as palliative care for adults. In "WHO Definition of Palliative Care" (2014, http://www.who.int/cancer/palliative/definition/en/), the World Health Organization's definition of palliative

FIGURE 6.5

Mortality rates for children aged 1–4, by race, 1935–2007

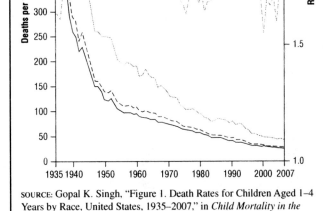

Black/white ratio — White --- All races ······ Black

Deaths per 100,000 population: 0, 50, 100, 150, 200, 250, 300, 350, 400, 450, 500, 550, 600, 650, 700

Rate ratio: 1.0, 1.5, 2.0, 2.5

1935 1940 1950 1960 1970 1980 1990 2000 2007

SOURCE: Gopal K. Singh, "Figure 1. Death Rates for Children Aged 1–4 Years by Race, United States, 1935–2007," in *Child Mortality in the United States, 1935–2007: Large Racial and Socioeconomic Disparities Have Persisted Over Time*, U.S. Department of Health and Human Services, Health Resources and Services Administration, Maternal and Child Health Bureau, 2010, http://www.hrsa.gov/healthit/images/mchb_child_mortality_pub.pdf (accessed January 23, 2014)

FIGURE 6.6

Mortality rates for children aged 5–14, by race, 1935–2007

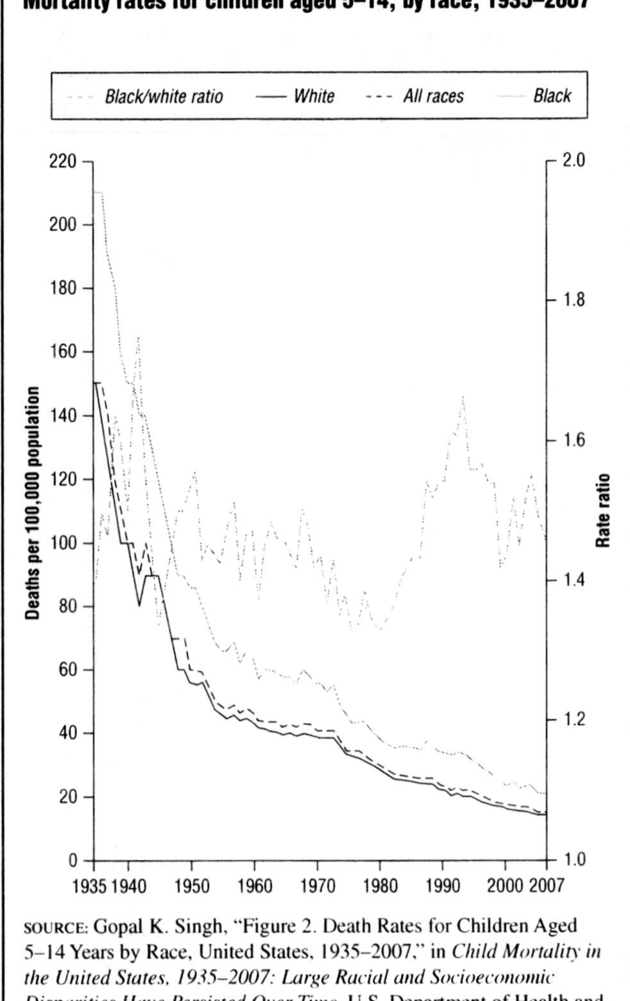

SOURCE: Gopal K. Singh, "Figure 2. Death Rates for Children Aged 5–14 Years by Race, United States, 1935–2007," in *Child Mortality in the United States, 1935–2007: Large Racial and Socioeconomic Disparities Have Persisted Over Time*, U.S. Department of Health and Human Services, Health Resources and Services Administration, Maternal and Child Health Bureau, 2010, http://www.hrsa.gov/healthit/images/mchb_child_mortality_pub.pdf (accessed January 23, 2014)

care for children is consistent with its definition of palliative care for adults, but with different emphases:

- Palliative care for children is the active total care of the child's body, mind, and spirit, and also involves giving support to the family.
- It begins when illness is diagnosed, and continues regardless of whether or not a child receives treatment directed at the disease.
- Health providers must evaluate and alleviate a child's physical, psychological, and social distress.
- Effective palliative care requires a broad multidisciplinary approach that includes the family and makes use of available community resources; it can be successfully implemented even if resources are limited.
- It can be provided in tertiary care facilities, in community health centres, and even in children's homes.

Parents play a major role in shaping end-of-life care for children. Although it is part of the caregiver's job to assess and respond to the needs of the patient's family members, parents must also be clear about their feelings, preferences, and concerns if caregivers are to provide the best possible care for the dying child.

Perhaps surprisingly, effective palliative care for children includes an emphasis on including the patient in discussions of care, including honest discussions about death. Michelson and Steinhorn reference studies suggesting that, difficult as it is for parents and caregivers to talk about death with dying children, parents typically do not regret doing so. Parents who do not speak with their dying children about death do, however, typically come to regret this approach. The American Society of Clinical Oncology notes in "Caring for a Terminally Ill Child: A Guide for Parents" (June 2013, http://www.cancer.net/coping/end-life-care/caring-terminally-ill-child-guide-parents)

FIGURE 6.7

Percentage distribution of five leading causes of death for children and young adults aged 1–24, 2011

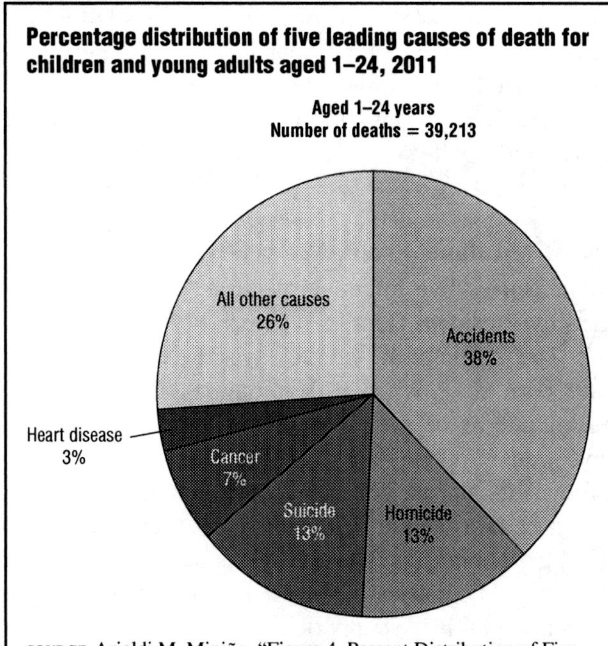

SOURCE: Arialdi M. Miniño, "Figure 4. Percent Distribution of Five Leading Causes of Death, by Age Group: United States, Preliminary 2011," in "Death in the United States, 2011," *NCHS Data Brief*, no. 115, Centers for Disease Control and Prevention, National Center for Health Statistics, March 2013, http://www.cdc.gov/nchs/data/databriefs/db115.pdf (accessed December 27, 2013)

that most children with advanced terminal illnesses are aware, either consciously or subconsciously, that they are dying. Even older children and adolescents who understand death fully may have large areas of uncertainty in their thinking, and the uncertainty can increase their levels of fear and anxiety. Health care professionals recommend that parents allow children to voice their own fears and concerns thoroughly, so that discussions can be shaped according to the individual child's understanding and needs. Parents are advised to speak clearly and directly, rather than obscuring the nature of death by using euphemisms. Sometimes, additionally, children feel that they need "permission" to die, because they are worried about their parents' and family members' well-being.

The relief of pain and discomfort is, as with adults, a primary concern of pediatric palliative caregivers. Pain is, of course, a highly subjective experience, and even with adults, its management varies from patient to patient and requires great sensitivity to the individual and his or her needs. With children, the complexity of pain management is further complicated by different experiences of pain depending on the child's developmental stage.

Another major focus of palliative care in both children and adults involves addressing patients' social, psychological, and spiritual concerns. As with pain management, caregivers' jobs in this realm are highly dependent on the child's stage of development. Infants and children up to the preschool level, for example, typically have little or no understanding of death. Often, then, the process of addressing mental and emotional needs involves acts of physical soothing, such as caressing or holding the child. Older children and adolescents typically understand death more fully, and they often benefit from being allowed to assume control whenever possible, such as by being included in medical discussions about their conditions and treatment options.

Children's inner needs may also be addressed outside of the medical setting, for example, by taking a vacation with parents, by being encouraged to continue engaging in "normal" activities for as long as possible, and by having the chance to say good-bye to friends, teachers, and other important people. Dealing sensitively with spiritual concerns and allowing for the comfort that religion or other forms of belief can provide is also part of the palliative caregiver's job. When parents communicate their religious beliefs to caregivers, these beliefs can be included in the overall process of making the child comfortable.

In cases where terminally ill children are expected to live less than six months and are no longer receiving treatment, palliative care gives way to hospice care. Hospice services, while similar to palliative care, often focus on increasing the comfort of the child and family in the home. Some families, however, find more comfort in the hospital setting as the end of life approaches. Hospice caregivers can typically accommodate families in either setting, provided that parents communicate their needs to the child's health care team.

MEDICAL DECISION MAKING FOR INFANTS

Before the 1980s U.S. courts were supportive of biological parents making decisions regarding the medical care of their newborns. Parents often made these decisions in consultation with pediatricians. Beginning in the 1980s medical advancements allowed for the survival of infants who would have not had a chance for survival before that time. Parents' and physicians' decisions became more challenging and complex.

The modern history of federal and state laws pertaining to the medical care of infants dates to 1982, when the Baby Doe regulations were issued. These regulations created a standard of medical care for infants: the possibility of future handicaps in a child should play no role in his or her medical treatment decisions.

The Baby Doe Rules

In April 1982 an infant with Down syndrome was born at Bloomington Hospital in Indiana. The infant also had esophageal atresia, an obstruction in the esophagus that prevents the passage of food from the mouth to the stomach. Following their obstetrician's recommendation, the parents decided to forgo surgery to repair the baby's esophagus. The baby would be kept pain-free with medication and allowed to die. The hospital, however, disagreed with the parents' decision and took the matter to the county court. The judge ruled that the parents had the legal right to their decision, which was based on a valid medical recommendation. The Indiana Supreme Court refused to hear the appeal. Before the county prosecutor could present the case to the U.S. Supreme Court, the six-day-old baby died.

The public outcry following the death of "Baby Doe" (the infant's court-designated name) brought immediate reaction from the administration of President Ronald Reagan (1911–2004). The U.S. Department of Health and Human Services (HHS) informed all hospitals receiving federal funding that discrimination against handicapped newborns would violate section 504 of the Rehabilitation Act of 1973. This section (nondiscrimination under federal grants and programs) states: "No otherwise qualified individual with a disability in the United States ... shall, solely by reason of her or his disability, be excluded from participation in, be denied the benefits of, or be subjected to discrimination under any program, service or activity receiving Federal financial assistance."

Furthermore, all hospitals receiving federal aid were required to post signs that read: "Discriminatory failure to feed and care for handicapped infants in this facility is prohibited by Federal law." The signs listed a toll-free hotline for anonymous reports of failure to comply.

Although government investigators (called Baby Doe squads) were summoned to many hospitals to verify claims of mistreatment (the hotline had 500 calls in its first three weeks alone), no violation of the law could be found. On the contrary, the investigators found doctors resuscitating babies who were beyond treatment because they feared legal actions. Finally, a group led by the American Academy of Pediatrics filed suit in March 1983 to have the Baby Doe rules overturned because they believed them to be harsh, unreasonably intrusive, and not necessarily in the best interests of the child. After various legal battles, in 1986 the U.S. Supreme Court ruled that the HHS did not have the authority to require such regulations and invalidated them.

Child Abuse Amendments and Their Legacy

As the Baby Doe regulations were being fought in the courts, President Reagan signed the Child Abuse Amendments (CAA) of 1984. The CAA extended and improved the provisions of the Child Abuse Prevention and Treatment Act (1974) and the Child Abuse Prevention and Treatment and Adoption Reform Act of 1978. The CAA established that states' child protection services systems would respond to complaints of medical neglect of children, including instances of withholding medically indicated treatment from disabled infants with life-threatening conditions. It noted that parents were the ones to make medical decisions for their disabled infants based on the advice of their physicians. These laws have been amended many times over the years, most recently by the Keeping Children and Families Safe Act of 2003, without voiding the states' and parents' responsibilities to disabled infants.

Born-Alive Infants Protection Act

The Born-Alive Infants Protection Act (BAIPA) was signed by President George W. Bush (1946–) in August 2002. The purpose of the law was to ensure that all infants born alive, whether developmentally able to survive long term or not, were given legal protection as people under federal law. The law did not prohibit or require medical care for newly born infants who were below a certain weight or developmental age, nor did it address gestational age. David Boyle et al. of the American Academy of Pediatrics Neonatal Resuscitation Program Steering Committee supported this point of view in "Born-Alive Infants Protection Act of 2001, Public Law No. 107-207" (*Pediatrics*, vol. 111, no. 3, March 1, 2003), stating that the law:

> Should not in any way affect the approach that physicians currently follow with respect to the extremely premature infant.... At the time of delivery, and regardless of the circumstances of the delivery, the medical condition and prognosis of the newly born infant should be assessed. At that point decisions about withholding or discontinuing medical treatment that is considered futile may be considered by the medical care providers in conjunction with the parents acting in the best interest of their child. Those newly born infants who are deemed appropriate to not resuscitate or to have medical support withdrawn should be treated with dignity and respect, and provided with "comfort care" measures.

By 2005, however, the opinion that the BAIPA should not affect physicians' approach to their care of premature infants was questioned. Sadath A. Sayeed of the University of California, San Francisco, notes in "Baby Doe Redux? The Department of Health and Human Services and the Born-Alive Infants Protection Act of 2002: A Cautionary Note on Normative Neonatal Practice" (*Pediatrics*, vol. 116, no. 4, October 1, 2005) that in 2005 the HHS announced that it would investigate circumstances in which medical care had been withheld from any born-alive infant. The agency also suggested, as with the Baby Doe regulations, that individuals in health care facilities should report any infractions of the law that they might notice.

Sayeed criticizes the law's "all-encompassing definition of born alive," reporting that it includes any fetus "'at any stage of development ... regardless of whether the expulsion or extraction occurs as a result of natural or induced labor, cesarean section, or induced abortion,' and it makes no reference to standards of care or best interests, nor does it specifically protect a parent's decision-making authority. Under the law's strict logic, an 18-week miscarried fetus with a detectable heart beat after delivery is entitled to the full protections of the law as determined by 'any Act of Congress, or any ruling, regulation, or interpretation of the various administrative bureaus and agencies.'"

In "Resuscitation of Likely Nonviable Newborns: Would Neonatology Practices in California Change if the Born-Alive Infants Protection Act Were Enforced?" (*Pediatrics*, vol. 123, no. 4, April 2009), J. Colin Partridge et al. of the University of California, San Francisco, address the effects of the BAIPA. The researchers note that in 2005 they conducted a survey of neonatologists in active practice in California. More than half of the respondents had neither heard of the BAIPA nor its enforcement guidelines. The physicians admitted rarely assessing the medical condition and prognosis of any fetus less than 23 weeks of gestation; 23 weeks of gestation appears to be the threshold for a fetus to have a chance of survival outside of the womb. Only 6% of the responding neonatologists thought the law should be enforced. Partridge et al. conclude that "until outcomes for infants of <24 weeks' gestation improve, legislation that changes resuscitation practices for extreme prematurity seems an unjustifiable restriction of physician practice and parental rights."

MEDICAL DECISION MAKING FOR CHILDREN

Under U.S. law, children under the age of 18 years cannot provide legally binding consent regarding their health care. Parents or guardians legally provide that consent, and, in most situations, physicians and the courts give parents wide latitude in the medical decisions they make for their children.

Religious Beliefs and Medical Treatment

Some parents refuse medical treatment for their children because of religious reasons. When such refusal is likely to result in death or undue suffering for a child, the government may step in. Although the U.S. Constitution prohibits government interference with religious practices and guarantees freedom of religion, the government concurrently has a responsibility to safeguard the health and well-being of its citizens.

Bruce Patsner of the University of Houston Law Center explains in "Faith versus Medicine: When a Parent Refuses a Child's Medical Care" (June 2009, http://www.law.uh.edu/Healthlaw/perspectives/2009/(BP)%20Faith.pdf) that the power of the government to intervene in the medical affairs of its citizens has limits, which are partly based on whether the intervention meets a "public health justification" criterion. For example, Patsner notes that the government's responsibility to protect the public health is the basis on which the government can implement mandatory vaccination programs. In cases that do not threaten public health, Patsner suggests that state family laws, rather than federal laws, should provide the standards for parental decision making. Nonetheless, Patsner explains, "while parents may be entitled to believe whatever they want to believe from a religious point of view, denials of life-saving medical care to their children quickly cross over from mere belief into conduct, and this is not protected to the same degree. Put another way, parents are generally not allowed to sacrifice the lives of their children whose health interests they are supposed to protect before the children are legally old enough to be able to make their own decisions."

WISCONSIN COURT CASE. In 2009 two cases came to state courts that tested governmental limits to intervene in the medical decisions for a minor child when the parents refused medical treatment. The first case concerned 11-year-old Kara Neumann, who died in March 2008 from diabetic ketoacidosis, a complication of her undiagnosed and untreated type 1 diabetes. In "Trials for Parents Who Chose Faith over Medicine" (NYTimes.com, January 20, 2009), Dirk Johnson reports that although Kara "had grown so weak that she could not walk or speak," her parents refused to obtain medical care for her and instead relied on prayer to heal her. About a month after her death, Jill Falstad, the state attorney of Marathon County, Wisconsin, filed charges against Kara's parents. Each was found guilty of second-degree reckless homicide in 2009 and sentenced to six months in prison along with 10 years of probation.

MINNESOTA COURT CASE. The second important 2009 court case involving parental decisions about a child's medical condition concerned 13-year-old Daniel Hauser, who had developed Hodgkin's lymphoma (a cancer of the immune system). Maura Lerner explains in "Sleepy Eye Parents, Teen Fight to Refuse Chemo" (StarTribune.com, May 7, 2009) that in January 2009 Hauser was diagnosed with the cancer and prescribed six rounds of chemotherapy and radiation. After undergoing the first round of chemotherapy to treat a tumor in his chest, Hauser became sick, as is common for chemotherapy patients. His parents responded by refusing any more treatments and chose instead to treat him themselves by changing his diet. Hauser and his parents belonged to the Nemenhah, an obscure Native American religious organization that favors natural healing processes over medical intervention. They cited religious reasons for their decision.

James Olson, the attorney for Brown County, Minnesota, learned of Hauser's refusal and filed a petition against his parents, citing child neglect and endangerment.

Olson asked the judge to order the boy into treatment for his highly curable cancer. Agreeing with the petition, the judge ordered the parents to have their son continue his chemotherapy and radiation treatments.

In May 2009 Hauser's mother took him to California to avoid the judge's order but returned a week later. Eventually, Hauser resumed treatments, and in November 2009 the judge closed the case after the court-ordered chemotherapy and radiation treatments put the cancer into remission.

End-of-Life Decisions for Adolescents

Although many laws concerning adolescents have changed since the mid-20th century, such as those allowing adolescents to seek medical treatment for reproductive health and birth control services without parental consent, most states have no laws for end-of-life decisions by adolescents. Caprice Knapp et al. indicate in "Adolescents with Life-Threatening Illnesses" (*American Journal of Hospice and Palliative Care*, vol. 27, no. 2, March 2010) that although U.S. laws do not consider adolescents under the age of 18 years to be competent to make their own health care decisions, health care practitioners often do. In a review of available studies, the researchers add, however, that practitioners from various medical fields differ on the question of how much to involve adolescents in life-altering decisions. For example, studies "suggest that adolescents do not have the capacity to make long-term decisions considering their stage of development," and that they are more likely than adults "to make decisions based on emotions rather than facts." Conversely, behaviorists note that "a portfolio of evidence suggests that adolescents are capable of consenting to procedures and have the capacity to make decisions."

CHAPTER 7

SUICIDE, EUTHANASIA, AND ASSISTED SUICIDE

SUICIDE

Suicide is a taboo subject for many people in the contemporary United States. Religious prohibitions against killing oneself, negative stereotypes about the mentally ill, and a general unwillingness to dwell on intractable emotional and physical pain may be among the factors that make suicide a topic to be avoided for most people. Nevertheless, suicide is a common occurrence in the United States, as in other countries, and it is in the interest of public health to be able to consider the phenomenon clearly.

As Table 4.1 in Chapter 4 shows, suicide was the 10th-leading cause of death nationally in 2011, accounting for 38,285 deaths. The age-adjusted rate of death by suicide, at 12 per 100,000 people in 2011, was consistent with historic rates of suicide. The age-adjusted rate of death by suicide has fluctuated within a fairly narrow range since 1950, from 13.2 in 1950 to 10.4 in 2000. (See Table 7.1.) In general, then, the likelihood that a person of any age in the United States will commit suicide has been consistent since the beginning of the post–World War II period.

Demographic Variations in the Suicide Rate

Although the overall rate of suicide in the United States since 1950 has been relatively steady, there have been sizable variations by demographic subgroups, and the suicide rates for different age groups have changed noticeably over time.

At all points between 1950 and 2010, U.S. males have been roughly four times as likely as females to commit suicide. (See Table 7.1.) The age-adjusted suicide rate for males was 21.2 deaths per 100,000 population in 1950 and 19.8 in 2010, and the age-adjusted suicide rate for females was 5.6 in 1950 and 5 in 2010. According to the Centers for Disease Control and Prevention (CDC), in "Suicide: Facts at a Glance" (2012, http://www.cdc.gov/violenceprevention/pdf/suicide_datasheet_2012-a.pdf), males accounted for 79% of all suicides in 2010, but females were more likely to have considered suicide and have historically attempted suicide more often than males. Females are the most likely to commit suicide by poisoning, the method used in 37.4% of female suicides in 2010, whereas men are the most likely to commit suicide by firearm, the method used in 56% of male suicides in 2010.

Table 7.2 shows the numbers of deaths and the death rates not only for suicide but also for other types of deaths stemming from external injuries, such as accidents and homicides, classified according to the mechanism of death. In 2010 the suicide rate was 12.4 deaths per 100,000 population, compared with 58.6 deaths per 100,000 from all injuries that year. The number of suicides, at 38,364, was nearly two and a half times greater than the number of homicides (16,259). Of particular note is the fact that, of the 31,672 firearm deaths in the United States that year, 19,392 (61.2%) were suicides, compared with 11,078 homicides (35%).

Many analysts suggest that the ease of obtaining firearms in the United States contributes significantly to the suicide rate. Whereas other methods of committing suicide, such as poisoning (which accounted for 6,599 suicides in 2010) and suffocation (9,493) are not always successful and in general take longer to complete, the use of a firearm minimizes the gap between the impulse and the act of suicide, and it is almost always fatal. Other observers note, however, that suicide rates in the United States are not disproportionately high compared with developed countries where firearms are less readily available.

Suicide rates have historically been higher for older people than for younger people, but the increase in rates as men age has typically been larger than the increase for women as they age. (See Table 7.1.) The trend for women, moreover, reverses past age 65, so that the oldest

TABLE 7.1

Death rates for suicide, by sex, race, Hispanic origin, and age, selected years 1950–2010

[Data are based on death certificates]

Sex, race, Hispanic origin, and age	1950[a,b]	1960[a,b]	1970[b]	1980[b]	1990[b]	2000[c]	2009[c]	2010[c]
All persons				Deaths per 100,000 resident population				
All ages, age-adjusted[d]	13.2	12.5	13.1	12.2	12.5	10.4	11.8	12.1
All ages, crude	11.4	10.6	11.6	11.9	12.4	10.4	12.0	12.4
Under 1 year	. . .	. . .	. . .	. . .	. . .	. . .	. . .	. . .
1–4 years	. . .	. . .	. . .	. . .	. . .	. . .	. . .	. . .
5–14 years	0.2	0.3	0.3	0.4	0.8	0.7	0.6	0.7
15–24 years	4.5	5.2	8.8	12.3	13.2	10.2	10.0	10.5
15–19 years	2.7	3.6	5.9	8.5	11.1	8.0	7.5	7.5
20–24 years	6.2	7.1	12.2	16.1	15.1	12.5	12.6	13.6
25–44 years	11.6	12.2	15.4	15.6	15.2	13.4	14.6	15.0
25–34 years	9.1	10.0	14.1	16.0	15.2	12.0	13.1	14.0
35–44 years	14.3	14.2	16.9	15.4	15.3	14.5	16.1	16.0
45–64 years	23.5	22.0	20.6	15.9	15.3	13.5	17.9	18.6
45–54 years	20.9	20.7	20.0	15.9	14.8	14.4	19.2	19.6
55–64 years	26.8	23.7	21.4	15.9	16.0	12.1	16.4	17.5
65 years and over	30.0	24.5	20.8	17.6	20.5	15.2	14.8	14.9
65–74 years	29.6	23.0	20.8	16.9	17.9	12.5	13.7	13.7
75–84 years	31.1	27.9	21.2	19.1	24.9	17.6	15.8	15.7
85 years and over	28.8	26.0	19.0	19.2	22.2	19.6	16.4	17.6
Male								
All ages, age-adjusted[d]	21.2	20.0	19.8	19.9	21.5	17.7	19.2	19.8
All ages, crude	17.8	16.5	16.8	18.6	20.4	17.1	19.3	19.9
Under 1 year	. . .	. . .	. . .	. . .	. . .	. . .	. . .	. . .
1–4 years	. . .	. . .	. . .	. . .	. . .	. . .	. . .	. . .
5–14 years	0.3	0.4	0.5	0.6	1.1	1.2	0.8	0.9
15–24 years	6.5	8.2	13.5	20.2	22.0	17.1	16.1	16.9
15–19 years	3.5	5.6	8.8	13.8	18.1	13.0	11.6	11.7
20–24 years	9.3	11.5	19.3	26.8	25.7	21.4	20.8	22.2
25–44 years	17.2	17.9	20.9	24.0	24.4	21.3	23.0	23.6
25–34 years	13.4	14.7	19.8	25.0	24.8	19.6	21.0	22.5
35–44 years	21.3	21.0	22.1	22.5	23.9	22.8	24.9	24.6
45–64 years	37.1	34.4	30.0	23.7	24.3	21.3	27.9	29.2
45–54 years	32.0	31.6	27.9	22.9	23.2	22.4	29.3	30.4
55–64 years	43.6	38.1	32.7	24.5	25.7	19.4	26.1	27.7
65 years and over	52.8	44.0	38.4	35.0	41.6	31.1	29.1	29.0
65–74 years	50.5	39.6	36.0	30.4	32.2	22.7	24.3	23.9
75–84 years	58.3	52.5	42.8	42.3	56.1	38.6	32.9	32.3
85 years and over	58.3	57.4	42.4	50.6	65.9	57.5	44.0	47.3
Female								
All ages, age-adjusted[d]	5.6	5.6	7.4	5.7	4.8	4.0	4.9	5.0
All ages, crude	5.1	4.9	6.6	5.5	4.8	4.0	5.0	5.2
Under 1 year	. . .	. . .	. . .	. . .	. . .	. . .	. . .	. . .
1–4 years	. . .	. . .	. . .	. . .	. . .	. . .	. . .	. . .
5–14 years	0.1	0.1	0.2	0.2	0.4	0.3	0.5	0.4
15–24 years	2.6	2.2	4.2	4.3	3.9	3.0	3.6	3.9
15–19 years	1.8	1.6	2.9	3.0	3.7	2.7	3.2	3.1
20–24 years	3.3	2.9	5.7	5.5	4.1	3.2	4.1	4.7
25–44 years	6.2	6.6	10.2	7.7	6.2	5.4	6.2	6.4
25–34 years	4.9	5.5	8.6	7.1	5.6	4.3	5.1	5.3
35–44 years	7.5	7.7	11.9	8.5	6.8	6.4	7.4	7.5
45–64 years	9.9	10.2	12.0	8.9	7.1	6.2	8.5	8.6
45–54 years	9.9	10.2	12.6	9.4	6.9	6.7	9.3	9.0
55–64 years	9.9	10.2	11.4	8.4	7.3	5.4	7.4	8.0
65 years and over	9.4	8.4	8.1	6.1	6.4	4.0	4.0	4.2
65–74 years	10.1	8.4	9.0	6.5	6.7	4.0	4.6	4.8
75–84 years	8.1	8.9	7.0	5.5	6.3	4.0	3.6	3.7
85 years and over	8.2	6.0	5.9	5.5	5.4	4.2	3.2	3.3
White male[e]								
All ages, age-adjusted[d]	22.3	21.1	20.8	20.9	22.8	19.1	21.4	22.0
All ages, crude	19.0	17.6	18.0	19.9	22.0	18.8	21.9	22.6
15–24 years	6.6	8.6	13.9	21.4	23.2	17.9	17.6	18.3
25–44 years	17.9	18.5	21.5	24.6	25.4	22.9	25.7	26.2
45–64 years	39.3	36.5	31.9	25.0	26.0	23.2	31.4	33.0
65 years and over	55.8	46.7	41.1	37.2	44.2	33.3	31.5	31.7
65–74 years	53.2	42.0	38.7	32.5	34.2	24.3	26.6	26.3
75–84 years	61.9	55.7	45.5	45.5	60.2	41.1	35.3	34.9
85 years and over	61.9	61.3	45.8	52.8	70.3	61.6	46.9	50.8

TABLE 7.1

Death rates for suicide, by sex, race, Hispanic origin, and age, selected years 1950–2010 [CONTINUED]

[Data are based on death certificates]

Sex, race, Hispanic origin, and age	1950[a,b]	1960[a,b]	1970[b]	1980[b]	1990[b]	2000[c]	2009[c]	2010[c]
Black or African American male[e]				Deaths per 100,000 resident population				
All ages, age-adjusted[d]	7.5	8.4	10.0	11.4	12.8	10.0	8.9	9.1
All ages, crude	6.3	6.4	8.0	10.3	12.0	9.4	8.5	8.7
15–24 years	4.9	4.1	10.5	12.3	15.1	14.2	10.4	11.1
25–44 years	9.8	12.6	16.1	19.2	19.6	14.3	13.2	14.5
45–64 years	12.7	13.0	12.4	11.8	13.1	9.9	9.6	9.5
65 years and over	9.0	9.9	8.7	11.4	14.9	11.5	9.6	8.3
65–74 years	10.0	11.3	8.7	11.1	14.7	11.1	8.0	7.6
75–84 years[f]	*	*	*	10.5	14.4	12.1	11.9	9.9
85 years and over	—	*	*	*	*	*	*	*
American Indian or Alaska Native male[e]								
All ages, age-adjusted[d]	—	—	—	19.3	20.1	16.0	14.6	15.5
All ages, crude	—	—	—	20.9	20.9	15.9	15.1	16.1
15–24 years	—	—	—	45.3	49.1	26.2	28.9	30.6
25–44 years	—	—	—	31.2	27.8	24.5	20.4	20.9
45–64 years	—	—	—	*	*	15.4	15.4	17.8
65 years and over	—	—	—	*	*	*	*	*
Asian or Pacific Islander male[e]								
All ages, age-adjusted[d]	—	—	—	10.7	9.6	8.6	8.7	9.5
All ages, crude	—	—	—	8.8	8.7	7.9	8.4	9.3
15–24 years	—	—	—	10.8	13.5	9.1	8.0	10.9
25–44 years	—	—	—	11.0	10.6	9.9	9.7	10.6
45–64 years	—	—	—	13.0	9.7	9.7	12.1	12.8
65 years and over	—	—	—	18.6	16.8	15.4	15.3	14.9
Hispanic or Latino male[e,g]								
All ages, age-adjusted[d]	—	—	—	—	13.7	10.3	9.9	9.9
All ages, crude	—	—	—	—	11.4	8.4	8.5	8.5
15–24 years	—	—	—	—	14.7	10.9	10.7	10.7
25–44 years	—	—	—	—	16.2	11.2	11.4	11.2
45–64 years	—	—	—	—	16.1	12.0	12.6	12.9
65 years and over	—	—	—	—	23.4	19.5	16.0	15.7
White, not Hispanic or Latino male[g]								
All ages, age-adjusted[d]	—	—	—	—	23.5	20.2	23.4	24.2
All ages, crude	—	—	—	—	23.1	20.4	24.7	25.7
15–24 years	—	—	—	—	24.4	19.5	19.4	20.4
25–44 years	—	—	—	—	26.4	25.1	29.5	30.3
45–64 years	—	—	—	—	26.8	24.0	33.6	35.4
65 years and over	—	—	—	—	45.4	33.9	32.5	32.7
White female[e]								
All ages, age-adjusted[d]	6.0	5.9	7.9	6.1	5.2	4.3	5.5	5.6
All ages, crude	5.5	5.3	7.1	5.9	5.3	4.4	5.7	5.9
15–24 years	2.7	2.3	4.2	4.6	4.2	3.1	3.8	4.2
25–44 years	6.6	7.0	11.0	8.1	6.6	6.0	7.1	7.3
45–64 years	10.6	10.9	13.0	9.6	7.7	6.9	9.6	9.9
65 years and over	9.9	8.8	8.5	6.4	6.8	4.3	4.4	4.5
Black or African American female[e]								
All ages, age-adjusted[d]	1.8	2.0	2.9	2.4	2.4	1.8	1.8	1.8
All ages, crude	1.5	1.6	2.6	2.2	2.3	1.7	1.8	1.8
15–24 years	1.8	*	3.8	2.3	2.3	2.2	2.1	2.0
25–44 years	2.3	3.0	4.8	4.3	3.8	2.6	2.7	2.8
45–64 years	2.7	3.1	2.9	2.5	2.9	2.1	2.5	2.1
65 years and over	*	*	2.6	*	1.9	1.3	1.0	*
American Indian or Alaska Native female[e]								
All ages, age-adjusted[d]	—	—	—	4.7	3.6	3.8	5.4	6.1
All ages, crude	—	—	—	4.7	3.7	4.0	5.6	5.9
15–24 years	—	—	—	*	*	*	11.1	10.4
25–44 years	—	—	—	10.7	*	7.2	7.5	7.4
45–64 years	—	—	—	*	*	*	5.9	6.2
65 years and over	—	—	—	*	*	*	*	*

women are among the least likely females to commit suicide, whereas the oldest men are the males most likely to commit suicide.

Specifically, boys and men aged 15 to 24 years had a suicide rate of 16.9 deaths per 100,000 population in 2010, men aged 25 to 44 years had a suicide rate of

TABLE 7.1

Death rates for suicide, by sex, race, Hispanic origin, and age, selected years 1950–2010 [CONTINUED]

[Data are based on death certificates]

Sex, race, Hispanic origin, and age	1950[a, b]	1960[a, b]	1970[b]	1980[b]	1990[b]	2000[c]	2009[c]	2010[c]
Asian or Pacific Islander female[e]				Deaths per 100,000 resident population				
All ages, age-adjusted[d]	—	—	—	5.5	4.1	2.8	3.5	3.4
All ages, crude	—	—	—	4.7	3.4	2.7	3.5	3.4
15–24 years	—	—	—	*	3.9	2.7	4.4	3.5
25–44 years	—	—	—	5.4	3.8	3.3	3.9	4.1
45–64 years	—	—	—	7.9	5.0	3.2	4.7	4.7
65 years and over	—	—	—	*	8.5	5.2	4.8	4.3
Hispanic or Latina female[e, g]								
All ages, age-adjusted[d]	—	—	—	—	2.3	1.7	2.0	2.1
All ages, crude	—	—	—	—	2.2	1.5	1.8	2.0
15–24 years	—	—	—	—	3.1	2.0	2.3	3.1
25–44 years	—	—	—	—	3.1	2.1	2.5	2.4
45–64 years	—	—	—	—	2.5	2.5	2.5	2.8
65 years and over	—	—	—	—	*	*	2.3	2.2
White, not Hispanic or Latina female[g]								
All ages, age-adjusted[d]	—	—	—	—	5.4	4.7	6.1	6.2
All ages, crude	—	—	—	—	5.6	4.9	6.5	6.7
15–24 years	—	—	—	—	4.3	3.3	4.1	4.4
25–44 years	—	—	—	—	7.0	6.7	8.3	8.6
45–64 years	—	—	—	—	8.0	7.3	10.5	10.7
65 years and over	—	—	—	—	7.0	4.4	4.5	4.7

. . . Category not applicable.
*Rates based on fewer than 20 deaths are considered unreliable and are not shown.
—Data not available.
[a]Includes deaths of persons who were not residents of the 50 states and the District of Columbia (D.C.).
[b]Underlying cause of death was coded according to the 6th Revision of the *International Classification of Diseases* (ICD) in 1950, 7th Revision in 1960, 8th Revision in 1970, and 9th Revision in 1980–1998.
[c]Starting with 1999 data, cause of death is coded according to ICD-10.
[d]Age-adjusted rates are calculated using the year 2000 standard population. Prior to 2001, age-adjusted rates were calculated using standard million proportions based on rounded population numbers. Starting with 2001 data, unrounded population numbers are used to calculate age-adjusted rates.
[e]The race groups, white, black, Asian or Pacific Islander, and American Indian or Alaska Native, include persons of Hispanic and non-Hispanic origin. Persons of Hispanic origin may be of any race. Death rates for the American Indian or Alaska Native, Asian or Pacific Islander, and Hispanic populations are known to be underestimated.
[f]In 1950, rate is for the age group 75 years and over.
[g]Prior to 1997, data from states that did not report Hispanic origin on the death certificate were excluded.
Notes: Starting with *Health, United States, 2003*, rates for 1991–1999 were revised using intercensal population estimates based on the 1990 and 2000 censuses. For 2000, population estimates are bridged-race April 1 census counts. Starting with *Health, United States, 2012*, rates for 2001–2009 were revised using intercensal population estimates based on the 2000 and 2010 censuses. For 2010, population estimates are bridged-race April 1 census counts. Figures for 2001 include September 11-related deaths for which death certificates were filed as of October 24, 2002. for terrorism-related ICD-10 codes. Age groups were selected to minimize the presentation of unstable age-specific death rates based on small numbers of deaths and for consistency among comparison groups. Starting with 2003 data, some states allowed the reporting of more than one race on the death certificate. The multiple-race data for these states were bridged to the single-race categories of the 1977 Office of Management and Budget standards, for comparability with other states. Data for additional years are available.

SOURCE: "Table 35. Death Rates for Suicide, by Sex, Race, Hispanic Origin, and Age: United States, Selected Years 1950–2010," in *Health, United States, 2012: With Special Feature on Emergency Care*, Centers for Disease Control and Prevention, National Center for Health Statistics, 2013, http://www.cdc.gov/nchs/data/hus/hus12.pdf (accessed December 27, 2013)

23.6, men aged 45 to 64 years had a suicide rate of 29.2, and men aged 65 years and older had a suicide rate of 29. By contrast, the suicide rate for girls and women aged 15 to 24 years was 3.9 deaths per 100,000 population, the rate for women aged 25 to 44 years was 6.4, the rate for women aged 45 to 64 years was 8.6, and the rate for women over the age of 65 years was 4.2. Among men, those aged 85 years and older had the highest suicide rate of any age-based subgroup (47.3 deaths per 100,000 population), whereas women aged 85 years and older had one of the lowest suicide rates of any subgroup (3.3 deaths per 100,000 population).

Although older men have significantly higher suicide rates than younger men, in general older people are less likely to commit suicide in the 21st century than in earlier decades. (See Table 7.1.) The suicide rate for men and women aged 65 years and older decreased by half between 1950 and 2010, falling from 30 deaths per 100,000 population to 14.9, and the suicide rate for men and women aged 45 to 64 years fell from 23.5 to 18.6. Meanwhile, the suicide rate for teenagers and young adults aged 15 to 24 years has more than doubled, from 4.5 in 1950 to 10.5 in 2010, and the rate for adults aged 25 to 44 years has risen from 11.6 in 1950 to 15 in 2010.

As Table 7.1 further shows, suicide rates vary significantly by race and ethnicity. Age-adjusted rates in 2010, as in prior decades, were highest for non-Hispanic white males (24.2 deaths per 100,000 population) and Native American males (15.5). African American males (9.1), Asian and Pacific Islander males (9.5), and Hispanic

TABLE 7.2

Number of deaths and death rates, by mechanism and intent of death, 2010

[Totals for selected causes of death differ from those shown in other tables that utilize standard mortality tabulation lists. Rates are per 100,000 population; age-adjusted rates are per 100,000 U.S. standard population. Rates are based on populations enumerated in the 2010 census as of April 1.]

Mechanism and intent of death	Number	Rate	Age-adjusted rate
All injury	**180,811**	**58.6**	**57.1**
Unintentional	120,859	39.1	38.0
Suicide	38,364	12.4	12.1
Homicide	16,259	5.3	5.3
Undetermined	4,908	1.6	1.6
Legal intervention/war	421	0.1	0.2
Cut/pierce	**2,598**	**0.8**	**0.8**
Unintentional	105	0.0	0.0
Suicide	673	0.2	0.2
Homicide	1,799	0.6	0.6
Undetermined	21	0.0	0.0
Legal intervention/war	—	a	a
Drowning	**4,521**	**1.5**	**1.4**
Unintentional	3,782	1.2	1.2
Suicide	409	0.1	0.1
Homicide	52	0.0	0.0
Undetermined	278	0.1	0.1
Fall	**26,852**	**8.7**	**8.1**
Unintentional	26,009	8.4	7.9
Suicide	781	0.3	0.3
Homicide	12	a	a
Undetermined	50	0.0	0.0
Fire/hot object or substance	**3,194**	**1.0**	**1.0**
Unintentional	2,845	0.9	0.9
Suicide	131	0.0	0.0
Homicide	92	0.0	0.0
Undetermined	126	0.0	0.0
Legal intervention/war	—	a	a
Fire/flame	**3,127**	**1.0**	**1.0**
Unintentional	2,782	0.9	0.9
Suicide	131	0.0	0.0
Homicide	89	0.0	0.0
Undetermined	125	0.0	0.0
Hot object/substance	**67**	**0.0**	**0.0**
Unintentional	63	0.0	0.0
Suicide	—	a	a
Homicide	3	a	a
Undetermined	1	a	a
Firearm	**31,672**	**10.3**	**10.1**
Unintentional	606	0.2	0.2
Suicide	19,392	6.3	6.1
Homicide	11,078	3.6	3.6
Undetermined	252	0.1	0.1
Legal intervention/war	344	0.1	0.1
Machinery[b]	**590**	**0.2**	**0.2**
All transport	**37,402**	**12.1**	**11.9**
Unintentional	37,236	12.1	11.8
Suicide	114	0.0	0.0
Homicide	39	0.0	0.0
Undetermined	13	a	a
Legal intervention/war	—	a	a
Motor vehicle traffic[b]	**33,687**	**10.9**	**10.7**
Occupant[b]	10,246	3.3	3.3
Motorcyclist[b]	4,177	1.4	1.3
Pedal cyclist[b]	551	0.2	0.2
Pedestrian[b]	4,383	1.4	1.4
Other[b]	10	a	a
Unspecified[b]	14,320	4.6	4.6
Pedal cyclist, other[b]	242	0.1	0.1
Pedestrian, other[b]	1,074	0.3	0.3
Other land transport	**1,524**	**0.5**	**0.5**
Unintentional	1,358	0.4	0.4
Suicide	114	0.0	0.0
Homicide	39	0.0	0.0
Undetermined	13	a	a
Other transport	**875**	**0.3**	**0.3**
Unintentional	875	0.3	0.3
Homicide	—	a	a
Legal intervention/war	—	a	a
Natural/environmental[b]	**1,576**	**0.5**	**0.5**
Overexertion[b]	**10**	**a**	**a**
Poisoning	**42,917**	**13.9**	**13.7**
Unintentional	33,041	10.7	10.6
Suicide	6,599	2.1	2.1
Homicide	79	0.0	0.0
Undetermined	3,197	1.0	1.0
Legal intervention/war	1	a	a
Struck by or against	**912**	**0.3**	**0.3**
Unintentional	788	0.3	0.2
Suicide	—	a	a
Homicide	123	0.0	0.0
Undetermined	1	a	a
Legal intervention/war	—	a	a
Suffocation	**16,362**	**5.3**	**5.2**
Unintentional	6,165	2.0	1.9
Suicide	9,493	3.1	3.1
Homicide	544	0.2	0.2
Undetermined	160	0.1	0.0
Other specified, classifiable	**2,002**	**0.6**	**0.7**
Unintentional	1,395	0.5	0.5
Suicide	337	0.1	0.1
Homicide	211	0.1	0.1
Undetermined	15	a	a
Legal intervention/war	44	0.0	0.0
Other specified, not elsewhere classified	**1,973**	**0.6**	**0.6**
Unintentional	1,023	0.3	0.3
Suicide	245	0.1	0.1
Homicide	495	0.2	0.2
Undetermined	184	0.1	0.1
Legal intervention/war	26	0.0	0.0
Unspecified	**8,230**	**2.7**	**2.5**
Unintentional	5,688	1.8	1.7
Suicide	190	0.1	0.1
Homicide	1,735	0.6	0.6
Undetermined	611	0.2	0.2
Legal intervention/war	6	a	a

males (9.9) were considerably less likely to commit suicide. Likewise, non-Hispanic white females (6.2) and Native American females (6.1) were more likely to commit suicide than their African American (1.8), Hispanic (2.1), and Asian and Pacific Islander (3.4) counterparts.

Cross-Cultural and Historical Attitudes toward Suicide

Attitudes about suicide, like rates of suicide, vary significantly across and within cultures. Although

TABLE 7.2

Number of deaths and death rates, by mechanism and intent of death, 2010 [CONTINUED]

[Totals for selected causes of death differ from those shown in other tables that utilize standard mortality tabulation lists. Rates are per 100,000 population; age-adjusted rates are per 100,000 U.S. standard population. Rates are based on populations enumerated in the 2010 census as of April 1.]

0.0 Quantity more than zero but less than 0.05.
—Quantity zero.
[a] Figure does not meet standards of reliability or precision.
[b] Intent of death is unintentional.

SOURCE: Adapted from Sherry L. Murphy, Jiaquan Xu, and Kenneth D. Kochanek, "Table 18. Number of Deaths, Death Rates, and Age-Adjusted Death Rates for Injury Deaths, by Mechanism and Intent of Death: United States, 2010," in "Deaths: Final Data for 2010," *National Vital Statistics Reports*, vol. 61, no. 4, May 8, 2013, http://www.cdc.gov/nchs/data/nvsr/nvsr61/nvsr61_04.pdf (accessed December 28, 2013)

cultural influences are notoriously difficult to isolate in scientific studies, a large body of literature exists testifying to the different ways that cultures and religions throughout history have understood the act of ending one's own life.

In ancient Greece, the suicides of those who had decided that their lives were no longer useful were considered acceptable and even rational acts, and there was no prohibition on their seeking help from others in the carrying out of their wishes. Similarly, ancient Romans who dishonored themselves or their families were expected to commit suicide to maintain their dignity and, frequently, the family property. Early Christians were quick to embrace martyrdom as a guarantee of eternal salvation, but during the fourth century St. Augustine of Hippo (354–430) discouraged the practice. He and later theologians were concerned that many Christians who were suffering in this world would see suicide as a reasonable and legitimate way to depart to a better place in the hereafter. The view of the Christian theologian St. Thomas Aquinas (c. 1225–1274) is reflected in *Catechism of the Catholic Church* (August 23, 2002, http://www.vatican.va/archive/ccc_css/archive/catechism/ccc_toc.htm), which states that "suicide contradicts the natural inclination of the human being to preserve and perpetuate his life [and] is contrary to love for the living God."

Islam and Judaism also condemn the taking of one's own life. By contrast, Buddhist monks and nuns have been known to commit suicide by self-immolation (burning themselves alive) as a form of social protest. In a ritual called *suttee*, which is now outlawed, widows in India showed devotion to their deceased husbands by being cremated with them, sometimes throwing themselves on the funeral pyres, although it was not always voluntary. Widowers (men whose wives had died) did not follow this custom.

The Japanese people have traditionally associated a certain idealism with suicide. During the 12th century samurai warriors practiced voluntary *seppuku* (ritual self-disembowelment) to avoid dishonor at the hands of their enemies. Some samurai committed this form of slow suicide to atone for wrongdoing or to express devotion to a superior who had died. As recently as 1970 the novelist Kimitake Hiraoka (1925–1970) publicly committed *seppuku*. During World War II (1939–1945) Japanese kamikaze pilots inflicted serious casualties by purposely crashing their planes into enemy ships, killing themselves along with enemy troops.

Quasi-religious reasons sometimes motivate mass suicide. In 1978 more than 900 members of a group known as the People's Temple killed themselves in Jonestown, Guyana. In 1997 a group called Heaven's Gate committed mass suicide in California. The devastating September 11, 2001, terrorist attacks against the United States were the result of a suicidal plot enacted by a religious extremist group. Suicide bombings in other parts of the world have also been attributed to extremist groups that have twisted or misinterpreted the fundamental tenets of Islam to further their political objectives.

CONTEMPORARY ATTITUDES TOWARD SUICIDE. In *In More Religious Countries, Lower Suicide Rates* (July 3, 2008, http://www.gallup.com/poll/108625/More-Religious-Countries-Lower-Suicide-Rates.aspx), Brett Pelham and Zsolt Nyiri of the Gallup Organization indicate that in 2008 the United States' suicide rate of 11.05 deaths per 100,000 population was near the median (the middle value) suicide rate when compared with other countries of the world. The United States also fell near the median level of scores on the Gallup Religiosity Index, which is a measure of the importance of religion in people's lives. Pelham and Nyiri determine that the suicide rates of countries worldwide tend to rise and fall with their level of religiosity: those having a higher level of religiosity (a higher score) often have a lower suicide rate. Conversely, those having a lower level of religiosity (a lower score) typically have a higher suicide rate. The religiosity score for the United States on the Gallup Religiosity Index was 61 and the suicide rate was 11.05 deaths per 100,000 population in 2008. In comparison, the religiosity score for Kuwait was 83 and the suicide rate was 1.95 deaths per 100,000 population, and the religiosity score for Russia was 28 and the suicide rate was 36.15 deaths per 100,000 population.

Sascha O. Becker and Ludger Woessmann show in *Knocking on Heaven's Door? Protestantism and Suicide* (June 10, 2011, http://www2.warwick.ac.uk/fac/soc/economics/research/workingpapers/2011/twerp_966.pdf) that suicide rates are higher in countries that are mainly Protestant than in countries that are mainly Catholic. The researchers compare data from the Prussian countries during the 19th century and more recent data from the

Organisation for Economic Co-operation and Development. The data clearly show that in all circumstances, more people committed suicide in Protestant countries than in Catholic countries. Becker and Woessmann suggest that "sociological and theological differences between Protestants and Catholics make suicide more likely among the former group."

In *Views on End-of-Life Medical Treatments* (November 21, 2013, http://www.pewforum.org/files/2013/11/end-of-life-survey-report-full-pdf.pdf), the Pew Research Center reports that a growing percentage of Americans believes that individuals have a moral right to kill themselves in certain circumstances. Nearly six out of 10 (62%) U.S. adults expressed a belief in an individual's right to end his or her life if that person "is suffering great pain with no hope of improvement," and 56% supported the individual's right to die if she or he "has an incurable disease." By contrast, in 1990 support for the right to suicide in cases involving great pain with no hope of improvement stood at 55%, and support for the right to suicide in cases involving incurable disease stood at 49%. Growing minorities of U.S. adults also supported an individual's right to suicide if he or she is "ready to die [because] living has become a burden" (38% of Americans, up from 27% in 1990) or if he or she "is an extremely heavy burden on his or her family" (32% of Americans, up from 29% in 1990).

Suicide among Teenagers and Young Adults

The suicide rate among young people aged 15 to 24 years nearly tripled between 1950 and 1990, from 4.5 suicides per 100,000 population to 13.2. (See Table 7.1.) Between 1990 and 2010 the teen and young adult suicide rate fell slightly, while remaining well above mid-20th-century levels. This increase in the youth suicide rate was historically unprecedented. Prior to the 1950s, suicide rates had always been observed to increase with age, in keeping with common assumptions about why a person might choose to end his or her life. Older people, faced with declining health and a shrinking sense of possibility, might be said to turn to suicide for reasons that can be rationally supported. By contrast, young people have a great deal of life and possibility ahead of them, and they cannot claim to know what they might make of their future. Accordingly, self-harm is not considered a rational decision for a teenager or young adult.

The reasons for the dramatic rise in the suicide rates for those aged 15 to 24 years have not been firmly established, partly because suicide in general resists sociological and scientific analysis. Kimberly A. Van Orden et al. explain in "The Interpersonal Theory of Suicide" (*Psychological Review*, vol. 117, no. 2, April 2010) that suicide is difficult to study because, although effective research requires large sample sizes, the number of people who commit or attempt suicide is low relative to the overall population. Additionally, suicidal people generally cannot be included in clinical study groups because of researchers' concerns about safety, and people who succeed in committing suicide are not, obviously, available for study after the fact. Finally, Van Orden et al. suggest that the study of suicide has been held back by a relative absence of comprehensive theories about the phenomenon.

One influential, if not universally accepted, explanation for the rise in youth suicide in the late 20th century is that of the economists David M. Cutler, Edward L. Glaeser, and Karen E. Norberg in "Explaining the Rise in Youth Suicide" (Jonathan Gruber, editor, *Risky Behavior among Youths: An Economic Analysis*, 2001). Cutler, Glaeser, and Norberg suggest that young people use suicide to attract attention from others because they have few other forms of power, and they find evidence that suicide functions virally among peer groups, elevating the overall numbers of suicide attempts among teens and young adults. In attempting to isolate the societal changes that may have triggered the sustained rise in teen suicides, the authors suggest that the most important variable is the rise of young people living in homes with a divorced parent. Although they do not discount the fact that this variable interacts with other variables, such as racial and ethnic background, access to firearms, and income, they maintain that no single factor influences the suicide rate among young people more powerfully than the divorce rate.

As with other age groups, male teens and young adults are far more likely to commit suicide than female teens and young adults. As Table 7.1 shows, the suicide rate for males aged 15 to 24 years was 16.9 in 2010, compared with 3.9 for females aged 15 to 24 years. According to the CDC, in "Suicide Prevention: Youth Suicide" (January 9, 2014, http://www.cdc.gov/violenceprevention/pub/youth_suicide.html), males accounted for 81% of all suicide deaths among young people aged 10 to 24 years.

However, the public-health concerns relating to suicide among young people go beyond deaths. Far more teens attempt suicide than successfully commit suicide. According to Cutler, Glaeser, and Norberg, for every teen who commits suicide, 400 other teens attempt suicide, 100 require medical treatment for their suicide attempts, and 30 are hospitalized in the aftermath of their suicide attempts. Moreover, the demographic characteristics of those teens and young adults who die from suicide differ considerably from the characteristics of those who attempt suicide but do not ultimately die.

TABLE 7.3

Percentage of students in grades 9–12 who seriously considered suicide, by sex, grade level, race, and Hispanic origin, 1991, 2001, and 2011

[Data are based on a national sample of high school students, grades 9–12]

Sex, grade level, race, and Hispanic origin	Seriously considered suicide		
	1991	2001	2011
Total	**29.0**	**19.0**	**15.8**
Male			
Total	**20.8**	**14.2**	**12.5**
9th grade	17.6	14.7	12.9
10th grade	19.5	13.8	11.4
11th grade	25.3	14.1	14.3
12th grade	20.7	13.7	11.5
Not Hispanic or Latino:			
White	21.7	14.9	12.8
Black or African American	13.3	9.2	9.0
Hispanic or Latino	18.0	12.2	12.6
Female			
Total	**37.2**	**23.6**	**19.3**
9th grade	40.3	26.2	21.5
10th grade	39.7	24.1	22.3
11th grade	38.4	23.6	16.7
12th grade	30.7	18.9	15.8
Not Hispanic or Latina:			
White	38.6	24.2	18.4
Black or African American	29.4	17.2	17.4
Hispanic or Latina	34.6	26.5	21.0

SOURCE: Adapted from "Table 61. Health Risk Behaviors among Students in Grades 9–12, by Sex, Grade Level, Race, and Hispanic Origin: United States, Selected Years 1991–2011," in *Health, United States, 2012: With Special Feature on Emergency Care*, Centers for Disease Control and Prevention, National Center for Health Statistics, 2013, http://www.cdc.gov/nchs/data/hus/hus12.pdf (accessed December 27, 2013)

Whereas young males are more likely to commit suicide, young females are more likely to consider and attempt it. As Table 7.3 shows, 15.8% of high school students reported seriously considering suicide in 2011, down from 19% in 2001 and 29% in 1991. More females (19.3%) than males (12.5%) seriously considered suicide in 2011, and the rates were highest among girls in the ninth and 10th grades. Among males, African Americans (9%) were less likely than non-Hispanic whites (12.8%) or Hispanics (12.6%) to have seriously considered suicide. Among females, Hispanics (21%) were more likely than either non-Hispanic whites (18.4%) or African Americans (17.4%) to have seriously considered self-harm.

Similar patterns applied to those high school students who attempted suicide in 2011. (See Table 7.4.) More female (9.8%) than male (5.8%) high school students attempted suicide, and girls in the ninth (11.8%) and 10th (11.6%) grades were the most likely age group to have attempted suicide. Among female students, Hispanics (13.5%) were far more likely to have attempted suicide than whites (7.9%) or African Americans (8.8%), while among male students African Americans (7.7%) were slightly more likely than Hispanics (6.9%) and whites (4.6%) to have attempted suicide. Among those suicide attempts that required medical treatment, there was more convergence between female and male numbers, but the numbers were still higher among females (2.9%) than males (1.9%). Likewise, Hispanic females (4.1%) and females in the ninth (3.7%) and 10th (3.4%) grades were significantly more likely than other subgroups to have made a suicide attempt that necessitated medical treatment.

Hispanic high school students' increased likelihood of considering and attempting suicide is not well under-

TABLE 7.4

Percentage of high school students who attempted suicide and whose suicide attempt resulted in the need for medical attention, by sex, race/ethnicity, and grade, 2011

	Attempted suicide			Suicide attempt treated by a doctor or nurse		
	Female	Male	Total	Female	Male	Total
Category	%	%	%	%	%	%
Race/ethnicity						
White*	7.9	4.6	6.2	2.2	1.5	1.9
Black*	8.8	7.7	8.3	2.4	2.4	2.4
Hispanic	13.5	6.9	10.2	4.1	2.2	3.2
Grade						
9	11.8	6.8	9.3	3.7	2.0	2.8
10	11.6	5.1	8.2	3.4	1.8	2.6
11	7.4	5.9	6.6	2.0	1.9	1.9
12	7.7	5.0	6.3	2.3	1.8	2.0
Total	**9.8**	**5.8**	**7.8**	**2.9**	**1.9**	**2.4**

*Non-Hispanic.
Note: Attempts during the 12 months before the survey.

SOURCE: Adapted from "Table 25. Percentage of High School Students Who Attempted Suicide and Whose Suicide Attempt Resulted in an Injury, Poisoning, or Overdose That Had to Be Treated by a Doctor or Nurse, by Sex, Race/Ethnicity, and Grade—United States, Youth Risk Behavior Survey, 2011," in *Youth Risk Behavior Surveillance—United States, 2011, Morbidity and Mortality Weekly Report*, vol. 61, no. 4, June 8, 2012, http://www.cdc.gov/mmwr/pdf/ss/ss6104.pdf (accessed December 28, 2013)

TABLE 7.5

Percentage of high school students who attempted suicide and whose suicide attempt resulted in the need for medical attention, by sex and selected U.S. sites, 2011

	Attempted suicide			Suicide attempt treated by a doctor or nurse		
	Female	Male	Total	Female	Male	Total
Site	%	%	%	%	%	%
State surveys						
Alabama	9.6	4.7	7.1	3.7	1.5	2.6
Alaska	9.9	7.4	8.7	2.4	2.7	2.7
Arizona	11.7	9.0	10.3	3.9	2.8	3.3
Arkansas	11.3	8.5	10.0	4.5	3.5	4.1
Colorado	8.4	3.8	6.1	2.7	1.7	2.2
Connecticut	8.2	5.2	6.7	—	—	—
Delaware	8.8	6.7	7.8	2.4	2.4	2.4
Florida	8.2	5.5	6.9	2.0	2.4	2.3
Georgia	10.9	10.0	10.8	3.2	3.8	3.6
Hawaii	10.5	6.5	8.6	4.1	2.6	3.4
Idaho	8.1	5.1	6.5	2.3	1.5	1.9
Illinois	9.4	6.3	8.0	2.8	2.4	2.6
Indiana	11.4	10.5	11.0	3.9	4.0	3.9
Iowa	7.7	4.1	6.0	2.0	1.8	1.9
Kansas	5.7	6.0	5.9	2.2	2.8	2.5
Kentucky	10.8	10.4	10.9	4.1	4.9	4.6
Louisiana	10.4	10.6	10.6	6.3	4.3	5.4
Maine	7.1	7.7	7.6	—	—	—
Maryland	11.1	10.1	10.9	4.9	5.2	5.2
Massachusetts	8.2	5.2	6.8	2.1	2.4	2.3
Michigan	9.2	7.0	8.1	3.3	2.1	2.7
Mississippi	9.5	7.2	8.5	2.8	3.1	3.1
Montana	6.9	6.0	6.5	2.4	2.2	2.4
Nebraska	8.5	6.8	7.7	2.5	2.6	2.6
New Hampshire	7.5	4.8	6.1	2.9	2.0	2.4
New Jersey	6.5	5.6	6.0	1.8	2.5	2.1
New Mexico	12.3	5.0	8.6	4.2	1.8	3.0
New York	8.0	6.1	7.1	2.7	2.4	2.6
North Carolina	—	—	—	3.8	6.1	5.0
North Dakota	12.0	9.6	10.8	—	—	—
Ohio	9.9	8.0	9.1	3.9	4.1	4.0
Oklahoma	9.1	3.4	6.3	1.4	0.9	1.1
Rhode Island	8.1	9.1	8.7	3.0	4.7	3.9
South Carolina	12.8	8.6	11.0	4.3	3.1	3.7
South Dakota	10.6	5.1	7.9	4.3	1.3	2.8
Tennessee	8.5	3.9	6.2	3.0	1.3	2.2
Texas	12.9	8.4	10.8	4.6	2.2	3.5
Utah	6.5	7.3	7.2	2.8	3.3	3.1
Vermont	4.5	2.7	3.6	—	—	—
Virginia	12.4	8.4	10.5	3.7	3.1	3.4
West Virginia	6.2	4.8	5.5	1.9	1.8	1.9
Wisconsin	7.8	5.5	6.7	3.0	2.3	2.6
Wyoming	12.0	10.5	11.3	6.0	3.7	4.9
Median	9.1	6.6	7.8	3.0	2.5	2.7
Range	4.5–12.9	2.7–10.6	3.6–11.3	1.4–6.3	0.9–6.1	1.1–5.4
Large urban school district surveys						
Boston, MA	9.7	7.6	8.6	2.9	4.3	3.6
Broward County, FL	7.5	4.4	6.0	2.1	2.3	2.2
Charlotte-Mecklenburg, NC	12.8	16.7	15.3	—	—	—
Chicago, IL	16.0	15.3	15.8	5.6	5.6	5.6
Dallas, TX	11.4	6.6	9.1	4.1	2.5	3.3
Detroit, MI	14.0	9.6	12.3	5.4	4.0	5.0
District of Columbia	10.6	12.5	11.5	4.7	5.0	4.8
Duval County, FL	12.9	12.1	12.7	4.5	5.2	4.9
Houston, TX	10.6	11.4	11.1	3.0	3.9	3.6
Los Angeles, CA	12.8	8.5	10.8	4.0	4.2	4.1
Memphis, TN	10.6	4.1	7.6	2.6	0.3	1.6
Miami-Dade County, FL	7.9	5.6	6.8	2.7	2.9	2.9
Milwaukee, WI	14.2	11.6	13.1	4.4	3.7	4.0

stood, but analysts have offered possible explanations for the phenomenon. As Jane Delgado, the president and chief executive officer of the National Alliance for Hispanic Health, tells Hope Gillette in "Attempted Suicide, Suicidal Fantasies More Common in Hispanic Teens" (VOXXI.com, January 29, 2013), the higher rates of suicidal thinking and attempted suicide are concentrated among a particular subset of Hispanic girls: first-generation immigrants who were born in the United States. Delgado observes, "Adolescence is

TABLE 7.5

Percentage of high school students who attempted suicide and whose suicide attempt resulted in the need for medical attention, by sex and selected U.S. sites, 2011 [CONTINUED]

	Attempted suicide			Suicide attempt treated by a doctor or nurse		
	Female	Male	Total	Female	Male	Total
Site	%	%	%	%	%	%
New York City, NY	9.4	7.0	8.4	2.8	1.9	2.5
Orange County, FL	11.2	4.9	8.1	3.1	1.2	2.2
Palm Beach County, FL	8.8	7.9	8.5	2.9	3.6	3.3
Philadelphia, PA	13.0	8.8	11.2	3.7	3.2	3.6
San Bernardino, CA	11.5	6.6	9.2	3.2	1.7	2.5
San Diego, CA	11.2	6.9	9.1	3.2	2.7	3.0
San Francisco, CA	8.1	9.7	9.4	3.0	4.4	3.8
Seattle, WA	6.5	8.0	7.3	2.4	3.0	2.7
Median	11.2	8.0	9.2	3.1	3.4	3.4
Range	6.5–16.0	4.1–16.7	6.0–15.8	2.1–5.6	0.3–5.6	1.6–5.6

—Not available.
Note: Attempts during the 12 months before the survey.

SOURCE: Adapted from "Table 26. Percentage of High School Students Who Attempted Suicide and Whose Suicide Attempt Resulted in an Injury, Poisoning, or Overdose That Had to Be Treated by a Doctor or Nurse, by Sex—Selected U.S. Sites, Youth Risk Behavior Survey, 2011," in *Youth Risk Behavior Surveillance—United States, 2011, Morbidity and Mortality Weekly Report*, vol. 61, no. 4, June 8, 2012, http://www.cdc.gov/mmwr/pdf/ss/ss6104.pdf (accessed December 28, 2013)

the transition from childhood to adulthood and while we know that is a difficult time for most young people, it is even more difficult when a person has to negotiate the cultural norms of their family with those of the larger society."

Youth suicide is, additionally, more prevalent in rural areas than in urban areas. Cutler, Glaeser, and Norberg point out that, although the period corresponding with the rise in teen suicide rates (1950 to 1990) was characterized by increasing poverty and crime in inner cities, the states that saw the largest increases in youth suicides were Idaho, Montana, New Mexico, South Dakota, and Wyoming. Meanwhile, a number of states whose populations were highly concentrated in troubled inner cities during that time—Delaware, Massachusetts, New Jersey, and New York—saw the smallest increases in the teen suicide rate. Similarly, the proportion of high school students who reported attempting suicide in 2011 was highest in a number of states that were largely rural. (See Table 7.5.) The states with the largest proportion of students who attempted suicide that year were Wyoming (11.3%), Indiana (11%), South Carolina (11%), Kentucky (10.9%), Maryland (10.9%), Georgia (10.8%), North Dakota (10.8%), Texas (10.8%), Louisiana (10.6%), Virginia (10.5%), Arizona (10.3%), and Arkansas (10%).

SUICIDE AMONG LESBIAN, GAY, BISEXUAL, AND TRANSGENDER ADOLESCENTS. Another possible reason for the elevated rate of suicide attempts and deaths among young people is that a significant number of teens find themselves, as newly sexual beings, struggling to come to terms with same-sex attraction. Although the 21st century has witnessed a rapid increase in the levels of public acceptance of gay, lesbian, bisexual, and transgender (LGBT) lifestyles, mainstream attitudes have not changed at the same rate in all parts of the United States. Additionally, even for adolescents in more obviously tolerant cities and towns, self-acceptance, peer-group acceptance, and parental acceptance can represent forbidding obstacles.

The CDC notes in "Lesbian, Gay, Bisexual and Transgender Health: Youth" (March 25, 2014, http://www.cdc.gov/lgbthealth/youth.htm) that a 2009 survey of LGBT young people aged 13 to 21 years found that 80% had been verbally harassed at school, 40% had been physically harassed at school, 60% felt unsafe at school, and 20% had been physically assaulted at school. The CDC also notes that studies find that, compared with LGBT teens whose parents support and accept them, LGBT teens who experience high levels of rejection from their parents are significantly more likely, as young adults, to suffer from depression, to use illegal drugs, to engage in unprotected sex, and to attempt suicide.

Because mortality data generally do not include information about sexual orientation, it is unclear what proportion of teen suicides might be related to sexuality. However, according to the Suicide Prevention Resource Center, in *Suicide Risk and Prevention for Lesbian, Gay, Bisexual, and Transgender Youth* (2008, http://www.sprc.org/sites/sprc.org/files/library/SPRC_LGBT_Youth.pdf), research indicates that gay and lesbian young people aged 15 to 24 years are between one and a half to three times more likely than their straight counterparts to consider suicide and are one and a half to seven times more likely to attempt suicide.

EUTHANASIA AND PHYSICIAN-ASSISTED SUICIDE

The word *euthanasia*, which is derived from a Greek word meaning "good death," is commonly used to describe situations in which a terminally ill person requests assistance in ending his or her life to prevent further pain and suffering. However, euthanasia has also been used to refer to the practice of killing people without their consent, supposedly for reasons of helping them or improving society. This latter form of the practice is linked in the public imagination with the Nazi regime of Adolf Hitler (1889–1945). The Nazis' version of euthanasia was a bizarre interpretation of an idea espoused by two German professors, the psychiatrist Alfred Hoche (1865–1943) and the jurist Karl Binding (1841–1920), in their 1920 book *Die Freigabe der Vernichtung lebensunwerten Lebens* (*The Permission to Destroy Life Unworthy of Life*). While initially maintaining that it was ethical for physicians to assist in the deaths of those who requested an end to their suffering, the authors later argued that it was also permissible to end the lives of the mentally retarded and the mentally ill. Besides targeting the mentally retarded and mentally ill, the Nazi euthanasia program attempted to wipe out the entire Jewish people, along with other peoples it considered undesirable. Some contemporary opponents of euthanasia fear that a society that allows the practice will embark on a slippery slope leading in the direction of a euthanasia program such as the Nazis'.

In reality, euthanasia has been an accepted part of many societies throughout history, without having led to any such programs of involuntary euthanasia. As mentioned at the outset of this chapter, in ancient Greece and Rome, suicide in cases when the individual had become a burden to himself, his family, or his society was considered a rational act. Moreover, the contemporary movement to legalize euthanasia is strongly rooted in humanist thinking, which prioritizes the autonomy of the individual. Although still unacceptable to many religious traditions that emphasize God's authority to determine matters of life and death, euthanasia is generally motivated by compassion for suffering and ideas maintaining that true liberty includes the freedom to determine the time and manner of one's own death.

The modern euthanasia movement began in England, with the 1935 founding of the Voluntary Euthanasia Society, whose membership included well-known figures such as the playwright George Bernard Shaw (1856–1950), the philosopher Bertrand Russell (1872–1970), and the novelist H. G. Wells (1866–1946). In 1936 the House of Lords (the house of the English Parliament historically composed of aristocratic landowners, officials from the Church of England, and others appointed by the monarch) defeated a bill that would have permitted euthanasia in cases of terminal illness. Nonetheless, it was common knowledge that physicians of the era practiced euthanasia. That same year it was rumored that King George V (1865–1936), who had been seriously ill for several years, was "relieved of his sufferings" by his physician, with the approval of his wife, Queen Mary (1867–1953).

Some people call the act of forgoing medical treatment in the knowledge that death will result as passive euthanasia. This action is relatively uncontroversial and even permitted by many religious traditions, because it is the underlying illness that causes death by running its natural course. Terminally ill individuals in the United States have a right to refuse medical treatment, as do those who are sick but not terminally ill.

Much more controversial in the United States and other parts of the developed world is the practice of active euthanasia, also commonly referred to as physician-assisted suicide. Currently legal (in different forms) in Belgium, Luxembourg, the Netherlands, and Switzerland as well as in the U.S. states of Oregon, Washington, and Vermont, physician-assisted suicide typically involves the hastening of death through the administration of lethal drugs, as requested by the patient or another competent individual who represents the patient's wishes.

DIFFERING VIEWPOINTS ON THE RIGHT TO DIE

Federal Law

The U.S. Constitution does not guarantee the right to choose to die. However, the U.S. Supreme Court recognizes that Americans have a fundamental right to privacy, or what is sometimes called the "right to be left alone." Although the right to privacy is not explicitly mentioned in the Constitution, the Supreme Court has interpreted several amendments as encompassing this right. For example, in *Roe v. Wade* (410 U.S. 113 [1973]), the court ruled that the 14th Amendment protects the right to privacy against state action, specifically a woman's right to abortion. Another example is the landmark Karen Ann Quinlan case, which was based on right-to-privacy rulings by the U.S. Supreme Court. In *In re Quinlan* (70 N.J. 10, 355 A.2d 647 [1976]), the New Jersey Supreme Court held that the right to privacy included the right to refuse unwanted medical treatment and, as a consequence, the right to die (see Chapter 9).

Public Opinion

In "When Is Physician Assisted Suicide or Euthanasia Acceptable?" (*Journal of Medical Ethics*, vol. 29, no. 6, December 2003), Stéphanie Frileux et al. examine the opinion of the general public on euthanasia and physician-assisted suicide. The researchers define these terms as follows: "In physician assisted suicide, the physician provides the patient with the means to end his or her own life. In euthanasia, the physician deliberately and directly intervenes to end the patient's life; this is sometimes called 'active euthanasia' to distinguish it from withholding or withdrawing treatment needed to sustain life." Their study posed the questions: "Should a terminally ill patient be allowed to die? Should the medical profession have the option of helping such a patient to die?" Frileux et al. find that acceptability of euthanasia and physician-assisted suicide by the general public appears to depend on four factors: the level of patient suffering, the extent to which the patient requested death, the age of the patient, and the degree of curability of the illness.

Meanwhile, Lydia Saad of the Gallup Organization finds that Americans' expressed views on the subject of physician-assisted suicide vary widely depending on how pollsters word their questions. In *U.S. Support for Euthanasia Hinges on How It's Described* (May 29, 2013, http://www.gallup.com/poll/162815/support-euthanasia-hinges-described.aspx), Saad reports that, based on polling conducted in May 2013, 70% of Americans expressed support for euthanasia in cases of terminal illness when it is described as allowing physicians to "end the patient's life by some painless means." (See Table 7.6.) When, however, the practice is described as assisting a patient to "commit suicide," only 51% of Americans supported it. Saad notes that another contributing factor in respondents' answers may have been that when posing the question in the first way, without using the word *suicide*, pollsters specified that the patient's family members were involved in the decision. When asking the version of the question that described the practice as suicide, pollsters only mentioned the patient's desires and not his or her family's.

Saad indicates that Gallup's polling using the "suicide" version of the question dates back to 1996 and that the 2013 levels of support for allowing the practice, 51%, were very similar to levels of support in 1996. (See Figure 7.1.) Support stood at 52% in 1996 and then

TABLE 7.6

Support for physician-assisted suicide, by wording of question, 2013

(FORM A) WHEN A PERSON HAS A DISEASE THAT CANNOT BE CURED, DO YOU THINK DOCTORS SHOULD BE ALLOWED BY LAW TO END THE PATIENT'S LIFE BY SOME PAINLESS MEANS IF THE PATIENT AND HIS OR HER FAMILY REQUEST IT?

(FORM B) WHEN A PERSON HAS A DISEASE THAT CANNOT BE CURED AND IS LIVING IN SEVERE PAIN, DO YOU THINK DOCTORS SHOULD OR SHOULD NOT BE ALLOWED BY LAW TO ASSIST THE PATIENT TO COMMIT SUICIDE IF THE PATIENT REQUESTS IT?

	"End the patient's life by some painless means"	"Assist the patient to commit suicide"
	%	%
Should be allowed	70	51
Should not be allowed	27	45
No opinion	3	4

SOURCE: Lydia Saad, "Support for Physician-Assisted Suicide—Two Question Wordings," in *U.S. Support for Euthanasia Hinges on How It's Described*, The Gallup Organization, May 29, 2013, http://www.gallup.com/poll/162815/support-euthanasia-hinges-described.aspx (accessed December 28, 2013).

FIGURE 7.1

Support for physician-assisted "suicide," 1996–2013

WHEN A PERSON HAS A DISEASE THAT CANNOT BE CURED AND IS LIVING IN SEVERE PAIN, DO YOU THINK DOCTORS SHOULD OR SHOULD NOT BE ALLOWED BY LAW TO ASSIST THE PATIENT TO COMMIT SUICIDE IF THE PATIENT REQUEST IT?

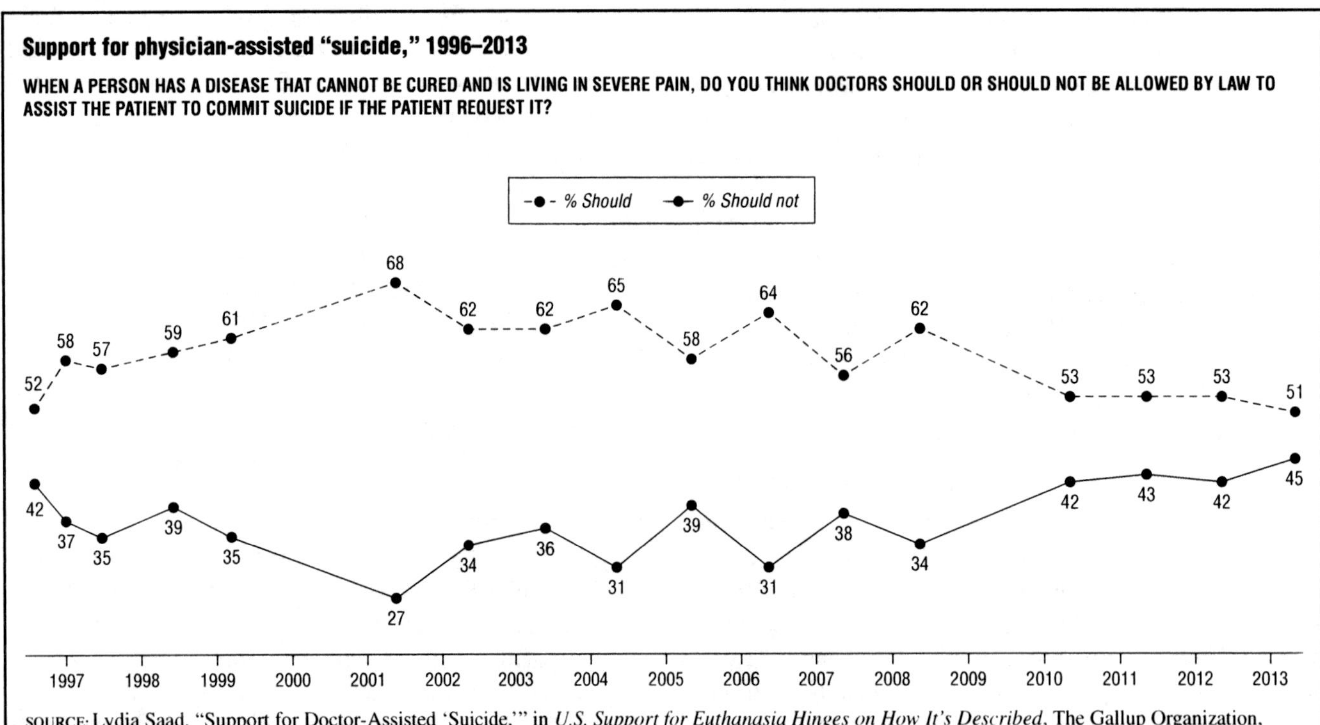

SOURCE: Lydia Saad, "Support for Doctor-Assisted 'Suicide,'" in *U.S. Support for Euthanasia Hinges on How It's Described*, The Gallup Organization, May 29, 2013, http://www.gallup.com/poll/162815/support-euthanasia-hinges-described.aspx (accessed December 28, 2013).

climbed steadily to 68% in 2001, before falling to 53% in 2010. Saad suggests that increasing support during the late 1990s may be largely attributable to the publicity surrounding Jack Kevorkian's (1928–2011) advocacy of physician-assisted suicide. Kevorkian, who was synonymous with the issue during the late 1990s, described euthanasia using the word *suicide*, effectively authorizing that description in the public sphere. He went to prison in 1999, however, and as his arguments and persona faded from public memory, no one with a similarly high profile continued his advocacy. Saad also suggests that increasing political polarization surrounding the issue of physician-assisted suicide in the early years of the new century explains part of the decrease in support for the practice. As Figure 7.2 shows, support among those who identify as Democrats or lean toward the Democratic Party fell by only 11 percentage points, from 71% in 2001 to 60% in 2013, whereas support among those who identify as Republicans or lean toward the Republican Party fell by 23 percentage points, from 64% in 2001 to 41% in 2013.

Finally, Saad notes that support for the practice of euthanasia when it is described as ending the life of a terminal patient by "some painless means" has been relatively steady since 1996. (See Figure 7.3.) Public support for the practice, when described in this way, rose from 37% in 1948 to 65% to a high of 75% in 1996. Between 1996 and 2013 support has remained consistently high, ranging between 64% and 75%.

The Medical Profession

Joris Gielen et al. interviewed 14 physicians and 13 nurses working in palliative care programs to determine what they thought about palliative sedation in end-of-life care and reported their findings in "The Attitudes of Indian Palliative-Care Nurses and Physicians to Pain Control and Palliative Sedation" (*Indian Journal of Palliative Care*, vol. 17, no. 1, January–April 2011). The health care providers all thought that palliative care painkillers were fine to administer, provided that they were titrated (gradually increased to achieve efficacy with the least amount of side effects) to the patient's pain. They thought that such light sedation was useful but disagreed whether deep sedation was acceptable.

In general, physician-assisted suicide is seen as being at odds with the work of doctors and nurses. In 2012 the American College of Physicians officially opposed physician-assisted suicide, reaffirming its statements of opposition from 2001 and 2005. The organization's formal position statement on this topic was published in the sixth edition of *Ethics Manual* (2012, http://www.acponline.org/running_practice/ethics/manual/manual6th.htm). The statement reads:

> The College does not support legalization of physician-assisted suicide or euthanasia. After much consideration, the College concluded that making physician-assisted suicide legal raised serious ethical, clinical, and social concerns and that the practice might undermine patient

FIGURE 7.2

Support for physician-assisted "suicide," by political party affiliation, 2001–13

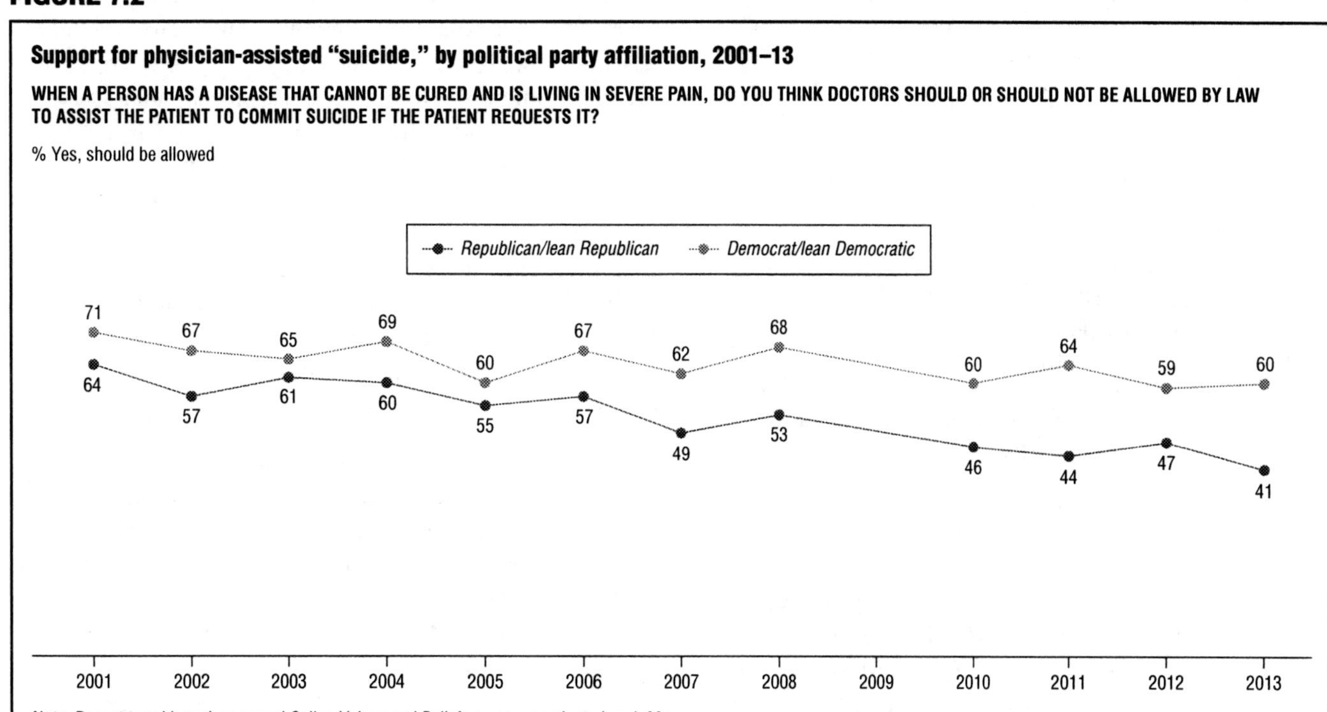

Note: Recent trend based on annual Gallup Values and Beliefs survey, conducted each May.

SOURCE: Lydia Saad, "Party Support for Doctor-Assisted 'Suicide,'" in *U.S. Support for Euthanasia Hinges on How It's Described*, The Gallup Organization, May 29, 2013, http://www.gallup.com/poll/162815/support-euthanasia-hinges-described.aspx (accessed December 28, 2013). Copyright © 2013 Gallup, Inc. All rights reserved. The content is used with permission; however, Gallup retains all rights of republication.

FIGURE 7.3

Support for physician ending a patient's life "by some painless means," 1948–2012

WHEN A PERSON HAS A DISEASE THAT CANNOT BE CURED, DO YOU THINK DOCTORS SHOULD BE ALLOWED BY LAW TO END THE PATIENT'S LIFE BY SOME PAINLESS MEANS IF THE PATIENT AND HIS OR HER FAMILY REQUEST IT?

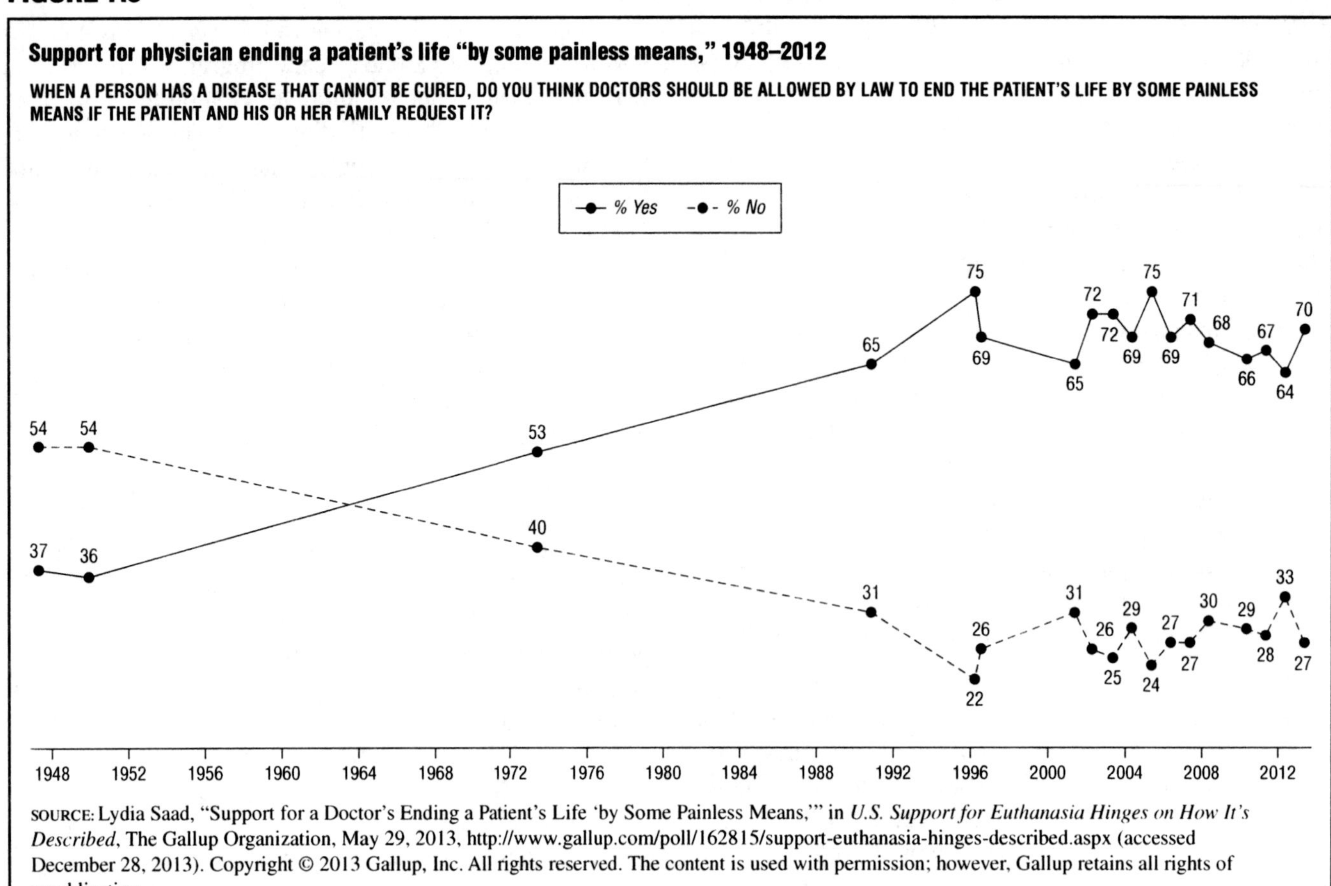

SOURCE: Lydia Saad, "Support for a Doctor's Ending a Patient's Life 'by Some Painless Means,'" in *U.S. Support for Euthanasia Hinges on How It's Described*, The Gallup Organization, May 29, 2013, http://www.gallup.com/poll/162815/support-euthanasia-hinges-described.aspx (accessed December 28, 2013).

> trust; distract from reform in end-of-life care; and be used in vulnerable patients, including those who are poor, are disabled, or are unable to speak for themselves or minority groups who have experienced discrimination. The major emphasis of the College and its members, including those who lawfully participate in the practice, should be ensuring that all persons can count on good care through to the end of life, with prevention or relief of suffering insofar as possible, an unwavering commitment to human dignity and relief of pain and other symptoms, and support for family and friends. Physicians and patients must continue to search together for answers to the problems posed by the difficulties of living with serious illness before death, neither violating the physician's personal and professional values, nor abandoning the patient to struggle alone.

The American Medical Association (AMA) updated its position statements on euthanasia and physician-assisted suicide in 1996. AMA policy "E-2.21 Euthanasia" (https://ssl3.ama-assn.org/apps/ecomm/PolicyFinderForm.pl?site=www.ama-assn.org&uri=/ama1/pub/upload/mm/PolicyFinder/policyfiles/HnE/E-2.21.HTM) states that "permitting physicians to engage in euthanasia would ultimately cause more harm than good. Euthanasia is fundamentally incompatible with the physician's role as healer, would be difficult or impossible to control, and would pose serious societal risks." The organization distinguishes between euthanasia, in which the physician takes an active role in the patient's death, and physician-assisted suicide. In AMA policy "E-2.211 Physician-Assisted Suicide" (June 1996, https://ssl3.ama-assn.org/apps/ecomm/PolicyFinderForm.pl?site=www.ama-assn.org&uri=/ama1/pub/upload/mm/PolicyFinder/policyfiles/HnE/E-2.211.HTM), the organization describes physician-assisted suicide as facilitating the death of a patient "by providing the necessary means and/or information to enable the patient to perform the life-ending act." The organization opposes physician-assisted suicide with language identical to that in its policy statement against euthanasia.

In April 2013 the American Nurses Association released the position statement "Euthanasia, Assisted Suicide, and Aid in Dying" (http://www.nursingworld.org/euthanasiaanddying), updating its 1994 statement prohibiting the practices. The statement reads: "The American Nurses Association (ANA) prohibits nurses' participation in assisted suicide and euthanasia because these acts are in direct violation of *Code of Ethics for Nurses with Interpretive Statements* (ANA, 2001; herein referred to as *The Code*), the ethical traditions and goals of the profession, and its covenant with society. Nurses have an obligation to provide humane, comprehensive, and compassionate care that respects the rights of patients but upholds the standards of the profession in the presence of chronic, debilitating illness and at end-of-life."

LEGAL PHYSICIAN-ASSISTED SUICIDE IN THE UNITED STATES

As of April 2014, Oregon, Washington, and Vermont were the only U.S. states that allowed physician-assisted suicide. In Montana, physician-assisted suicide has been in legal limbo since 2009, when the state supreme court ruled that the practice was legal under Montana law. The state legislature has not, however, formally created laws allowing and regulating the practice. In all three states that currently allow physician-assisted suicide, the option is available only to patients who have been given a prognosis of six months or less to live.

Oregon was the first state to legalize assisted suicide or, as the state and many advocates for the practice call it, "death with dignity." The Oregon Death with Dignity Act (DWDA) was passed in 1994 but was held up by legal challenges until 1997, when it was officially enacted. Oregon created strict limits and procedures for the practice of assisted suicide, intending to address concerns about physicians' roles in the process and about overuse of the procedure. Terminally ill Oregonians with six months or less to live are allowed to request prescriptions for lethal doses of drugs. They then must take the drugs on their own, without the help of a physician. Physicians who write prescriptions for life-ending medication must file paperwork with the state within seven days of doing so. In some cases, psychiatric evaluation is required. Thus, the approval of individual prescriptions is subject to medical review and monitored by the state. Physicians may not take an active role in the actual death, ensuring that the motivation for the act comes from the patient. As part of the Oregon law, detailed data are collected on those who request life-ending medication, and the state issues annual reports describing the extent of its reach and the characteristics of participating patients. These annual data releases indicate that since the law's implementation very few people have actually used it to end their suffering and that it has been used only in the sorts of cases for which it was intended.

The constitutionality of Oregon's law was ultimately decided by the U.S. Supreme Court in 2006, as described in further detail below. Following the Supreme Court's decision that Oregon was acting within its authority in implementing the practice of assisted suicide, voters in the neighboring state of Washington passed their own Death with Dignity Act, modeled closely on Oregon's, in 2008. Facing no serious legal challenges, Washington's law went into effect the following year. Vermont followed suit in 2013, again naming its own law the Death with Dignity Act and using the well-regarded Oregon template. As in Washington, the act met with no serious legal challenges and was implemented soon after being signed by the governor in mid-2013.

Conflict with Federal Law

As mentioned earlier, Oregon's DWDA was kept on hold due to legal challenges for three years after voters passed it in 1994, and in November 1997 a ballot measure to repeal the law was put before voters statewide. Oregonians voted to defeat the measure.

Immediately after this voter reaffirmation of the DWDA, the U.S. Drug Enforcement Administration (DEA) warned Oregon doctors that they could be arrested or have their medical licenses revoked for prescribing lethal doses of drugs. The DEA administrator Thomas A. Constantine (1938–), who was under pressure from some members of Congress, stated that prescribing a drug for suicide would be a violation of the Controlled Substances Act (CSA) of 1970 because assisted suicide was not a "legitimate medical purpose." Janet Reno (1938–), the U.S. attorney general, overruled Constantine in 1998 and decided that that portion of the CSA would not apply to states that legalize assisted suicide. Those opposed to the practice observed that Reno's ruling was inconsistent with other rulings, citing the government's opposite ruling in states that have legalized marijuana for medical use. (Reno maintained that the prescription of marijuana was still illegal, regardless of its medicinal value.)

In response to the DEA decision, Congress moved toward the passage of the Pain Relief Promotion Act. This law would promote the use of federally controlled drugs for the purpose of palliative care but would prevent their use for euthanasia and assisted suicide. In 2000 the U.S. House of Representatives passed the bill, but the U.S. Senate did not. The act never became law.

On November 6, 2001, John D. Ashcroft (1942–), who succeeded Reno as the U.S. attorney general, overturned Reno's 1998 ruling that prohibited the DEA from acting against physicians who administer drugs under the DWDA. Ashcroft said that taking the life of terminally ill patients was not a "legitimate medical purpose" for federally controlled drugs. The Oregon Medical Association and the Washington State Medical Association opposed Ashcroft's ruling. Even physicians who were opposed to assisted suicide expressed concern that the ruling might compromise patient care and that any DEA investigation might discourage physicians from prescribing pain medication to patients in need.

The state of Oregon disagreed so vehemently with Ashcroft's interpretation of the CSA that on November 7, 2001, the attorney general of Oregon filed suit, claiming that Ashcroft was acting unconstitutionally. A November 8, 2001, restraining order allowed the DWDA to remain in effect while the case was tried.

On April 17, 2002, in *State of Oregon and Peter A. Rasmussen et al. v. John Ashcroft* (Civil No. 01-1647-JO), Judge Robert E. Jones (1927–) of the U.S. District Court for the District of Oregon ruled in favor of the DWDA. His decision read, in part:

> State statutes, state medical boards, and state regulations control the practice of medicine. The CSA was never intended, and the [U.S. Department of Justice] and DEA were never authorized, to establish a national medical practice or act as a national medical board. To allow an attorney general—an appointed executive whose tenure depends entirely on whatever administration occupies the White House—to determine the legitimacy of a particular medical practice without a specific congressional grant of such authority would be unprecedented and extraordinary.... Without doubt there is tremendous disagreement among highly respected medical practitioners as to whether assisted suicide or hastened death is a legitimate medical practice, but opponents have been heard and, absent a specific prohibitive federal statute, the Oregon voters have made the legal, albeit controversial, decision that such a practice is legitimate in this sovereign state.

The U.S. Department of Justice appealed the ruling to the U.S. Court of Appeals for the Ninth Circuit in San Francisco. On May 26, 2004, the court stopped Ashcroft's attempts to override the Oregon law. The divided three-judge panel ruled that Ashcroft overstepped his authority when he declared that physicians who prescribe lethal drug doses are in violation of the CSA and when he instructed the DEA to prosecute the physicians. In addition, the court noted that Ashcroft's interpretation of the CSA violated Congress's intent.

The administration of George W. Bush (1946–) appealed the case to the U.S. Supreme Court, and in February 2005 the high court agreed to hear the DWDA challenge. On January 17, 2006, the court ruled in favor of Oregon in *Gonzales v. Oregon* (546 U.S. 243), holding that the CSA "does not allow the Attorney General to prohibit doctors from prescribing regulated drugs for use in physician-assisted suicide under state law permitting the procedure." Justice Anthony M. Kennedy (1936–), writing for the majority, stated that the U.S. attorney general did not have the power to override the Oregon physician-assisted suicide law. Kennedy also added that it should not be the attorney general who determines what is a "legitimate medical purpose" for the administration of drugs, because the job description for the attorney general does not include making health and medical policy.

DWDA Patients and Their Characteristics

Oregon, Washington, and Vermont each collect and release data about those who request prescriptions and die under the auspices of their DWD laws. Oregon's data, as mentioned earlier, have been instrumental in establishing that its DWDA has functioned as designed and not been subject to abuse or unforeseen problems. Washington's 2009 through 2012 data releases have in general reinforced this picture of how such a law functions in practice. As of April 2014, Vermont had not yet released numbers for 2013, the first year during which patients could request life-ending medication under its DWDA.

OREGON. Between 1998, when Oregon's DWDA was implemented, and 2012, prescriptions for life-ending medication were written for 1,050 people, 673 of whom are known to have died from ingesting these medications. (See Figure 7.4.) The number of prescriptions as well as the number of deaths has risen steadily since 1998.

In 2012, 115 Oregonians (out of a population of approximately 3.9 million) requested prescriptions to end their lives, and 77 of these patients' deaths were confirmed as being caused by the prescriptions. (See Figure 7.4 and Figure 7.5.) The gap between the number of prescriptions and the number of deaths accounts for several subsets of patients: those who have not taken their prescriptions by year's end but who go on to do so in the following year; those who choose not to take their life-ending medications and die of other causes; and those who die but whose paperwork has not been received by the state or is incomplete at the time of the data release. Figure 7.5 summarizes the outcomes for those patients who received medication under the DWDA in 2012, including those who received medication in 2011 and those who did not take the medication they were prescribed in 2012.

The median age for those 77 Oregonians who died from ingesting life-ending medication in 2012 was 69, slightly lower than the median age of 71 over the life of the DWDA's implementation. (See Table 7.7.) So far, men and women have been almost equally likely to use life-ending prescriptions under the terms of the DWDA. Among racial and ethnic groups, use of DWDA prescriptions has been confined almost exclusively to white Oregonians, who account for 654 (97.6%) of the total 673 deaths under the program from 1998 to 2012. (Non-Hispanic whites accounted for 77.8% of Oregon's total population in 2012.) DWDA participants in 2012 tended to be well-educated relative to the population at large. Over 80% had either attended (37.7%) or graduated from (42.9%) college, and only two participants (2.6%) had less than a high school diploma. In comparison, in 2012 college graduates accounted for 29.2% of Oregon's population, and 10.8% of the state's population had less than a high school diploma.

As Table 7.7 shows, almost all DWDA participants (97% in 2012 and 90.4% since 1998) were in hospice care prior to requesting life-ending medication. (Hospice care generally begins when a patient's remaining life expectancy is six months or less.) The overwhelming majority of DWDA participants had cancer (75.3% in 2012 and 80.3% since 1998).

FIGURE 7.4

Death with Dignity Act prescription recipients and known deaths, Oregon, 1998–2012

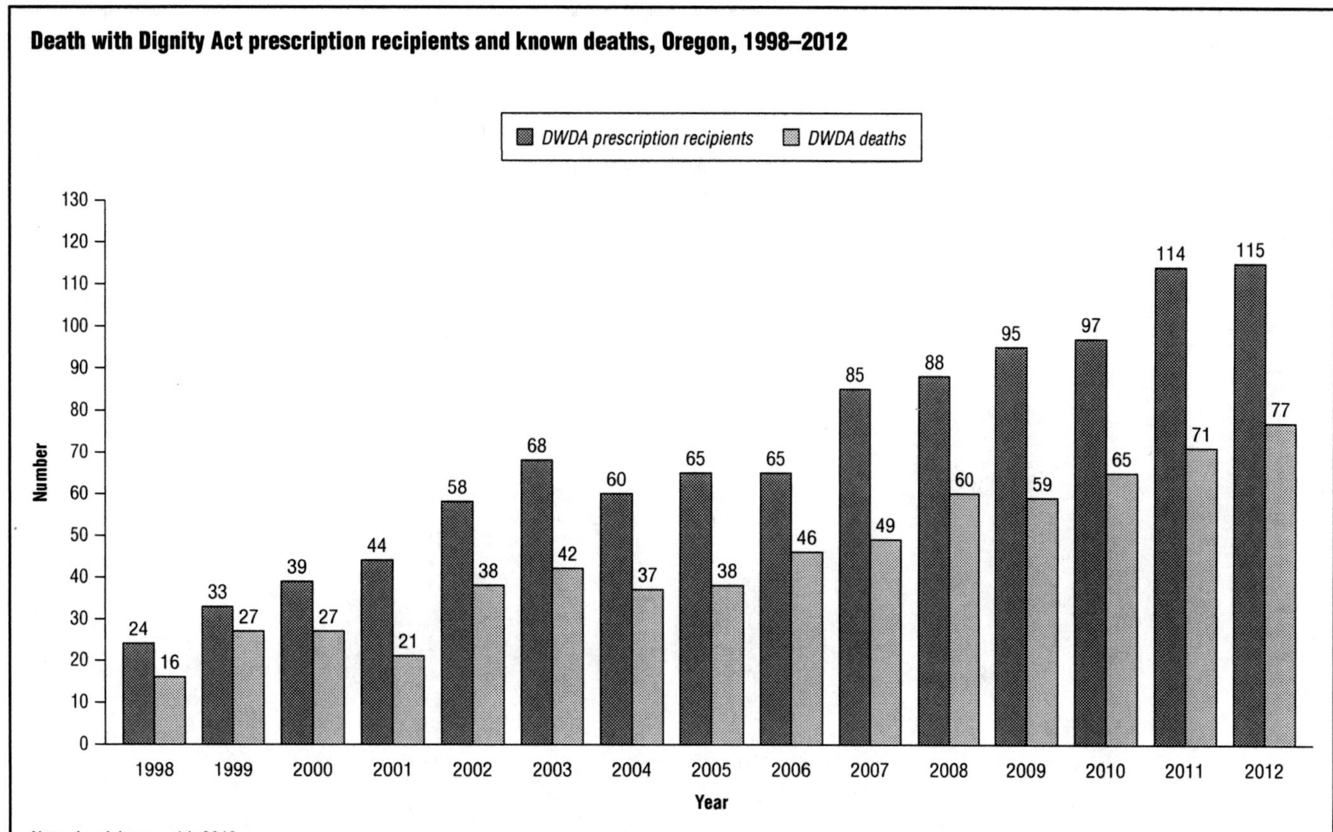

Note: As of January 14, 2013.

SOURCE: "Figure 1. DWDA Prescription Recipients and Deaths, by Year, Oregon, 1998–2012," in *Oregon's Death with Dignity Act–2012*, Oregon Public Health Division, 2013, http://public.health.oregon.gov/ProviderPartnerResources/EvaluationResearch/DeathwithDignityAct/Documents/year15.pdf (accessed December 28, 2013)

FIGURE 7.5

Outcomes for Death with Dignity Act patients who had prescriptions written, Oregon, 2012

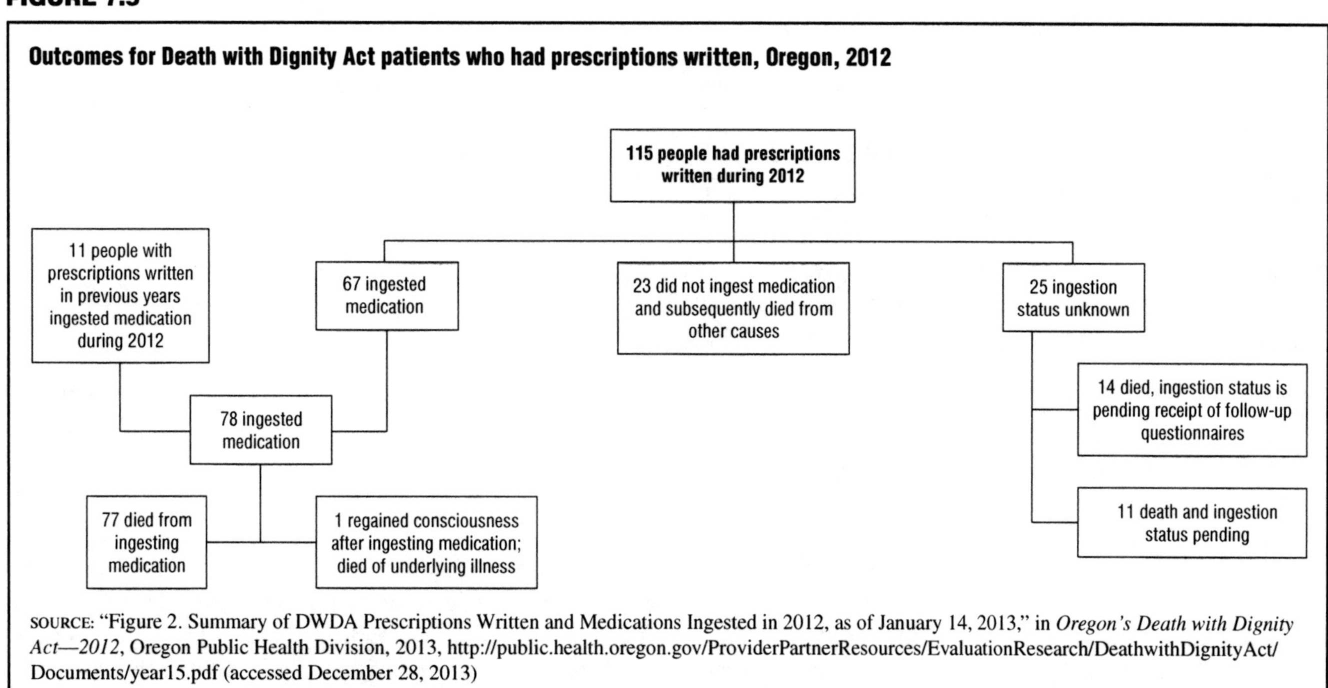

SOURCE: "Figure 2. Summary of DWDA Prescriptions Written and Medications Ingested in 2012, as of January 14, 2013," in *Oregon's Death with Dignity Act—2012*, Oregon Public Health Division, 2013, http://public.health.oregon.gov/ProviderPartnerResources/EvaluationResearch/DeathwithDignityAct/Documents/year15.pdf (accessed December 28, 2013)

TABLE 7.7

Characteristics and end-of-life care of Death with Dignity Act patients who ingested lethal medication and have died, Oregon, 1998–2012

Characteristics	2012 (Population = 77)	1998–2011 (Population = 596)	Total (Population = 673)
Sex	**Population (%)[a]**	**Population (%)[a]**	**Population (%)[a]**
Male (%)	39 (50.6)	308 (51.7)	347 (51.6)
Female (%)	38 (49.4)	288 (48.3)	326 (48.4)
Age			
18–34 (%)	0 (0.0)	6 (1.0)	6 (0.9)
35–44 (%)	1 (1.3)	14 (2.3)	15 (2.2)
45–54 (%)	8 (10.4)	44 (7.4)	52 (7.7)
55–64 (%)	16 (20.8)	123 (20.6)	139 (20.7)
65–74 (%)	23 (29.9)	170 (28.5)	193 (28.7)
75–84 (%)	18 (23.4)	168 (28.2)	186 (27.6)
85+ (%)	11 (14.3)	71 (11.9)	82 (12.2)
Median years (range)	69 (42–96)	71 (25–96)	71 (25–96)
Race			
White (%)	75 (97.4)	579 (97.6)	654 (97.6)
African American (%)	0 (0.0)	1 (0.2)	1 (0.1)
American Indian (%)	0 (0.0)	1 (0.2)	1 (0.1)
Asian (%)	1 (1.3)	7 (1.2)	8 (1.2)
Pacific Islander (%)	0 (0.0)	1 (0.2)	1 (0.1)
Other (%)	0 (0.0)	0 (0.0)	0 (0.0)
Two or more races (%)	0 (0.0)	0 (0.0)	0 (0.0)
Hispanic (%)	1 (1.3)	4 (0.7)	5 (0.7)
Unknown	0	3	3
Marital status			
Married (%)[b]	33 (42.9)	271 (45.7)	304 (45.4)
Widowed (%)	23 (29.9)	134 (22.6)	157 (23.4)
Never married (%)	6 (7.8)	49 (8.3)	55 (8.2)
Divorced (%)	15 (19.5)	139 (23.4)	154 (23.0)
Unknown	0	3	3
Education			
Less than high school (%)	2 (2.6)	40 (6.8)	42 (6.3)
High school graduate (%)	13 (16.9)	139 (23.5)	152 (22.8)
Some college (%)	29 (37.7)	148 (25.0)	177 (26.5)
Baccalaureate or higher (%)	33 (42.9)	264 (44.7)	297 (44.5)
Unknown	0	5	5
Residence			
Metro counties (%)[c]	34 (44.2)	253 (42.7)	287 (42.8)
Coastal counties (%)	4 (5.2)	47 (7.9)	51 (7.6)
Other western counties (%)	37 (48.1)	250 (42.2)	287 (42.8)
East of the Cascades (%)	2 (2.6)	43 (7.3)	45 (6.7)
Unknown	0	3	3
End of life care			
Hospice			
Enrolled (%)[d]	64 (97.0)	522 (89.7)	586 (90.4)
Not enrolled (%)	2 (3.0)	60 (10.3)	62 (9.6)
Unknown	11	14	25
Insurance			
Private (%)[e]	36 (51.4)	382 (66.2)	418 (64.6)
Medicare, Medicaid or other governmental (%)	34 (48.6)	185 (32.1)	219 (33.8)
None (%)	0 (0.0)	10 (1.7)	10 (1.5)
Unknown	7	19	26
Underlying illness			
Malignant neoplasms (%)	58 (75.3)	480 (80.9)	538 (80.3)
Lung and bronchus (%)	14 (18.2)	112 (18.9)	126 (18.8)
Breast (%)	4 (5.2)	52 (8.8)	56 (8.4)
Colon (%)	7 (9.1)	36 (6.1)	43 (6.4)
Pancreas (%)	2 (2.6)	42 (7.1)	44 (6.6)
Prostate (%)	5 (6.5)	26 (4.4)	31 (4.6)
Ovary (%)	2 (2.6)	25 (4.2)	27 (4.0)
Other (%)	24 (31.2)	187 (31.5)	211 (31.5)

Almost all Oregonians who have died under the terms of the DWDA informed their families of their decision (92.2% in 2012 and 94.2% since 1998) and died at home (97.4% in 2012 and 95.1% since 1998). (See Table 7.7.) Almost all 2012 DWDA patients cited the loss of autonomy (93.5%) and the decreasing ability to engage in activities that make life enjoyable (92.2%) as their reasons for choosing to end their life. Slightly fewer (77.9%) cited loss of dignity, and a majority (57.1%) cited the feeling of being a burden on family, friends,

TABLE 7.7

Characteristics and end-of-life care of Death with Dignity Act patients who ingested lethal medication and have died, Oregon, 1998–2012

[CONTINUED]

Characteristics	2012 (Population = 77)	1998–2011 (Population = 596)	Total (Population = 673)
Amyotrophic lateral sclerosis (%)	5 (6.5)	44 (7.4)	49 (7.3)
Chronic lower respiratory disease (%)	2 (2.6)	25 (4.2)	27 (4.0)
Heart disease (%)	2 (2.6)	10 (1.7)	12 (1.8)
HIV/AIDS (%)	1 (1.3)	8 (1.3)	9 (1.3)
Other illnesses (%)[f]	9 (11.7)	26 (4.4)	35 (5.2)
Unknown	0	3	3
DWDA process			
Referred for psychiatric evaluation (%)	2 (2.6)	40 (6.7)	42 (6.2)
Patient informed family of decision (%)[g]	71 (92.2)	493 (94.4)	564 (94.2)
Patient died at			
Home (patient, family or friend) (%)	75 (97.4)	562 (94.8)	637 (95.1)
Long term care, assisted living or foster care facility (%)	2 (2.6)	25 (4.2)	27 (4.0)
Hospital (%)	0 (0.0)	1 (0.2)	1 (0.1)
Other (%)	0 (0.0)	5 (0.8)	5 (0.7)
Unknown	0	3	3
Lethal medication			
Secobarbital (%)	20 (26.0)	374 (62.8)	394 (58.5)
Pentobarbital (%)	57 (74.0)	215 (36.1)	272 (40.4)
Other (%)[h]	0 (0.0)	7 (1.2)	7 (1.0)
End of life concerns[i]	**(Population = 77)**	**(Population = 592)**	**(Population = 669)**
Losing autonomy (%)	72 (93.5)	538 (90.9)	610 (91.2)
Less able to engage in activities making life enjoyable (%)	71 (92.2)	523 (88.3)	594 (88.8)
Loss of dignity (%)[j]	60 (77.9)	386 (82.7)	446 (82.0)
Losing control of bodily functions (%)	27 (35.1)	318 (53.7)	345 (51.6)
Burden on family, friends/caregivers (%)	44 (57.1)	214 (36.1)	258 (38.6)
Inadequate pain control or concern about it (%)	23 (29.9)	134 (22.6)	157 (23.5)
Financial implications of treatment (%)	3 (3.9)	15 (2.5)	18 (2.7)
Health-care provider present[k]	**(Population = 77)**	**(Population = 526)**	**(Population = 603)**
When medication was ingested[l]			
Prescribing physician	8	100	108
Other provider, prescribing physician not present	4	231	235
No provider	1	72	73
Unknown	64	123	187
At time of death			
Prescribing physician (%)	7 (9.1)	89 (17.3)	96 (16.2)
Other provider, prescribing physician not present (%)	4 (5.2)	254 (49.4)	258 (43.7)
No provider (%)	66 (85.7)	171 (33.3)	237 (40.1)
Unknown	0	12	12
Complications[l]	**(Population = 77)**	**(Population = 596)**	**(Population = 673)**
Regurgitated	0	22	22
Seizures	0	0	0
None	11	463	474
Unknown	66	111	177
Other outcomes			
Regained consciousness after ingesting DWDA medications[m]	1	5	6
Timing of DWDA event			
Duration (weeks) of patient-physician relationship[n]			
Median	19	12	12
Range	0–1,640	0–1,905	0–1,905
Number of patients with information available	77	594	671
Number of patients with information unknown	0	2	2
Duration (days) between 1st request and death			
Median	47	46	46
Range	16–388	15–1,009	15–1,009
Number of patients with information available	77	596	673
Number of patients with information unknown	0	0	0
Minutes between ingestion and unconsciousness[k]			
Median	5	5	5
Range	3–15	1–38	1–38
Number of patients with information available	11	462	473
Number of patients with information unknown	66	134	200
Minutes between ingestion and death[k]			
Median	20	25	25
Range (minutes–hours)	10 min–3.5 hrs	1 min–104 hrs	1 min–104 hrs
Number of patients with information available	11	467	478
Number of patients with information unknown	66	129	195

TABLE 7.7

Characteristics and end-of-life care of Death with Dignity Act patients who ingested lethal medication and have died, Oregon, 1998–2012

[CONTINUED]

[a]Unknowns are excluded when calculating percentages.
[b]Includes Oregon Registered Domestic Partnerships.
[c]Clackamas, Multnomah, and Washington counties.
[d]Includes patients that were enrolled in hospice at the time the prescription was written or at time of death.
[e]Private insurance category includes those with private insurance alone or in combination with other insurance.
[f]Includes deaths due to benign and uncertain neoplasms, other respiratory diseases, diseases of the nervous system (including multiple sclerosis, Parkinson's disease and Huntington's disease), musculoskeletal and connective tissue diseases, viral hepatitis, diabetes mellitus, cerebrovascular disease, and alcoholic liver disease.
[g]First recorded beginning in 2001. Since then, 24 patients (4.0%) have chosen not to inform their families, and 11 patients (1.8%) have had no family to inform. There was one unknown case in 2002, two in 2005, and one in 2009.
[h]Other includes combinations of secobarbital, pentobarbital, and/or morphine.
[i]Affirmative answers only ("Don't know" included in negative answers). Categories are not mutually exclusive. Data unavailable for four patients in 2001.
[j]First asked in 2003. Data available for all 77 patients in 2012, 467 patients between 1998–2011, and 544 patients for all years.
[k]The data shown are for 2001–2012 since information about the presence of a health care provider/volunteer, in the absence of the prescribing physician, was first collected in 2001.
[l]A procedure revision was made mid-year in 2010 to standardize reporting on the follow-up questionnaire. The new procedure accepts information about time of death and circumstances surrounding death only when the physician or another health care provider is present at the time of death. This resulted in a larger number of unknowns beginning in 2010.
[m]There have been a total of six patients who regained consciousness after ingesting prescribed lethal medications. These patients are not included in the total number of DWDA deaths. These deaths occurred in 2005 (1 death), 2010 (2 deaths), 2011 (2 deaths) and 2012 (1 death).
[n]Previous reports listed 20 records missing the date care began with the attending physician. Further research with these cases has reduced the number of unknowns.

SOURCE: "Table 1. Characteristics and End-of-Life Care of 673 DWDA Patients Who Have Died from Ingesting a Lethal Dose of Medication as of January 14, 2013, by Year, Oregon, 1998–2012," in *Oregon's Death with Dignity Act—2012*, Oregon Public Health Division, 2013, http://public.health.oregon.gov/ProviderPartnerResources/EvaluationResearch/DeathwithDignityAct/Documents/year15.pdf (accessed December 28, 2013)

and/or caregivers. Loss of control over bodily functions (35.1%), pain (29.9%), and financial concerns (3.9%) were cited by a minority of participants. The proportions of patients citing these reasons have been roughly constant since 1998.

WASHINGTON. Between 2009, when Washington's DWDA was implemented, and 2012, prescriptions for life-ending medication were written for 376 people in the state, and 353 are known to have died from ingesting these medications. (See Figure 7.6.) As in Oregon, the number of prescriptions and the number of deaths rose in each year after the law's passage.

In 2012, 121 Washingtonians (out of a population of 7.9 million) requested prescriptions to end their lives, and 104 of these patients' deaths were confirmed as being caused by the prescriptions. (See Figure 7.6 and Figure 7.7.) The gap between the number of prescriptions and the number of deaths was smaller than in Oregon, but the reasons for the gap are similar. Figure 7.7 summarizes the outcomes for those patients who received medications under Washington's DWDA in 2012.

The demographic characteristics of those who ended their life under Washington's DWDA in 2012 are similar to those who did so in Oregon. Roughly equal numbers of men and women died, and 96% of participants were over the age of 55 years. (See Table 7.8.) Participants were more likely to be non-Hispanic white than in the state at large, and they were more likely to have some advanced education and to have graduated from college.

Of the 104 Washingtonians who died under the terms of the DWDA, 76 had cancer. (See Table 7.8.) Washington DWDA patients' top end-of-life concerns were similar to those of their counterparts in Oregon: 94% cited the loss of autonomy as one of their reasons for choosing to end their life, and 90% cited the decreasing ability to engage in activities that make life enjoyable. (See Table 7.9.) The loss of dignity was a factor for 84% of patients, loss of control over bodily functions was a factor for 56%, and worries about burdening family,

FIGURE 7.6

Death with Dignity Act participants and known deaths, Washington, 2009–12

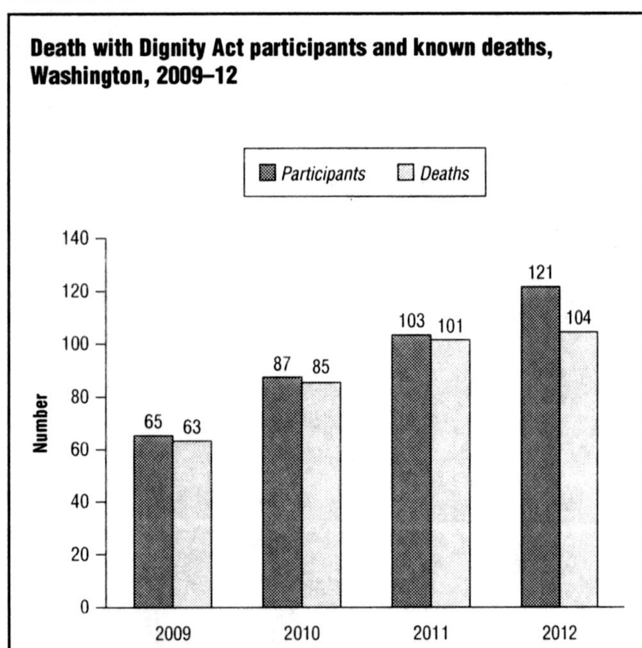

SOURCE: "Figure 2. Number of Death with Dignity Participants and Known Deaths, 2009–2012," in *Washington State Department of Health 2012 Death with Dignity Act Report: Executive Summary*, Washington State Department of Health, 2013, http://www.doh.wa.gov/portals/1/Documents/Pubs/422-109-DeathWithDignityAct2012.pdf (accessed December 28, 2013)

FIGURE 7.7

Outcomes for Death with Dignity Act patients who received medication, Washington, 2012

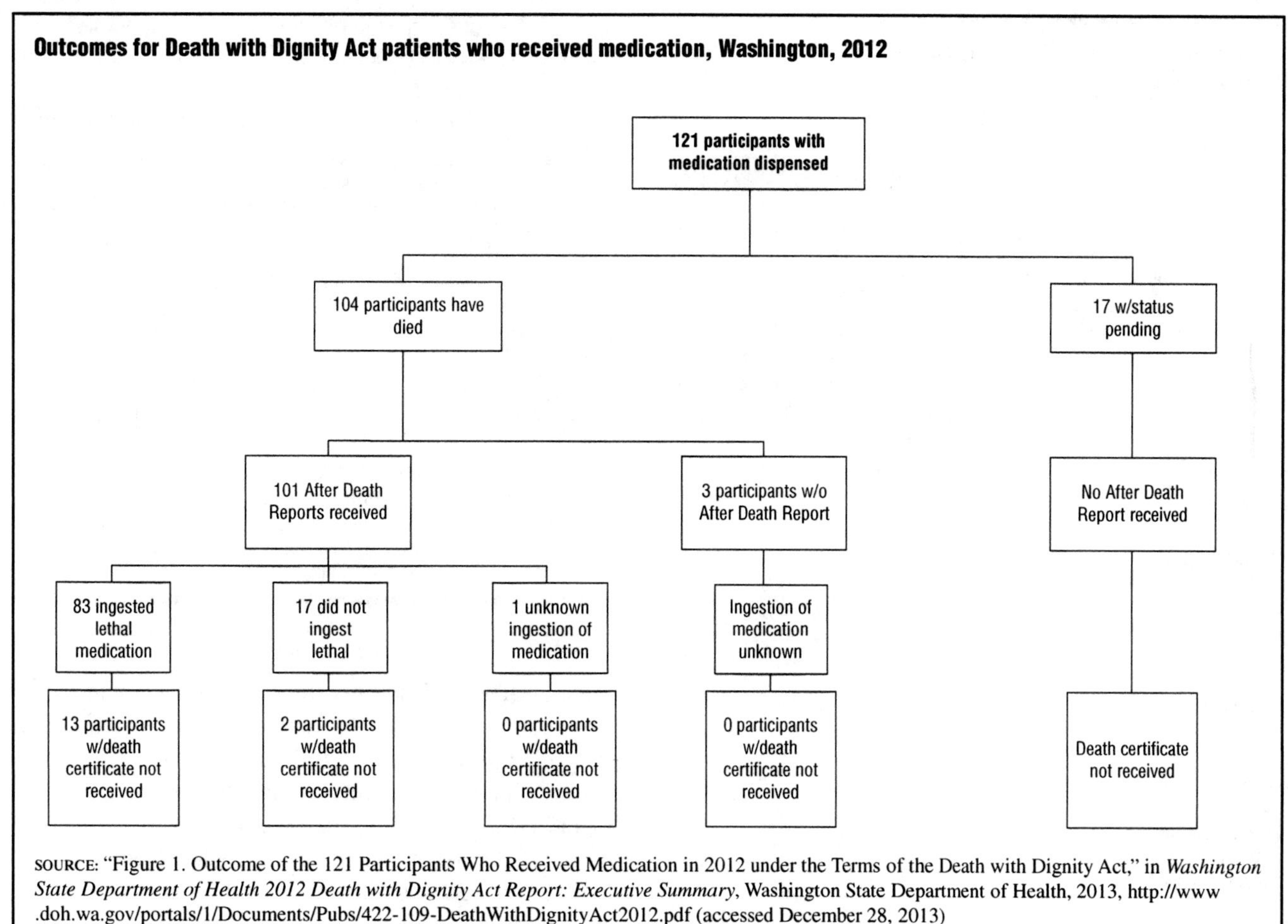

SOURCE: "Figure 1. Outcome of the 121 Participants Who Received Medication in 2012 under the Terms of the Death with Dignity Act," in *Washington State Department of Health 2012 Death with Dignity Act Report: Executive Summary*, Washington State Department of Health, 2013, http://www.doh.wa.gov/portals/1/Documents/Pubs/422-109-DeathWithDignityAct2012.pdf (accessed December 28, 2013)

friends, and/or caregivers were a factor for 63%. Pain (33%) and financial concerns (5%) were, as in Oregon, much less often cited.

EUTHANASIA AND ASSISTED SUICIDE AROUND THE WORLD

Switzerland

Active euthanasia is illegal in Switzerland, but assisted suicide has been legal since 1940, provided that no selfish motive is involved. All assisted suicides in Switzerland must be videotaped and reported to the police. Following the patient's death, the police are contacted so that they can begin an investigation. If no selfish motive is established, the death is recorded and the case is closed.

The Swiss Academy of Medical Sciences has historically been opposed to physicians' involvement in assisted suicide, but a number of private groups of nonphysicians have been established to provide accompaniment and assistance for those who choose to die in the country. The most prominent of these organizations are DIGNITAS and EXIT-Deutsche Schweiz, which also provide a range of end-of-life services and advocate on behalf of right-to-die and end-of-life issues.

The Netherlands

Legal euthanasia in the Netherlands became gradually decriminalized between the 1970s and the early years of the new century. In 1971 a Dutch physician who helped her terminally ill 78-year-old mother die was found guilty of murder but sentenced extremely lightly, to a one-week suspended jail sentence and one-year probation. This sentence encouraged other physicians to come forward, admitting that they had also assisted in patients' suicides. Two years later the Royal Dutch Medical Association announced that, should a physician assist in the death of a terminally ill patient, it was up to the court to decide if the physician's action could be justified by "a conflict of duties." In 1984 the Dutch Supreme Court, ruling on a well-known 1982 case, found the physician involved not guilty of murder. Thereafter, each euthanasia case brought under prosecution was judged on its individual circumstances. Compliance with certain guidelines for performing euthanasia laid down by the Royal Dutch Medical Association and the Dutch courts in 1984 protected physicians from prosecution.

On April 10, 2001, the Dutch Parliament systematized the practice of euthanasia, voting 46–28 in favor of the Termination of Life on Request and Assisted Suicide

TABLE 7.8

Characteristics of Death with Dignity Act participants who have died, Washington, 2011–12

	2012		2011[a]	
	Number	(%)	Number	(%)
Sex[b]				
Male	45	43	49	52
Female	44	42	45	48
Unknown (death certificate not received)	15	15		
Age (years)[b]				
18–44	1	1	3	3
45–54	3	2	9	10
55–64	31	30	22	23
65–74	35	33	27	29
75–84	24	23	19	20
85+	10	10	14	15
Range (min–max)	35–95		41–101	
Race and ethnicity[c]				
Non-Hispanic white	86	83	82	94
Hispanic and/or non-white	3	3	5	6
Unknown (death certificate not received)	15	14		
Marital status[c]				
Married	38	37	40	46
Widowed	12	12	13	15
Divorced	28	27	24	28
Domestic partner	3	3		
Never married	8	8	10	11
Unknown (death certificate not received)	15	13		
Education[c]				
Less than high school	2	2	4	5
High school graduate	13	13	17	20
Some college	23	22	24	28
Baccalaureate or higher	50	48	41	46
Missing	1	1	1	1
Unknown (death certificate not received)	15	14		
Residence[b, d]				
West of the Cascades	94	90	89	95
East of the Cascades	10	10	5	5
Underlying illness[d]				
Cancer	76	73	73	78
Neuro-degenerative disease (incl. ALS[e])	10	10	11	12
Respiratory disease (incl. COPD[f])	10	10	4	4
Heart disease	5	4	4	4
Other illnesses	3	3	2	2
Insurance status[g]				
Private only	22	22	31	34
Medicare or Medicaid only	55	55	36	40
Combination of private and Medicare/Medicaid	12	12	12	13
None	0	0	3	3
Unknown	11	11	9	10

TABLE 7.8

Characteristics of Death with Dignity Act participants who have died, Washington, 2011–12 [CONTINUED]

[a]Data published in 2011 Data and Statistical Report (Vital Statistics Data, Death with Dignity Data).
[b]Data are collected from multiple documents. At time of publication, data are available for all 104 of the participants in 2012 who died.
[c]Data are collected from the Death Certificate. At time of publication, data are available for 89 of the 104 participants in 2012 who died.
[d]Counties west of the Cascades include: Clallam, Clark, Cowlitz, Grays Harbor, Island, Jefferson, King, Kitsap, Lewis, Mason, Pacific, Pierce, San Juan, Skagit, Skamania, Snohomish, Thurston, Wahkiakum, and Whatcom. Counties east of the Cascades include: Adams, Asotin, Benton, Chelan, Columbia, Douglas, Ferry, Franklin, Garfield, Grant, Kittitas, Klickitat, Lincoln, Okanogan, Pend Oreille, Spokane, Stevens, Walla Walla, Whitman, and Yakima.
[e]Amyotrophic Lateral Sclerosis (ALS).
[f]Chronic Obstructive Pulmonary Disease (COPD).
[g]Data are collected from the After Death Reporting form. At the time of publication, data are available for 101 of the 104 participants in 2012 who died.

SOURCE: "Table 2. Characteristics of the Participants of the Death with Dignity Act Who Have Died," in *Washington State Department of Health 2012 Death with Dignity Act Report: Executive Summary*, Washington State Department of Health, 2013, http://www.doh.wa.gov/portals/1/Documents/Pubs/422-109-DeathWithDignityAct2012.pdf (accessed December 28, 2013)

(Review Procedures) Act. Arguments in favor of the bill included public approval ratings of 90%. In May 2001 the results of a Dutch public opinion poll revealed that nearly half of respondents favored making lethal drugs available to older adults who no longer wanted to live.

Belgium

The Belgian Act on Euthanasia passed in 2002, following the passage of the 2001 law in the Netherlands. The Belgian law applies to competent adults who have an incurable illness causing unbearable, constant suffering and to patients in a persistent vegetative state who made their wishes known within the previous five years in front of two witnesses. It allows someone to terminate the life of another at his or her "voluntary, well-considered, and repeated" request, but does not allow physician-assisted suicide. All acts of euthanasia must be reported. Belgium also offers all patients in the country free medication for pain relief in order to ensure that people do not choose to end their life because they cannot afford to alleviate their suffering.

Luxembourg

In February 2008 the Parliament of the Grand Duchy of Luxembourg passed a bill that decriminalized euthanasia. However, Henri Guillaume (1955–), the grand duke of Luxembourg, refused to sign the bill into law. In 2009 his power was curtailed by the parliament, and his signature is no longer required for bills to become law. In April of that year the bill that decriminalized euthanasia officially went into force.

The United Kingdom and Canada

As of April 2014, neither the United Kingdom nor Canada had passed laws allowing for the practice of any form of euthanasia or assisted suicide, but in both countries large majorities of citizens approved of allowing mentally competent people with terminal illnesses to end their life with medical assistance. In both countries, as well, debate and legal actions related to right-to-die issues suggested the possibility of change in the near future.

Parts of the United Kingdom measurably eased their prohibitions on assisted suicide in early 2010, when Keir Starmer (1962–), the director of public prosecutions for the country's Crown Prosecution Service (the legal office responsible for criminal prosecutions in England and

TABLE 7.9

End of life concerns of Death with Dignity Act participants who have died, Washington, 2011–12

	2012		2011[a]	
	Number	(%)	Number	(%)
End of life concerns[b, c]				
Losing autonomy	94	94	79	87
Less able to engage in activities making life enjoyable	90	90	81	89
Loss of dignity	84	84	72	79
Losing control of bodily functions	56	56	52	57
Burden on family, friends/caregivers	63	63	49	54
Inadequate pain control or concern about it	33	33	35	38
Financial implications of treatment	5	5	4	4

[a]Data published in 2011 Data and Statistical Report (Vital Statistics Data, Death with Dignity Data).
[b]Data are collected from the After Death Reporting form. At the time of publication, data are available for 101 of the 104 participants in 2012 who died.
[c]Participants may have selected more than one end of life concern. Thus the totals are greater than 100 percent.

SOURCE: "Table 3. End of Life Concerns of Participants of the Death with Dignity Act Who Have Died," in *Washington State Department of Health 2012 Death with Dignity Act Report: Executive Summary*, Washington State Department of Health, 2013, http://www.doh.wa.gov/portals/1/Documents/Pubs/422-109-DeathWithDignityAct2012.pdf (accessed December 28, 2013)

Wales), announced new guidelines for the prosecution of those who assisted loved ones in ending their life. Although assisting in a suicide carried a possible prison sentence of 14 years in the United Kingdom, the new guidelines suggested that in cases meeting certain conditions—conditions that showed that the act was one of compassion carried out at the clear request of a person with an incurable illness or disability—loved ones who assisted in a suicide would not be prosecuted. Subsequent cases of assisted suicide, some of which occurred in England and Wales and some of which involved loved ones traveling with terminally ill people to commit suicide in Switzerland, have not typically resulted in prosecutions since 2010. Bonnie Gardner notes in "Support for Doctor-Assisted Suicide" (YouGov.co.uk, July 5, 2012), public opinion polls conducted by YouGov find that in 2012, 69% of the population of the United Kingdom supported the legalization of assisted suicide in cases where the patient is terminally ill.

Canada, whose ban on euthanasia and assisted suicide was last affirmed by a Canadian Supreme Court ruling in 1993, saw a reopening of the debate on this in 2011. In that year a daughter who accompanied her terminally ill 89-year-old mother to Switzerland to end her life and a woman suffering from advanced amyotrophic lateral sclerosis (ALS; a degenerative neurologic condition commonly known as Lou Gehrig's disease) filed suit in British Columbia, challenging the Canadian law that made assisted suicide illegal. Represented by the British Columbia Civil Liberties Association (BCCLA), the case made it to the British Columbia Supreme Court (the second-highest court at the provincial level). The court ruled in 2012 that the Criminal Code of Canada violated the rights of the terminally ill, and it granted the ALS patient the right to an assisted suicide. The federal government, however, appealed the ruling, which was subsequently overturned by the British Columbia Court of Appeals. The ALS patient died in 2012 from her underlying illness, but the BCCLA appealed to the Canadian Supreme Court. In January 2014 the high court agreed to hear the case. Adrian Morrow reports in "Majority of Canadians Approve of Assisted Suicide: Poll" (GlobeandMail.com, October 11, 2013) that approximately 70% of Canadians (with variations depending on the wording of the question) approved of legalizing assisted suicide in 2013.

CHAPTER 8
ADVANCE CARE PLANNING

As patients in the United States have come to enjoy more autonomy in their medical decision making, as medical technologies for extending life indefinitely have become common, and as the number of elderly Americans has skyrocketed, advance planning for the medical care that one will receive at the end of life has become increasingly important. The likelihood that a given person might one day be chronically or terminally ill and unable to make decisions about his or her own medical treatments is much higher for people who are alive today than for people in prior generations. Other decisions that need to be made as the end of life approaches involve the circumstances in which patients would like to spend their final weeks and days in the event that an underlying illness has reached its terminal stages.

When a patient's own wishes about such matters are unknown, the responsibility for making decisions falls to loved ones. In many cases, this responsibility is an unwelcome and forbidding one, requiring sons and daughters, for example, to make choices that may or may not correspond with their parents' wishes. This may disrupt the loved ones' attempts to grieve appropriately, and it may add unnecessary guilt to their feelings of loss. Additionally, patients who are incapacitated as they approach the end of life may consign themselves to unnecessary suffering and a diminishment in the quality of their lives if they have not made their wishes known in advance. Artificial nutrition and hydration (ANH) is believed, for example, to cause excess discomfort in those whose bodies are naturally shutting down. Likewise, medical procedures intended to prolong life but that result in only an additional week or month of life may cause so much pain and stress that the additional time may not seem worthwhile.

For those patients who do not want their lives extended regardless of the cost to their comfort and quality of life, advance care planning is particularly crucial. In U.S. hospitals, illness is treated aggressively and life is prolonged at all costs unless doctors and staff are given specific requests indicating otherwise. In the absence of specific requests not to treat all illnesses aggressively, doctors are likely to keep even the oldest and sickest patients alive for as long as possible.

Advance care planning involves thinking through one's preferences about the end of life, ideally in consultation with medical professionals who can provide guidance about what the trajectory of a disease or chronic condition may look like. The most thorough plans for the end of life foresee the maximum number of possible scenarios in which a medical decision might be necessary. Advance directives are also dependent on the individual's religious and ethical beliefs. In thinking through end-of-life options, some people find it helpful to discuss their decisions with spiritual counselors, mental-health professionals, and others.

Once an individual has come to conclusions about how medical decisions should be made on his or her behalf in the event of incapacitation, the resulting wishes must be clearly expressed in legal documents known as advance directives.

ADVANCE DIRECTIVES

Advance directives are legal documents that help protect patients' rights of self-determination (the right to make one's own medical decisions, including the right to accept or refuse treatment). These documents are a person's requests concerning health care should he or she be unable to communicate them when the need arises due to physical or mental disabilities. There are two primary types of advance directives: a living will and a durable power of attorney for health care.

A living will should not be confused with a last will and testament, a legal document detailing how a deceased person's property is to be allocated after his or her death. A living will is, instead, a legal document that states a person's wishes for dealing with life-sustaining medical procedures and other issues associated with end-of-life care. It applies to decisions made while the individual is alive but unable to speak or reason clearly in the moment, due to his or her medical condition. Living wills commonly address the following issues: to what extent life-sustaining treatments and technologies such as ventilators, respirators, and dialysis machines will be used; whether or not cardiopulmonary resuscitation should be used if the heartbeat or breathing stops; whether and to what extent ANH will be supplied; and whether, following death, one's organs and tissues will be donated.

A medical power of attorney (also called a health care proxy, durable power of attorney, or appointment of health care agent) is the other primary type of advance directive. It is a legal document in which one person gives another the legal authority to act or speak on his or her behalf should he or she become debilitated and not able to make decisions. While especially important in end-of-life care, a medical power of attorney can also be useful to those who are not on the point of death but who are temporarily unable to make medical decisions for themselves. Physicians determine when a patient is unable to make decisions, and at the point that the physician's determination has been made, the medical power of attorney goes into effect.

The purposes of these two types of advance directives may seem to overlap because both are attempts to provide ways of making decisions on behalf of the patient once he or she is unable to do so. Legal and medical professionals, however, usually advise individuals to craft both forms of advance directive. A living will might cover all medical decisions that can be foreseen, but medical situations are inherently complicated, and as a situation changes, it may be necessary to have someone present to make decisions under the terms of a medical power of attorney.

The Patient Self-Determination Act

In 1990 Congress enacted the Patient Self-Determination Act (PSDA) as part of the Omnibus Budget Reconciliation Act of 1990. This legislation was intended to "reinforce individuals' constitutional right to determine their final health care."

The PSDA took effect on December 1, 1991. It requires most health care institutions to provide patients, on admission, with a summary of their health care decision-making rights and to ask them if they have an advance directive. Health care institutions must also inform the patient of the facility's policies with respect to honoring advance directives. The PSDA requires health care providers to educate their staff and the community about advance directives. It also prohibits hospital personnel from discriminating against patients based on whether they have an advance directive, and patients are informed that having an advance directive is not a prerequisite to receiving medical care.

Advance Directives and State Law

All 50 states and the District of Columbia have laws recognizing the use of living wills and durable powers of attorney for health care, but the provisions of these laws vary from state to state. Charles P. Sabatino of the American Bar Association conducted an extensive literature review of health care advance planning and published his findings in "The Evolution of Health Care Advance Planning Law and Policy" (*Milbank Quarterly*, vol. 88, no. 2, June 2010). He indicates that in the 30 years since advance health care planning had been available as of 2010, laws from various states had evolved in a heterogeneous manner but with important points of convergence. Sabatino notes that one convergent point is the movement from a "legal transactional approach" to a "communications approach." The latter is evolving into Physician Orders for Life-Sustaining Treatment (POLST), and the communications approach and its evolution toward POLST help translate patients' wishes and desires in end-of-life care into "visible and portable medical orders."

Because of the heterogeneity of state laws regarding advance directives, it is important for individuals to understand their own states' requirements prior to crafting an advance directive. Advance directives that meet one state's guidelines may not be honored by hospitals in another state. The National Hospice and Palliative Care Organization (NHPCO) maintains a database of advance directive forms meeting the legal requirements of all U.S. states. Individuals can access the database at http://www.caringinfo.org/i4a/pages/index.cfm?pageid=3289.

Since the 1980s the Uniform Law Commission (also known as the National Conference of Commissioners on Uniform State Laws), a nonprofit group that advocates for consistency among the laws of individual states in the United States, has urged state legislatures to adopt uniform laws regarding patient autonomy, advance directives, and medical decision making. In 1993 the organization created a law called the Uniform Health-Care Decisions Act (UHCDA; http://www.uniformlaws.org/ActSummary.aspx?title=Health-Care%20Decisions%20Act), intended to serve as a model for state legislative bills. Endorsed by the American Bar Association and adopted by a number of states since first being introduced, the UHCDA remains one of the best standardized approaches to advance directives and other issues, in the opinion of many legal experts. The act includes a model advance directive, reprinted here as Table 8.1.

TABLE 8.1

Advance health-care directive

Optional Form

The following form may, but need not, be used to create an advance health-care directive. The other sections of this [Act] govern the effect of this or any other writing used to create an advance health-care directive. An individual may complete or modify all or any part of the following form:

ADVANCE HEALTH-CARE DIRECTIVE

Explanation

You have the right to give instructions about your own health care. You also have the right to name someone else to make health-care decisions for you. This form lets you do either or both of these things. It also lets you express your wishes regarding donation of organs and the designation of your primary physician. If you use this form, you may complete or modify all or any part of it. You are free to use a different form.

Part 1 of this form is a power of attorney for health care. Part 1 lets you name another individual as agent to make health-care decisions for you if you become incapable of making your own decisions or if you want someone else to make those decisions for you now even though you are still capable. You may also name an alternate agent to act for you if your first choice is not willing, able, or reasonably available to make decisions for you. Unless related to you, your agent may not be an owner, operator, or employee of [a residential long-term health-care institution] at which you are receiving care.

Unless the form you sign limits the authority of your agent, your agent may make all health-care decisions for you. This form has a place for you to limit the authority of your agent. You need not limit the authority of your agent if you wish to rely on your agent for all health-care decisions that may have to be made. If you choose not to limit the authority of your agent, your agent will have the right to:

(a) consent or refuse consent to any care, treatment, service, or procedure to maintain, diagnose, or otherwise affect a physical or mental condition;
(b) select or discharge health-care providers and institution;
(c) approve or disapprove diagnostic tests, surgical procedures, programs of medication, and orders not to resuscitate; and
(d) direct the provision, withholding, or withdrawal of artificial nutrition and hydration and all other forms of health care.

Part 2 of this form lets you give specific instructions about any aspect of your health care. Choices are provided for you to express your wishes regarding the provision, withholding, or withdrawal of treatment to keep you alive, including the provision of artificial nutrition and hydration, as well as the provision of pain relief. Space is also provided for you to add to the choices you have made or for you to write out any additional wishes.

Part 3 of this form lets you express an intention to donate your bodily organs and tissues following your death.

Part 4 of this form lets you designate a physician to have primary responsibility for your health care.

After completing this form, sign and date the form at the end. It is recommended but not required that you request two other individuals to sign as witnesses. Give a copy of the signed and completed form to your physician, to any other health-care providers you may have, to any health-care institution at which you are receiving care, and to any health-care agents you have named. You should talk to the person you have named as agent to make sure that he or she understands your wishes and is willing to take the responsibility.

You have the right to revoke this advance health-care directive or replace this form at any time.

* * * * * * * * *

PART 1

POWER OF ATTORNEY FOR HEALTH CARE

1. DESIGNATION OF AGENT: I designate the following individual as my agent to make health-care decisions for me:

____

(name of individual you choose as agent)

____

(address) (city) (state) (zip code)

____

(home phone) (work phone)

OPTIONAL: If I revoke my agent's authority or if my agent is not willing, able, or reasonably available to make a health-care decision for me, I designate as my first alternate agent:

____

(name of individual you choose as first alternate agent)

____

(address) (city) (state) (zip code)

____

(home phone) (work phone)

OPTIONAL: If I revoke the authority of my agent and first alternate agent or if neither is willing, able, or reasonably available to make a health-care decision for me, I designate as my second alternate agent:

____

(name of individual you choose as first alternate agent)

____

(address) (city) (state) (zip code)

____

(home phone) (work phone)

(Add additional sheets if needed.)

Another commonly used template for advance directives, called "Five Wishes," was developed in Florida by the nonprofit organization Aging with Dignity. The document probes legal and medical issues as well as spiritual and emotional ones. It even outlines small details, such as requests for favorite music to be played and poems to be read, and provides space for individuals to record their wishes for funeral arrangements. Free of legal and medical jargon, the "Five Wishes" form is comparatively easy to complete. As of early 2014, "Five Wishes" met

TABLE 8.1

Advance health-care directive [CONTINUED]

2. AGENT'S AUTHORITY: My agent is authorized to make all health-care decisions for me, including decisions to provide, withhold, or withdraw artificial nutrition and hydration and other forms of health care to keep me alive, except as I state here:

____

____

____

3. WHEN AGENT'S AUTHORITY BECOMES EFFECTIVE: My agent's authority becomes effective when my primary physician determines that I am unable to make my own health-care decisions unless I mark the following box. If I mark this box [ ], my agent's authority to make health-care decisions for me takes effect immediately.

4. AGENT'S OBLIGATION: My agent shall make health-care decisions for me in accordance with this power of attorney for health care, any instructions I give in Part 2 of this form, and my other wishes to the extent known to my agent. To the extent my wishes are unknown, my agent shall make health-care decisions for me in accordance with what my agent determines to be in my best interest. In determining my best interest, my agent shall consider my personal values to the extent known to my agent.

NOMINATION OF GUARDIAN: If a guardian of my person needs to be appointed for me by a court, I nominate the agent designated in this form. If that agent is not willing, able, or reasonably available to act as guardian, I nominate the alternate agents whom I have named, in the order designated.

PART 2

INSTRUCTIONS FOR HEALTH CARE

If you are satisfied to allow your agent to determine what is best for you in making end-of-life decisions, you need not fill out this part of the form. If you do fill out this part of the form, you may strike any wording you do not want.

6. END-OF-LIFE DECISIONS: I direct that my health-care providers and others involved in my care provide, withhold, or withdraw treatment in accordance with the choice I have marked below:

[ ] (a) Choice Not To Prolong Life
I do not want my life to be prolonged if (i) I have an incurable and irreversible condition that will result in my death within a relatively short time, (ii) I become unconscious and, to a reasonable degree of medical certainty, I will not regain consciousness, or (iii) the likely risks and burdens of treatment would outweigh the expected benefits, OR

[ ] (b) Choice To Prolong Life
I want my life to be prolonged as long as possible within the limits of generally accepted health-care standards.

7. ARTIFICIAL NUTRITION AND HYDRATION: Artificial nutrition and hydration must be provided, withheld, or withdrawn in accordance with the choice I have made in paragraph (6) unless I mark the following box. If I mark this box [ ], artificial nutrition and hydration must be provided regardless of my condition and regardless of the choice I have made in paragraph (6).

8. RELIEF FROM PAIN: Except as I state in the following space, I direct that treatment for alleviation of pain or discomfort be provided at all times, even if it hastens my death:

____

____

9. OTHER WISHES: (If you do not agree with any of the optional choices above and wish to write your own, or if you wish to add to the instructions you have given above, you may do so here.) I direct that:

____

____

(Add additional sheets if needed.)

PART 3

DONATION OF ORGANS AT DEATH (OPTIONAL)

10. Upon my death (mark applicable box)

[ ] (a) I give any needed organs, tissues, or parts, OR
[ ] (b) I give the following organs, tissues, or parts only

____

[ ] (c) My gift is for the following purposes (strike any of the following you do not want)

(i) Transplant
(ii) Therapy
(iii) Research
(iv) Education

living will or advance directive criteria in 42 states and the District of Columbia. It did not meet advance directive criteria in eight states: Alabama, Indiana, Kansas, New Hampshire, Ohio, Oregon, Texas, and Utah. Other forms were necessary in these states, although the "Five Wishes" document could still serve as a guide for family and physicians and could be attached to the state's required form. The "Five Wishes" form can be filled out online (or a blank form can be printed) at https://fivewishesonline.agingwithdignity.org/.

TABLE 8.1

Advance health-care directive [CONTINUED]

PART 4

PRIMARY PHYSICIAN (OPTIONAL)

11. I designate the following physician as my primary physician:

(name of physician)

(address) (city) (state) (zip code)

(phone)

OPTIONAL: If the physician I have designated above is not willing, able, or reasonably available to act as my primary physician, I designate the following physician as my primary physician:

(name of physician)

(address) (city) (state) (zip code)

(phone)

* * * * * * * * * *

EFFECT OF COPY: A copy of this form has the same effect as the original.

12. SIGNATURES: Sign and date the form here:

(date) (sign your name)

(address) (print name)

(city) (state)

Optional SIGNATURES OF WITNESSES:

(First witness)	(Second witness)
(print name)	(print name)
(address)	(address)
(city) (state)	(city) (state)
(signature of witness)	(signature of witness)
(date)	(date)

SOURCE: "Advance Health-Care Directive," in *Patient Self-Determination Act: Providers Offer Information on Advance Directives but Effectiveness Uncertain,* U.S. General Accounting Office, August 1995, http://www.gao.gov/archive/1995/he95135.pdf (accessed January 28, 2014)

PRO-LIFE ALTERNATIVE TO LIVING WILLS. The National Right to Life Committee opposes active and passive euthanasia and seeks to define all life as equally worthy of preservation. In the interest of promoting its viewpoint, the organization offers an alternative to standard living wills. Called the "Will to Live" (http://www.nrlc.org/medethics/willtolive/), it does not consider ANH as forms of medical treatment but as basic necessities for the preservation of life.

In the Absence of a Durable Power of Attorney for Health Care

Physicians usually involve family members in medical decisions when the patient has not designated a proxy or surrogate in advance. Many states have surrogate consent laws for this purpose. Some have laws that designate the order in which family members may assume the role of surrogate decision maker. For example, the spouse may be the prime surrogate, followed by an adult child, then the patient's parent, and so on.

Most states specify a decision-making standard for surrogates: either a substituted judgment standard, a best interests standard, or a combination of the two. A substituted judgment standard requires the surrogate to do what the patient would do in the situation were the patient competent. A best interests standard requires the surrogate to weigh health care options for the patient and then decide what is in the patient's best interest.

The Importance of Communicating Wishes

The completion of an advance directive should be the start of an ongoing discussion among the individual, family members, and the family doctor about end-of-life health care. Discussions about one's advance directive do not have to be limited to treatment preferences and medical circumstances. Sometimes knowing things such as the patient's religious beliefs and values can be important for the proxy when speaking for the patient's interests. The Institute for Ethics at the University of New Mexico has devised a values history form (http://hsc.unm.edu/ethics/docs/Values_History.pdf) to help people examine their attitudes about issues related to illness, health care, and dying. It may serve as a valuable tool to guide discussions between the patient and the proxy, as well as among family members.

When preparing an advance directive, it is vitally important for the family and proxy to have a thorough understanding of the patient's desires for end-of-life care. Even when a patient has a living will calling for no "heroic measures," the family's demands may carry more weight with physicians. If a dying person's family demands continued medical intervention, it is likely that the hospital or doctor will comply, absent unambiguous and widely known evidence of the patient's wishes, rather than risk a lawsuit. To ensure that one's wishes are carried out at the end of life, then, one must supplement an advance directive with effective communication.

Advance Directives and the Cost of End-of-Life Care

In "Regional Variation in the Association between Advance Directives and End-of-Life Medicare Expenditures" (*Journal of the American Medical Association*, vol. 306, no. 13, October 5, 2011), Lauren Hersch Nicholas et al. of the University of Michigan seek to determine if there is a connection between advance directives and Medicare costs for end-of-life care. The researchers find that there is a variability of Medicare costs nationally in end-of-life care and that there are some regions of the country in which end-of-life care costs much more than in other regions. These are the regions in which there appears to be a connection between end-of-life care costs and advance directives.

By using a variety of statistical methods, Nicholas et al. note that "advance directives are associated with important differences in treatment during the last six months of life for patients who live in areas of high medical expenditures but not in other regions." The researchers also indicate, "This suggests that the clinical effect of advance directives is critically dependent on the context in which a patient receives care. Advance directives may be especially important for ensuring treatment consistent with patients' preferences for those who prefer less aggressive treatment at the end of life but are patients in systems characterized by high intensity of treatment." What Nicholas et al. mean is that Medicare payments might go down in areas of the country in which high-intensity care is given at the end of life. Many people in their advance directives indicate whether they want certain high-intensity care.

The Prevalence of Advance Directives

The Centers for Disease Control and Prevention (CDC) notes in *Advance Care Planning: Ensuring Your Wishes Are Known and Honored if You Are Unable to Speak for Yourself* (2012, http://www.cdc.gov/aging/pdf/advanced-care-planning-critical-issue-brief.pdf) that polling organizations and other surveyors routinely find that most people would prefer to die at home rather than in a hospital, nursing home, or other facility. Nevertheless, a majority of people die in medical facilities each year. Only about one-third of adults have an advance directive, according to the CDC. The prevalence of advance directives is low even among the severely or terminally ill, less than half of whom have legal documents in their medical files to guide their end-of-life treatment. The CDC further notes that even when patients have advance directives, their doctors are usually unaware of this fact.

There are a number of explanations for the low prevalence of advance directives in the United States. One of the leading explanations is that a lack of clarity surrounds the process for crafting an advance directive and communicating with a physician about it. The differences in state laws, together with the fact that the process varies from hospital to hospital and physician to physician, make it hard for patients to know the right way to communicate their end-of-life desires. Another key reason for the low utilization of advance directives is the more general unwillingness in American society to consider death honestly. The idea of thinking through the end of one's life and dwelling on circumstances in which one might be near death and unable to speak or make decisions is actively discouraged by some societal norms.

Many Americans also worry that prioritizing palliative care or otherwise expressing wishes about quality of life will come into conflict with doctors' commitment to saving their lives. In reality there is no conflict between the two priorities, as medical ethics demands that a shift from prolongation of life to quality of life would only occur after there was no hope for a meaningful prolongation of life. The areas of confusion and denial surrounding the end of life obscure this reality, however; as a result, most people approve of prioritizing quality of life and comfort in the abstract, but when faced with concrete scenarios involving their own lives, they are less certain.

FIGURE 8.1

Percentage of home health care patients, nursing home residents, and discharged hospice care patients with any advanced directive, 2004 and 2007

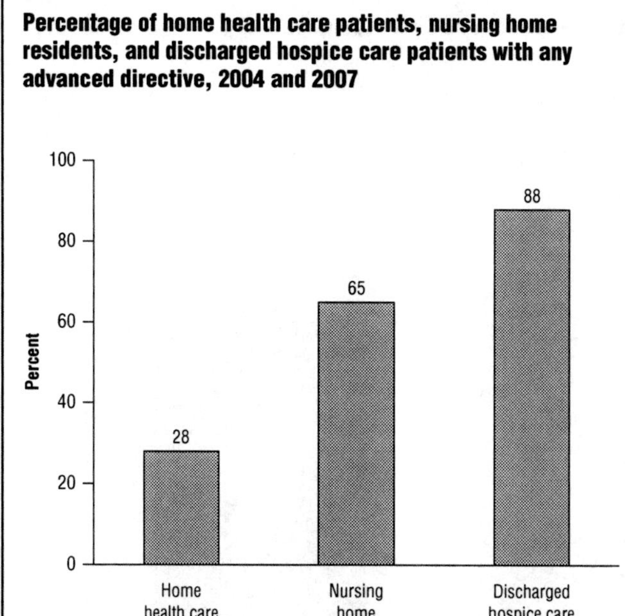

SOURCE: Adrienne L. Jones, Abigail J. Moss, and Lauren D. Harris-Kojetin, "Figure 1. Percentage of Home Health Care Patients, Nursing Home Residents, and Discharged Hospice Care Patients with Any Advance Directive: United States, 2004 and 2007," in "Use of Advance Directives in Long-term Care Populations," *NCHS Data Brief*, no. 54, Centers for Disease Control and Prevention, National Center for Health Care Statistics, January 2011, http://www.cdc.gov/nchs/data/databriefs/db54.pdf (accessed January 27, 2014)

The low prevalence of advance directives is, finally, partly a function of cultural attitudes. A number of surveys have found that African American and Hispanic patients are more likely than non-Hispanic white patients to prioritize life-extending interventions, which are the norm in U.S. hospitals in the absence of advance directives. These groups are, accordingly, less likely to craft advance directives stating a preference for other approaches to treatment.

In *Use of Advance Directives in Long-Term Care Populations* (January 2011, http://www.cdc.gov/nchs/data/databriefs/db54.pdf), which provided the most recent available national data on the prevalence of advance directives as of early 2014, Adrienne L. Jones, Abigail J. Moss, and Lauren D. Harris-Kojetin of the National Center for Health Statistics describe the prevalence of advance care planning in three populations whose need for advance care planning is generally seen to be more acute than that of other subgroups: people receiving home health care, people receiving hospice care, and people residing in nursing homes. Based on a survey of nursing home patients conducted in 2004 and surveys of home health and hospice patients conducted in 2007, the authors find that 28% of home health patients had advance directives. (See Figure 8.1.) Advance directives were more prevalent among residents of nursing homes (65%) and discharged hospice patients (88%; patients can be discharged from hospice either due to death or due to the determination that, contrary to previous diagnoses, they have more than six months to live).

These variations are logical, in the authors' view, given that among the three populations, those receiving home health care can generally expect to live the longest and thus to put off making decisions about their end-of-life care. Residents of nursing homes have in many cases seen a progression of their diseases and conditions beyond the point at which they can be adequately cared for in the home, and hospice patients are typically in the final six months of life.

As would be expected, the rates of advance directive prevalence varied by age within each of the three populations. (See Figure 8.2.) In each group, those under the age of 65 years were the least likely to have completed an advance directive, whereas those aged 85 years and older were the most likely to have completed an advance directive. The least variation by age was among hospice patients: 81% of those under the age of 65 years had advance directives, compared with 93% of those aged 85 years and older. Cultural factors may be more determinative of the prevalence of advance care directives than age, as Figure 8.3 suggests. African Americans in home health care or nursing homes were approximately half as likely as their white counterparts to have completed advance directives. In hospice care, however, where all patients understand that death is imminent, the gap between African American and white patients with advance directives narrowed considerably.

The most common type of advance directive among the three populations surveyed by Jones, Moss, and Harris-Kojetin was a do-not-resuscitate order, typically considered only one of numerous elements a living will comprises. (See Figure 8.4.) The second most-common type of advance directive among the three populations surveyed was a living will. (See Figure 8.5.) A comparison of Figure 8.4 and Figure 8.5 shows that a much smaller percentage of nursing home residents and hospice patients had living wills than do-not-resuscitate orders, whereas home health care patients were more likely to have a living will than a do-not-resuscitate order.

FIGURE 8.2

Percentage of home health care patients, nursing home residents, and discharged hospice care patients with any advanced directive, by age, 2004 and 2007

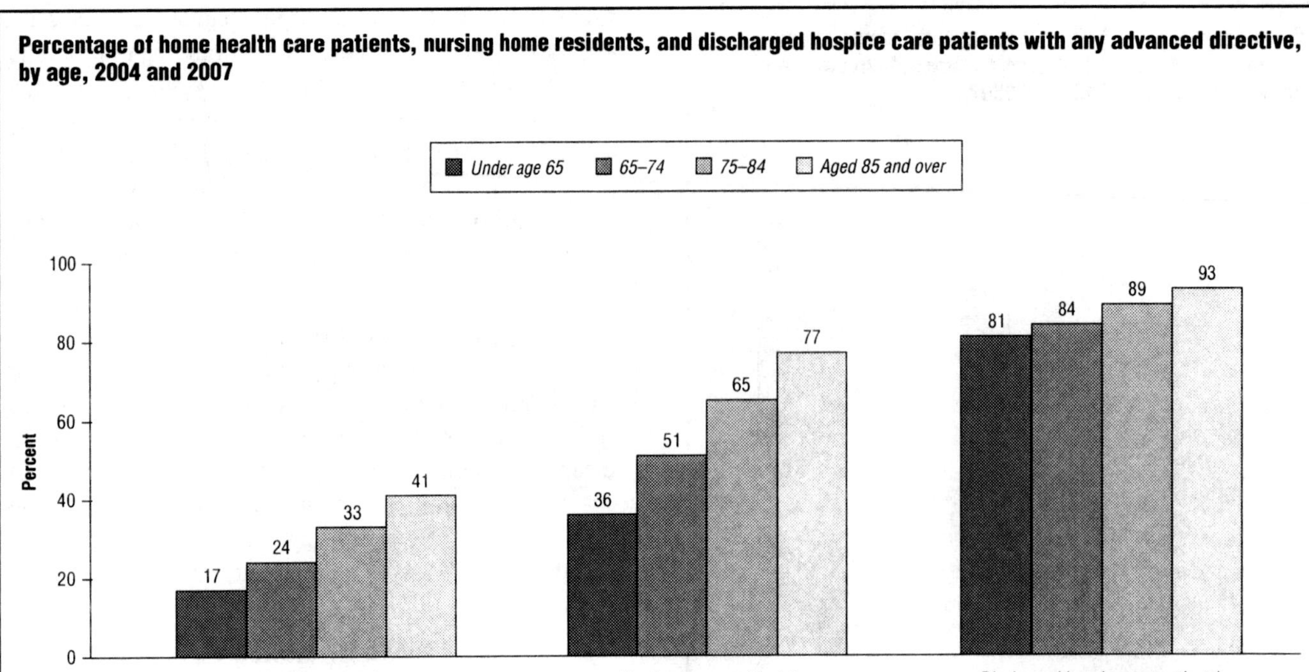

[a]Age at interview.
[b]Age at discharge.

SOURCE: Adrienne L. Jones, Abigail J. Moss, and Lauren D. Harris-Kojetin, "Figure 2. Percentage of Home Health Care Patients, Nursing Home Residents, and Discharged Hospice Care Patients with Any Advance Directive, by Age: United States, 2004 and 2007," in "Use of Advance Directives in Long-term Care Populations," *NCHS Data Brief*, no. 54, Centers for Disease Control and Prevention, National Center for Health Care Statistics, January 2011, http://www.cdc.gov/nchs/data/databriefs/db54.pdf (accessed January 27, 2014)

FIGURE 8.3

Percentage of home health care patients, nursing home residents, and discharged hospice care patients with any advanced directive, by race, 2004 and 2007

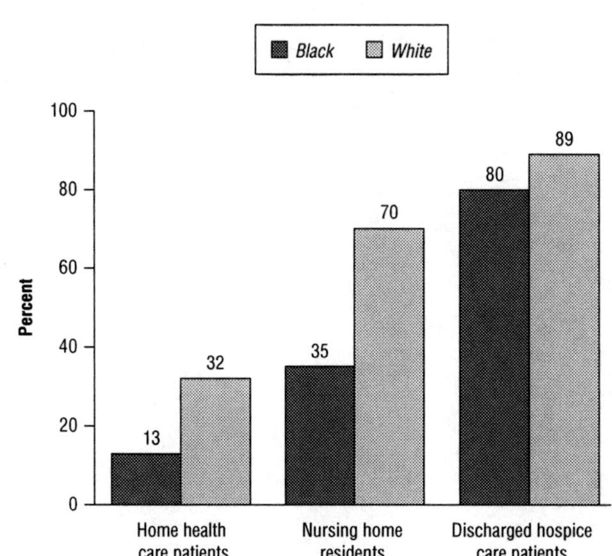

SOURCE: Adrienne L. Jones, Abigail J. Moss, and Lauren D. Harris-Kojetin, "Figure 3. Percentage of Home Health Care Patients, Nursing Home Residents, and Discharged Hospice Care Patients with Any Advance Directive, by Race: United States, 2004 and 2007," in "Use of Advance Directives in Long-term Care Populations," *NCHS Data Brief*, no. 54, Centers for Disease Control and Prevention, National Center for Health Care Statistics, January 2011, http://www.cdc.gov/nchs/data/databriefs/db54.pdf (accessed January 27, 2014)

FIGURE 8.4

Percentage of home health care patients, nursing home residents, and discharged hospice care patients with a do not resuscitate order, by age, 2004 and 2007

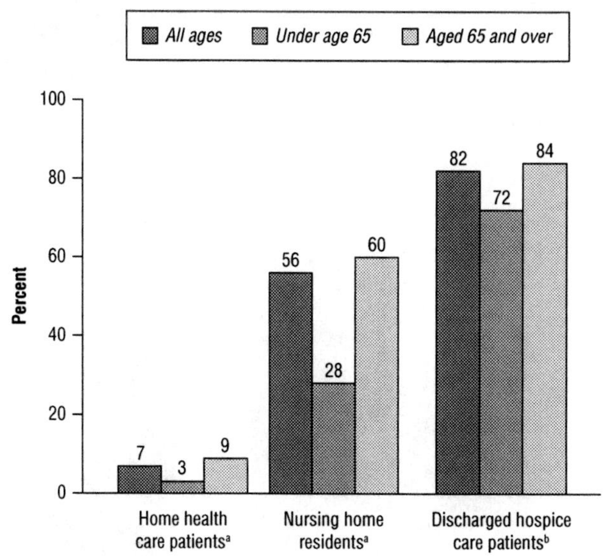

[a]Age at interview.
[b]Age at discharge.

SOURCE: Adrienne L. Jones, Abigail J. Moss, and Lauren D. Harris-Kojetin, "Figure 5. Percentage of Home Health Care Patients, Nursing Home Residents, and Discharged Hospice Care Patients with a Do Not Resuscitate Order, by Age: United States, 2004 and 2007," in "Use of Advance Directives in Long-term Care Populations," *NCHS Data Brief*, no. 54, Centers for Disease Control and Prevention, National Center for Health Care Statistics, January 2011, http://www.cdc.gov/nchs/data/databriefs/db54.pdf (accessed January 27, 2014)

FIGURE 8.5

Percentage of home health care patients, nursing home residents, and discharged hospice care patients with a living will, by age, 2004 and 2007

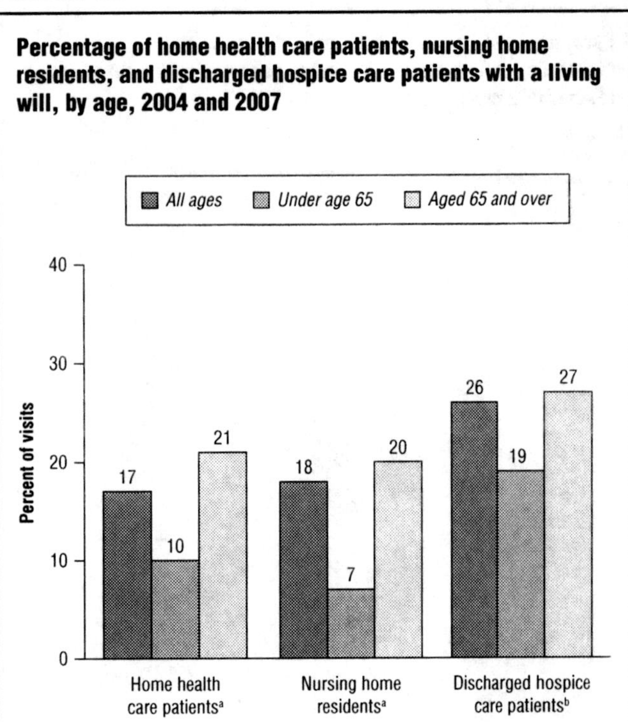

[a]Age at interview.
[b]Age at discharge.

SOURCE: Adrienne L. Jones, Abigail J. Moss, and Lauren D. Harris-Kojetin, "Figure 4. Percentage of Home Health Care Patients, Nursing Home Residents, and Discharged Hospice Care Patients with a Living Will, by Age: United States, 2004 and 2007," in "Use of Advance Directives in Long-term Care Populations," *NCHS Data Brief*, no. 54, Centers for Disease Control and Prevention, National Center for Health Care Statistics, January 2011, http://www.cdc.gov/nchs/data/databriefs/db54.pdf (accessed January 27, 2014)

CHAPTER 9
COURTS AND THE END OF LIFE

The Ad Hoc Committee of the Harvard Medical School's redefinition of death, in 1968, as brain death rather than the cessation of circulation and respiration, was an early attempt to clarify the new physiological and ethical issues raised by advances in medical technology. Such issues were not settled with the redefinition of death, however, as the foregoing chapters have made clear.

There are many patients near the end of life whose bodies cannot function but who are nevertheless not legally brain dead, and many of these people can be kept alive through artificial respiration and artificial nutrition and hydration (ANH) for months or even years. Debate frequently arises in cases when such patients can be kept alive but are in a permanent vegetative state (PVS) with no hope for recovery. Should they be kept alive for decades even though they will never be fully conscious again? Who is entitled to make such decisions?

Debate also arises in situations when patients are conscious but are able to remain alive only with the help of a ventilator and ANH. Should such people be allowed to end their own lives? What role should doctors and hospitals play in such situations? What if such people are not mentally competent to make such decisions? Decisions about these and other complex life and death situations have frequently ended up in state and federal courts, and the resulting decisions have gradually accumulated into the evolving body of law that now governs end-of-life issues.

THE RIGHT TO PRIVACY: KAREN ANN QUINLAN

The landmark case of Karen Ann Quinlan (1954–1985) was the first to deal with the dilemma of withdrawing life-sustaining treatment from a patient who was not terminally ill but who was not really "alive." The decision to terminate life support, which was once a private matter between the patient's family and doctor, became an issue to be decided by the courts. The New Jersey Supreme Court ruling on this case became the precedent for nearly all right-to-die cases nationwide.

In 1975, 21-year-old Karen Ann Quinlan suffered cardiopulmonary arrest after ingesting a combination of alcohol and drugs. She subsequently went into a PVS. Fred Plum (1924–2010), a world-renowned neurologist who had coined the term *persistent vegetative state*, described her as no longer having any cognitive function but retaining the capacity to maintain the vegetative parts of neurological function. She grimaced, made chewing movements, uttered sounds, and maintained a normal blood pressure, but she was entirely unaware of anyone or anything. The medical opinion was that Quinlan had some brain stem function, but that it could not support breathing. She had been on a respirator since her admission to the hospital.

Quinlan's parents asked that her respirator be removed and that she be allowed to die. Quinlan's doctor refused, claiming that his patient did not meet the Harvard Criteria for brain death. Joseph Quinlan (1925–1996), Quinlan's father, went to court to seek appointment as his daughter's guardian (because she was of legal age) and to gain the power to authorize "the discontinuance of all extraordinary medical procedures now allegedly sustaining Karen's vital processes." The court refused to grant him guardianship over his daughter and denied his petition to have Quinlan's respirator turned off.

First and Eighth Amendments Are Irrelevant to the Case

Joseph Quinlan subsequently appealed to the New Jersey Supreme Court. He requested, as a parent, to have Quinlan's life support removed based on the U.S. Constitution's First Amendment (the right to religious freedom). In *In re Quinlan* (70 N.J. 10, 355 A.2d 647 [1976]), the court rejected his request. It also indicated that the Eighth Amendment (protection against cruel and unusual punishment) did not apply to Quinlan's case, explaining that this amendment applied to protection from excessive criminal punishment. The court considered Quinlan's cruel and unusual circumstances not punishment inflicted by the law or state, but the result of "an accident of fate and nature."

The Right to Privacy

The New Jersey Supreme Court, however, stated that an individual's right to privacy was most relevant to the case. Although the Constitution does not expressly indicate a right to privacy, U.S. Supreme Court rulings in past cases had not only recognized this right but had also determined that some areas of the right to privacy are guaranteed by the Constitution. The New Jersey Supreme Court ruled that "Karen's right of privacy may be asserted in her behalf, in this respect, by her guardian and family under the particular circumstances presented by this record," and further noted, "We have no doubt ... that if Karen were herself miraculously lucid for an interval (not altering the existing prognosis of the condition to which she would soon return) and perceptive of her irreversible condition, she could effectively decide upon discontinuance of the life-support apparatus, even if it meant the prospect of natural death."

The State's Interest

Balanced against Quinlan's constitutional right to privacy was the state's interest in preserving life. Judge Richard J. Hughes (1909–1992) of the New Jersey Supreme Court noted that in many cases the court had ordered medical treatment continued because the minimal bodily invasion (usually blood transfusion) resulted in recovery. He indicated that in Quinlan's case bodily invasion was far greater than minimal, consisting of 24-hour nursing care, antibiotics, respirator, catheter, and feeding tube. Judge Hughes further noted, "We think that the State's interest ... weakens and the individual's right to privacy grows as the degree of bodily invasion increases and the prognosis dims. Ultimately there comes a point at which the individual's rights overcome the State's interest."

Prevailing Medical Standards and Practices

Quinlan's physicians had refused to remove the respirator because they did not want to violate the prevailing medical standards and practices. Although Quinlan's physicians assured the court that the possibility of lawsuits and criminal sanctions did not influence their decision in this specific case, the court believed that the threat of legal ramifications strongly influenced the existing medical standards and practices of health care providers.

The court also observed that life-prolongation advances had rendered the existing medical standards ambiguous, leaving doctors in a quandary. Moreover, modern devices used for prolonging life, such as respirators, had confused the issue of "ordinary" and "extraordinary" measures. Therefore, the court suggested that respirators could be considered "ordinary" care for a curable patient, but "extraordinary" care for irreversibly unconscious patients.

The court also suggested that hospitals should form ethics committees to assist physicians with difficult cases such as Quinlan's. These committees would be similar to a multi-judge panel exploring different solutions to an appeal. The committees would not only diffuse professional responsibility but would also eliminate any possibly unscrupulous motives of physicians or families. The justices considered the court's intervention on medical decisions an infringement on the physicians' field of competence.

The state had promised to prosecute anyone who terminated Quinlan's life support because such an act would constitute homicide. The New Jersey Supreme Court, however, rejected this consequence because the resulting death would be from natural causes.

After Quinlan's Respirator Was Removed

In March 1976 the New Jersey Supreme Court ruled that, if the hospital ethics committee agreed that Quinlan would not recover from irreversible coma, her respirator could be removed. Furthermore, all parties involved would be legally immune from criminal and civil prosecution. After Quinlan's respirator was removed, however, she continued to breathe on her own and remained in a PVS until she died of multiple infections in 1985.

Some people wondered why the Quinlans did not request permission to discontinue Karen's ANH. In *Karen Ann: The Quinlans Tell Their Story* (1977), the Quinlans state that they had moral problems with depriving their daughter of food and antibiotics.

SUBSTITUTED JUDGMENT

Superintendent of Belchertown State School et al. v. Joseph Saikewicz

Joseph Saikewicz was a mentally incompetent resident of the Belchertown State School of the Massachusetts Department of Mental Health. In April 1976 Saikewicz was diagnosed with acute myeloblastic monocytic leukemia (cancer of the blood). He was 67 years old but had the mental age of about two years and eight months. The superintendent of the mental institution petitioned the court for a guardian ad litem (a temporary guardian for the duration of the trial). The court-appointed guardian recommended that it would be in the patient's best interests that he not undergo chemotherapy.

In May 1976 the probate judge ordered nontreatment of the disease based in part on findings of medical experts, who indicated that chemotherapy might produce remission of leukemia in 30% to 50% of the cases. If remission occurred, it would last between two and 13 months. Chemotherapy, however, would make Saikewicz suffer adverse side effects that he would not understand. Without chemotherapy, the patient might live for several weeks or months, but would die without the pain or discomfort associated with chemotherapy.

Saikewicz died on September 4, 1976, from pneumonia, a complication of the leukemia. Nevertheless, his case, *Superintendent of Belchertown State School et al. v. Joseph Saikewicz* (Mass., 370 N.E.2d 417 [1977]), was heard by the Massachusetts Supreme Court to establish a precedent on the question of substituted judgment (letting another entity, such as a court, ethics committee, surrogate, or guardian, determine what the patient would do in the situation were the patient competent).

The court agreed that extraordinary measures should not be used if the patient will not recover from the disease. The court also ruled that a person has a right to the preservation of his or her bodily integrity and can refuse medical invasion. The Massachusetts Supreme Court turned to *In re Quinlan* for support of its right of privacy argument.

THE RIGHTS OF AN INCOMPETENT PATIENT. Once the right to refuse treatment had been established, the court declared that everyone, including an incompetent person, has the right of choice. Referring to *Quinlan*, the court recommended that the patient not receive the treatment most people with leukemia would choose. (Unlike some later courts, the *Quinlan* court accepted the premise that a vegetative patient would not want to remain "alive.") The *Saikewicz* court believed that the "substituted judgment" standard would best preserve respect for the integrity and autonomy of the patient. In other words, the decision maker (in this case, the court) would put itself in Saikewicz's position and make the treatment decision the patient most likely would make were he competent. The court believed Saikewicz would have refused treatment.

In evaluating the role of the hospital and the guardian in the decision-making process, the *Saikewicz* court rejected the *Quinlan* court's recommendation that an ethics committee should be the source of the decision. The court instead concluded that the judicial branch of government was the proper venue.

Charles S. Soper, as Director of Newark Developmental Center et al. v. Dorothy Storar

John Storar, a 52-year-old mentally retarded man with a mental age of about 18 months, was diagnosed with terminal cancer in 1980. His mother, Dorothy Storar, petitioned the court to discontinue blood transfusions that were delaying her son's death, which would probably occur within three to six months.

At the time of the hearing, Storar required two units of blood about every one to two weeks. He found the transfusions disagreeable and had to be given a sedative before the procedure. He also had to be restrained during the transfusions. Storar's physician reported that after the transfusions, however, Storar had more energy and was able to resume most of his normal activities. Without the blood transfusions there would be insufficient oxygen in his blood, causing his heart to beat faster and his respiratory rate to increase, impeding normal activities.

The probate court granted Dorothy Storar the right to terminate the treatments, but the order was stayed and treatment continued pending an appeal to the New York Appellate Division (or appellate court). Storar died before the case, *Charles S. Soper, as Director of Newark Developmental Center et al. v. Dorothy Storar* (N.Y., 420 N.E.2d 64 [1981]), could be heard, rendering the decision moot, but because the issue was considered to be of public importance, the appellate court proceeded to hear the case.

The appellate court agreed with the probate court that a guardian can make medical decisions for an incompetent patient. Nevertheless, the parent/guardian "may not deprive a child of life-saving treatment." In this case there were two threats to Storar's life: the incurable cancer and the loss of blood that could be remedied with transfusions. Because the transfusions did not, in the eyes of the majority opinion written by Judge Sol Wachtler (1930–), cause much pain, the appellate court overturned the probate court's ruling.

Dissenting from this determination, Judge Hugh R. Jones (1914–2001) believed the treatments did not serve Storar's best interests. They did not relieve his pain and, in fact, caused him additional pain. Because the blood transfusions would not cure his cancer, they could be considered extraordinary treatments. Finally, Judge Jones reasoned that Storar's mother had cared for him for a long time and knew best how he felt, and therefore the court should respect her decision.

COMPETENT PATIENTS' WISHES

Michael J. Satz etc. v. Abe Perlmutter

Not all the cases of patients seeking to terminate life support concern incompetent people. Abe Perlmutter, aged 73, was suffering from amyotrophic lateral sclerosis (ALS; a degenerative neurologic condition commonly known as Lou Gehrig's disease). ALS is always fatal after prolonged physical degeneration, but it does not affect mental function.

Perlmutter's 1978 request to have his respirator removed was approved by the Circuit Court of Broward County, Florida. At a bedside hearing, the court questioned whether the patient truly understood the consequences of his request. Perlmutter told the judge that if the respirator were removed, "It can't be worse than what I'm going through now."

The state appealed the case before the Florida District Court of Appeals (appellate court), citing the state's duty to preserve life and to prevent the unlawful killing of a human being. The state also noted the hospital's and the doctors' fear of criminal prosecution and civil liability. In *Michael J. Satz, State Attorney for Broward County, Florida v. Abe Perlmutter* (Fla. App., 362 So.2d, 160 [1978]), the appellate court concluded that Perlmutter's right to refuse treatment overrode the state's interests and found in Perlmutter's favor.

THE STATE'S INTERESTS. An individual's right to refuse medical treatment is generally honored as long as it is consistent with the state's interests, which include:

- Interest in the preservation of life
- Need to protect innocent third parties
- Duty to prevent suicide
- Requirement that it help maintain the ethical integrity of medical practice

In the *Perlmutter* case, the Florida District Court of Appeals found that the preservation of life is an important goal, but not when the disease is incurable and causes the patient to suffer. The need to protect innocent third parties refers to cases in which a parent refuses treatment for him- or herself and a third party suffers, such as the abandonment of a minor child when the parent dies. Perlmutter's children were all adults and Perlmutter was not committing suicide. Were it not for the respirator, he would be dead; therefore, disconnecting it would not cause his death but would result in the disease running its natural course. Finally, the court turned to *Quinlan* and *Saikewicz* to support its finding that there are times when medical ethics dictates that a dying person needs comfort more than treatment. The court concluded:

> Abe Perlmutter should be allowed to make his choice to die with dignity.... It is all very convenient to insist on continuing Mr. Perlmutter's life so that there can be no question of foul play, no resulting civil liability and no possible trespass on medical ethics. However, it is quite another matter to do so at the patient's sole expense and against his competent will, thus inflicting never-ending physical torture on his body until the inevitable, but artificially suspended, moment of death. Such a course of conduct invades the patient's constitutional right of privacy, removes his freedom of choice and invades his right to self-determine.

The state again appealed the case, this time to the Supreme Court of Florida, which, in *Michael J. Satz etc. v. Abe Perlmutter* (Fla., 379 So.2d 359 [1980]), supported the decision by the Florida District Court of Appeals. Shortly after this ruling, Perlmutter's respirator was disconnected, and he died of his disease on October 6, 1978.

THE SUBJECTIVE, LIMITED-OBJECTIVE, AND PURE-OBJECTIVE TESTS

In the Matter of Claire C. Conroy

Claire Conroy was an 84-year-old nursing-home patient suffering from "serious and irreversible mental and physical impairments with a limited life expectancy." In March 1984 her nephew (her guardian and only living relative) petitioned the Superior Court of Essex County, New Jersey, to remove her nasogastric feeding tube (a tube running from her nose into her stomach). Conroy's court-appointed guardian ad litem opposed the petition. The superior court approved the nephew's request, and the guardian ad litem appealed. Conroy died with the nasogastric tube in place while the appeal was pending. Nonetheless, the appellate court chose to hear the case *In the Matter of Claire C. Conroy* (486 A.2d 1209 [N.J. 1985]). The court reasoned that this was an important case and that its ruling could influence future cases with comparable circumstances.

Conroy suffered from heart disease, hypertension, and diabetes. She also had a gangrenous leg, bedsores, and an eye problem that required irrigation. She lacked bowel control, could not speak, and had a limited swallowing ability. In the appeals trial one medical expert testified that Conroy, although awake, was seriously demented. Another doctor testified that "although she was confused and unaware, 'she responds somehow.'"

Neither expert was sure if Conroy could feel pain, although she had moaned when subjected to painful stimuli. They agreed, however, that if the nasogastric tube were removed, Conroy would die a painful death.

Conroy's nephew testified that his aunt would never have wanted to be maintained in this manner. She feared doctors and had avoided them all her life. Because she was Roman Catholic, a priest was brought in to testify. In his judgment the removal of the tube would be ethical and moral even though her death might be painful.

The appeals court held that "the right to terminate life-sustaining treatment based on a guardian's judgment was limited to incurable and terminally ill patients who are brain dead, irreversibly comatose, or vegetative, and who would gain no medical benefit from continued treatment."

Furthermore, a guardian's decision did not apply to food withdrawal, which hastens death. The court deemed this active euthanasia, which it did not consider ethically permissible.

THE THREE TESTS. The court proposed three tests to determine if Conroy's feeding tube should have been removed. The subjective test served to clarify what Conroy would have decided about her tube feeding if she were able to do so. The court listed acceptable expressions of intent that should be considered by surrogates or by the court: spoken expressions, living wills, durable power of attorney, oral directives, prior behavior, and religious beliefs.

If the court determines that patients in Conroy's circumstance have not explicitly expressed their wishes, two other "best interests" tests may be used: the limited-objective and the pure-objective tests. The limited-objective test permits discontinuing life-sustaining treatment if medical evidence shows that the patient would reject treatment that would only prolong suffering and that medication would not alleviate pain. Under this test, the court requires the additional evidence from the subjective test. The pure-objective test applies when there is no trustworthy evidence, or any evidence at all, to help guide a decision. The burden imposed on the patient's life by the treatment should outweigh whatever benefit would result from the treatment.

In January 1985 the court concluded that Conroy failed the tests. Her intentions, while perhaps clear enough to help support a limited-objective test (she had shown some evidence of a desire to reject treatment), were not strong enough for the subjective test (clear expressions of her intent). In addition, the information on her possible pain versus benefits of remaining alive was not sufficient for either the limited-objective test (her pain might outweigh her pleasure in life) or the pure-objective test (her pain would be so great it would be inhumane to continue treatment). Had Conroy survived the appellate court's decision, the court would have required her guardian to investigate these matters further before reaching a decision.

Justice Alan B. Handler (1931–), dissenting in part, disagreed with the majority's decision to measure Conroy's "best interests" in terms of the possible pain she could have been experiencing. First, in many cases pain can be controlled through medication. Second, pain levels cannot always be determined, as was shown in Conroy's case. Finally, not all patients decide based on pain. Some fear being dependent on others, especially when their bodily functions deteriorate; others value personal privacy and dignity.

CAN DOCTORS BE HELD LIABLE?

Barber v. Superior Court of the State of California

Historically, physicians have been free from prosecution for terminating life support. A precedent, however, was set in 1983, when two doctors (Neil Barber and Robert Nejdl) were charged with murder and conspiracy to commit murder after agreeing to requests from a patient's family to discontinue life support.

Clarence Herbert suffered cardiorespiratory arrest following surgery. He was revived and placed on a respirator. Three days later his doctors diagnosed him as deeply comatose. The prognosis was that he would likely never recover. The family requested in writing that Herbert's respirator and other life-sustaining equipment be removed. The doctors complied, but Herbert continued to breathe on his own. After two days the family asked the doctors to remove the intravenous tubes that provided nutrition and hydration. The request was honored. From that point until his death, Herbert received care that provided a clean and hygienic environment and allowed for the preservation of his dignity.

A superior court judge ruled that because the doctors' behavior intentionally shortened the patient's life, they had committed murder. However, the court of appeals found in *Barber v. Superior Court of the State of California* (195 Cal.Rptr. 484 [Cal.App. 2 Dist. 1983]) that a patient's right to refuse treatment, and a surrogate's right to refuse treatment for an incompetent, superseded any liability that could be attributed to the physicians.

In ruling that the physicians' compliance with the request of Herbert's family did not constitute murder, the court of appeals stated that "cessation of 'heroic' life support measures is not an affirmative act but rather a withdrawal or omission of further treatment." In addition, ANH also constituted a medical treatment.

WHAT ARE THE HOSPITAL'S RIGHTS?

Patricia E. Brophy v. New England Sinai Hospital

In 1983 Paul E. Brophy Sr. (1937–1986) suffered the rupture of an aneurysm (a part of an artery wall that weakens, causing it to balloon outward with blood) that left him in a PVS. He was neither brain dead nor terminal. He had been a fireman and an emergency medical technician and often expressed the opinion that he never wanted to be kept alive artificially.

Brophy's wife, Patricia Brophy, brought suit when physicians refused to remove or clamp a gastrostomy tube (g-tube) that supplied nutrition and hydration to her husband. The Massachusetts Appeals Court ruled against Brophy, but in *Patricia E. Brophy v. New England Sinai Hospital* (497 N.E.2d 626 [Mass. 1986]) the Massachusetts Supreme Court allowed substituted judgment for a comatose patient who had previously made his intentions clear.

However, the Massachusetts Supreme Court did agree with the Massachusetts Appeals Court ruling that the hospital could not be forced to withhold food and water, which went against the hospital's ethical beliefs.

Consequently, the Massachusetts Supreme Court ordered New England Sinai Hospital to facilitate Brophy's transfer to another facility or to his home, where his wife could carry out his wishes.

In October 1986 Brophy was moved to Emerson Hospital in Concord, Massachusetts. He died there on October 23 after eight days with no food. The official cause of death was pneumonia.

VITALIST DISSENSIONS. In *Brophy*, Justices Joseph Richard Nolan (1925–2013) and Neil L. Lynch (1930–) of the Massachusetts Supreme Court strongly disagreed with the majority opinion to allow withdrawal of nutrition and hydration. Justice Nolan argued that food and water were not medical treatments that could be refused. In his view, food and water are basic human needs, and by permitting the removal of the g-tube, the court gave its stamp of approval to euthanasia and suicide.

Justice Lynch believed the Massachusetts Supreme Court majority had ignored what he considered to be valid findings by the Massachusetts Appeals Court, which found that Brophy's wishes, as expressed in his wife's substituted-judgment decision of withholding food and water, did not concern intrusive medical treatment. Rather, Brophy's decision, if he were competent to make it, was to knowingly terminate his life by declining food and water. This was suicide and the state was, therefore, condoning suicide.

In the Matter of Beverly Requena

Beverly Requena was a competent 55-year-old woman with ALS. She informed St. Clare's/Riverside Medical Center, a Roman Catholic hospital, that when she lost the ability to swallow, she would refuse artificial feeding. The hospital filed a suit to force Requena to leave the hospital, citing its policy against withholding food or fluids from a patient.

Requena was paralyzed from the neck down and was unable to make sounds, although she could form words with her lips. At the time of the hearing, she could not eat but could suck some nutrient liquids through a straw. Her abilities were quickly deteriorating, however.

The court did not question Requena's right to refuse nutrition, nor did the hospital question that right. That was a right that had been upheld in many previous cases. Nevertheless, reasserting its policy of refusing to participate in the withholding or withdrawal of ANH, the hospital offered to help transfer Requena to another facility that was willing to fulfill her wishes.

Requena did not want to transfer to another hospital. In the last 17 months, she had formed a relationship of trust in, and affection for, the staff. She also liked the familiar surroundings. The court found that being forced to leave would upset her emotionally and psychologically. The hospital staff was feeling stress as well. It was fond of Requena and did not want to see her die a presumably painful death from dehydration.

Judge Reginald Stanton ruled in *In the Matter of Beverly Requena* (517 A.2d 869 [N.J.Super.A.D. 1986]) that Requena could not be removed from the hospital without her consent and that the hospital would have to comply with her wishes. He stressed the importance of preserving the personal worth, dignity, and integrity of the patient. The hospital may provide her information about her prognosis and treatment options, but Requena alone had the right to decide what was best for her. Following the ruling, the hospital honored Requena's request and stopped giving her artificial nutrition. She died in December 1987.

Bouvia v. Superior Court of Los Angeles County

In 1983, 26-year-old Elizabeth Bouvia, a mentally competent college-educated quadriplegic with cerebral palsy and painful arthritis, could neither support nor feed herself and required ANH to remain alive. Completely bedridden, Bouvia could not sit up, relied on other people for every need, was in significant pain, was unable to find any enjoyment, and could find no permanent place to live where her needs could be met. Citing the torment that her condition imposed on her, Bouvia wanted to cease being artificially fed and hydrated, and she wanted to be allowed to do so in a California public hospital so that doctors could manage her pain while she died.

The hospital refused Bouvia's request, and she continued to be fed through a nasogastric tube against her will as she pursued her cause in court. A Los Angeles County trial court upheld the hospital's refusal, denying Bouvia's request to be allowed to die in the hospital and mandating that she continue being force-fed rather than be allowed to refuse medical treatment "motivated not by a bona fide exercise of her right of privacy but by a desire to terminate her life." Bouvia's life expectancy, provided that she be fed either mechanically or by hand, was likely to exceed 15 years, and the court reasoned that the state's interest in preserving her life for such a substantial period outweighed Bouvia's right to determine her own fate.

Bouvia appealed the decision, and in 1986 a California appeals court reversed the trial court's ruling. By the time of this second trial, Bouvia had attempted to live in a number of different housing settings and was currently residing in a second public hospital in Los Angeles County. The appellate judges reasoned that Bouvia was exercising the well-established right to refuse medical treatment, that her motives were not relevant, and that removal of the feeding tube would not constitute assisted suicide. The appeals court further argued that the trial court mistakenly emphasized the duration of time Bouvia could expect to live given continued medical intervention, while ignoring her concerns about the quality of her life during that time. The court ordered that the hospital remove Bouvia's feeding tube and prohibited doctors, nurses, and other hospital staff from replacing it or equipping her with any similar device.

Bouvia's feeding tube was removed. She lost weight and suffered from severe discomfort, but she reportedly found the process of starvation too painful to carry out, even with the help of medication. She began accepting nutrition and hydration again, and she lived well beyond even the 15 years of life expectancy predicted at the time of her first court case. Nine years after first requesting the right to die, Bouvia told Beverly Beyette, in "The Reluctant Survivor: Nine Years after Helping Her Fight for the Right to Die, Elizabeth Bouvia's Lawyer and Confidante Killed Himself—Leaving Her Shaken and Living the Life She Dreaded" (LATimes.com, September 13, 1992), "I'm very bitter that in 1983 the decision was against me because in 1983 physically I was strong enough and was ready to go through (with starving herself)." As of 2014, although she avoided media attention, Bouvia was still believed to be alive.

WHAT ARE THE NURSING HOME'S RIGHTS?

In the Matter of Nancy Ellen Jobes

In 1980, 24-year-old Nancy Ellen Jobes was in a car accident. At the time, she was four-and-a-half months pregnant. Doctors who treated her determined that her fetus was dead. During the surgery to remove the fetus, Jobes suffered a loss of oxygen and blood flow to the brain. Never regaining consciousness, she was moved to the Lincoln Park Nursing Home several months later.

The nursing home provided nourishment to Jobes through a jejunostomy tube (j-tube) that was inserted into the jejunum (midsection) of her small intestine. Five years later Jobes's husband, John Jobes, asked the nursing home to stop his wife's artificial feeding. The nursing home refused, citing moral considerations.

The trial court appointed a guardian ad litem, who, after reviewing the case, filed in favor of John Jobes. The nursing home moved to appoint a life advocate (a person who would support retaining the feeding tube), which was turned down by the trial court. The New Jersey Supreme Court heard the case *In the Matter of Nancy Ellen Jobes* (529 A.2d 434 [N.J. 1987]).

DIFFERING INTERPRETATIONS OF PVS. Whether Jobes was in a PVS was hotly debated, which revealed how different medical interpretations of the same patient's condition can produce different conclusions. After John Jobes initiated the suit, his wife was transferred to Cornell Medical Center for four days of observation and testing. The neurologist Fred Plum (1924–2010) and his associate David Levy concluded, after extensive examination and testing, that Jobes was indeed in a PVS and would never recover.

On the contrary, the neurologists Maurice Victor (1920–2001) and Allan Ropper testified for the nursing home. Having examined Jobes for about one-and-a-half hours, Victor reported that although the patient was severely brain damaged, he did not believe she was in a PVS. She had responded to his commands, such as to pick up her head or to stick out her tongue. However, he could not back up his testimony with any written record of his examination.

Ropper had also examined Jobes for about an hour and a half. He testified that some of the patient's motions, such as lifting an arm off the bed, excluded her from his definition of PVS. (His definition of PVS differed from Plum's in that it excluded patients who made reflexive responses to outside stimuli, a definition that would have also excluded Quinlan.) Testimony from the nurses who had cared for Jobes over the past years was also contradictory, with some asserting she smiled or responded to their care and others saying they saw no cognitive responses.

The New Jersey Supreme Court concluded that the neurological experts, especially Plum and Levy, "offered sufficiently clear and convincing evidence to support the trial court's finding that Jobes is in an irreversibly vegetative state." However, the court could find no "clear and convincing" evidence that Jobes, if she were competent, would want the j-tube removed. Jobes's family and friends, including her minister, had testified that in general conversation she had mentioned that she would not want to be kept alive with artificial life-support measures. The court did not accept these past remarks as clear evidence of the patient's intent.

With no clear and convincing evidence of Jobes's beliefs about artificial feeding, the New Jersey Supreme Court turned to *In re Quinlan* for guidance. The court stated, "Our review of these cases and medical authorities confirms our conclusion that we should continue to defer, as we did in *Quinlan*, to family members' substituted judgments about medical treatment for irreversibly vegetative patients who did not clearly express their medical preferences while they were competent. Those decisions are best made by the family because the family is best able to decide what the patient would want."

THE NURSING HOME'S RESPONSIBILITY. The New Jersey Supreme Court reversed the trial court decision that had allowed the nursing home to refuse to participate in the withdrawal of the feeding tube. The court noted, "Mrs. Jobes's family had no reason to believe that they were surrendering the right to choose among medical alternatives when they placed her in the nursing home."

The court pointed out that it was not until 1985, five years after Jobes's admission to the Lincoln Park Nursing Home, and only after her family requested the removal of her feeding tube, that her family learned of the nursing home's policy. The court ordered the nursing home to comply with the family's request. Jobes died in August 1987 after the court ruling allowed her husband to have the feeding tube removed.

Justice Daniel J. O'Hern (1930–2009) dissented on both issues. He claimed that not all families may be as loving as Jobes's. He was concerned for other individuals whose families might not be so caring but who would still have the authority to order the withdrawal of life-sustaining treatments. He also disagreed with the order given the nursing home to comply with the family's request to discontinue Jobes's feeding. "I believe a proper balance could be obtained by adhering to the procedure adopted [in] *In re Quinlan*, that would have allowed the nonconsenting physician not to participate in the life-terminating process."

CLEAR AND CONVINCING EVIDENCE

Throughout the history of right-to-die cases, there has been considerable debate about how to determine a patient's wishes. How clearly must a patient have expressed his or her wishes before becoming incompetent? Does a parent or other family member best represent the patient? Are casual conversations sufficient to reveal intentions, or must there be written instructions?

In the Matter of Philip K. Eichner, on Behalf of Joseph C. Fox v. Denis Dillon, as District Attorney of Nassau County

Eighty-three-year-old Joseph C. Fox went into a PVS after a hernia operation. He was a member of the Society of Mary, a Roman Catholic religious order. The local director of the society, Philip K. Eichner, filed suit, asking for permission to have Fox's respirator removed.

In *In the Matter of Philip K. Eichner, on Behalf of Joseph C. Fox v. Denis Dillon, as District Attorney of Nassau County* (N.Y., 420 N.E.2d 64 [1981]), the court reasoned that "the highest burden of proof beyond a reasonable doubt should be required when granting the relief that may result in the patient's death." The need for high standards "forbids relief whenever the evidence is loose, equivocal, or contradictory." Fox, however, had discussed his feelings in the context of formal religious conversations. Only two months before his final hospitalization, he had stated that he did not want his life prolonged if his condition became hopeless. The court argued, "These were obviously solemn pronouncements and not casual remarks made at some social gathering, nor can it be said that he was too young to realize or feel the consequences of his statements." Following the ruling, Fox's respirator was removed, and he died from congestive heart failure on January 24, 1980.

Fox's case was the first where the reported attitudes of an incompetent patient were accepted as "clear and convincing."

In the Matter of Westchester County Medical Center, on Behalf of Mary O'Connor

Not all patients express their attitudes about the use of life-sustaining treatments in serious religious discussions as did Fox. Nonetheless, courts have accepted evidence of "best interests" or "substituted judgments" in allowing the termination of life-sustaining treatments.

In 1985 Mary O'Connor had a stroke that rendered her mentally and physically incompetent. More than two years later she suffered a second major stroke, after which she had additional disabilities and difficulty swallowing. O'Connor's two daughters moved her to a long-term geriatric facility that was associated with the Westchester County Medical Center. During her hospital admission, her daughters submitted a signed statement to be added to her medical records. The document stated that O'Connor had indicated in many conversations that "no artificial life support be started or maintained in order to continue to sustain her life."

In June 1988, when O'Connor's condition deteriorated, she was admitted to Westchester County Medical Center. Because she was unable to swallow, her physician prescribed a nasogastric tube. The daughters objected to the procedure, citing their mother's expressed wish. The hospital petitioned the court for permission to provide artificial feeding, without which O'Connor would starve to death within seven to 10 days. The lower court found in favor of O'Connor's daughters. The hospital subsequently brought the case *In the Matter of Westchester County Medical Center, on Behalf of Mary O'Connor* (531 N.E.2d 607 [N.Y. 1988]) before the New York Court of Appeals.

O'Connor's physician testified that she was not in a coma. Although he anticipated that O'Connor's awareness might improve in the future, he believed she would never regain the mental ability to understand complex matters. This included the issue of her medical condition and treatment. The physician further indicated that, if his patient were allowed to starve to death, she would experience pain and "extreme, intense discomfort."

A neurologist testifying for the daughters reported that O'Connor's brain damage would keep her from experiencing pain. If she did have pain in the process of starving to death, she could be given medication. The doctor admitted, however, that he could not be "medically certain" because he had never had a patient die under the same circumstances.

The New York Court of Appeals majority concluded that although family and friends testified that O'Connor "felt that nature should take its course and not use further artificial means" and that it is "monstrous" to keep someone alive by "machinery," these expressions did not constitute clear and convincing evidence of her present desire to die. Also, she had never specifically discussed the issue of ANH. Nor had she ever expressed her wish to refuse artificial medical treatment should such refusal result in a painful death.

The court further noted that O'Connor's statements about refusing artificial treatments had generally been made in situations involving terminal illness, specifically cancer: her husband, two of her brothers, her stepmother, and a close friend had all died of cancer. Speaking for the court of appeals majority, Judge Wachtler stressed that O'Connor was not terminally ill, was conscious, and could interact with others, albeit minimally. Her main problem was that she could not eat on her own, and her physician could help her with that. Writing for the majority, Judge Wachtler stated, "Every person has a right to life, and no one should be denied essential medical care unless the evidence clearly and convincingly shows that the patient intended to decline the treatment under some particular circumstances. This is a demanding standard, the most rigorous burden of proof in civil cases. It is appropriate here because if an error occurs it should be made on the side of life."

THIS IS TOO RESTRICTIVE. Judge Richard D. Simons (1927–) of the New York Court of Appeals differed from the majority in his opinion of O'Connor's condition. O'Connor's "conversations" were actually limited to saying her name and words such as "okay," "all right," and "yes." Neither the hospital doctor nor the neurologist who testified for her daughters could say for sure that she understood their questions. The court majority mentioned the patient squeezing her doctor's hand in response to some questions, but failed to add that she did not respond to most questions.

Although O'Connor was not terminally ill, her severe mental and physical injuries (should nature take its course) would result in her death. Judge Simons believed the artificial feeding would not cure or improve her deteriorating condition.

Judge Wachtler noted that O'Connor had talked about refusing artificial treatment in the aftermath of the deaths of loved ones from cancer. He claimed this had no bearing on her present condition, which was not terminal. Judge Simons pointed out that O'Connor had worked for 20 years in a hospital emergency room and pathology laboratory. She was no casual observer of death, and her "remarks" about not wanting artificial treatment for herself carried a lot of weight. Her expressed wishes to her daughters, who were nurses and coworkers in the same hospital, could not be considered "casual," as the majority observed. Judge Simons stated that "Judges, the persons least qualified by training, experience or affinity to reject the patient's instructions, have overridden Mrs. O'Connor's wishes, negated her long held values on life and death, and imposed on her and her family their ideas of what her best interests require." O'Connor died 10 months later with the feeding tube still in place.

Daniel Gindes suggests in "Judicial Postponement of Death Recognition: The Tragic Case of Mary O'Connor" (*American Journal of Law and Medicine*, vol. 15, nos. 2–3, 1989) that the court made an error in its judgment. He concludes by stating that "artificial hydration and nutrition is not 'food.' It is a desperate treatment best used as a transition from acute crisis to normal functioning. This miraculous technology, misused, harms the very patients medicine purports to help. One can argue that the 'sanctity of life' is more offended by warehousing bodies, than by cessation of treatment. Incompetent patients, who have suffered structural damage to necessary nerve centers, do not get better. Feeding tubes cannot regenerate this fragile tissue. Perhaps one day doctors will be able to make people like Mary O'Connor well. Until then, they should leave them alone."

THE CASE OF NANCY BETH CRUZAN

Although *O'Connor* set a rigorous standard of proof for the state of New York, *Cruzan* was the first right-to-die case to be heard by the U.S. Supreme Court. It confirmed the legality of such strict standards for the entire country.

Nancy Beth Cruzan, by Co-guardians, Lester L. Cruzan Jr. and Joyce Cruzan v. Robert Harmon

In January 1983, 25-year-old Nancy Beth Cruzan (1957–1990) lost control of her car. A state trooper found her lying facedown in a ditch. She was in cardiac and respiratory arrest. Paramedics were able to revive her, but a neurosurgeon indicated that she had "a probable cerebral contusion compounded by significant anoxia." The final diagnosis estimated that she had suffered anoxia (deprivation of oxygen) for 12 to 14 minutes. After six minutes of oxygen deprivation, the brain generally suffers permanent damage.

Doctors surgically implanted a feeding tube about a month after the accident, following the consent of her husband. Within a year of the accident, however, Cruzan's husband had their marriage dissolved. In January 1986 Cruzan became a ward of the state of Missouri.

Medical experts diagnosed Cruzan to be in a PVS and indicated that she was capable of living another 30 years. Cruzan's parents, Joyce and Lester Cruzan Jr., believed that their daughter would not want to live in a PVS sustained by a feeding tube and asked the hospital to remove the tube; hospital employees refused to do so. Because Cruzan was an adult, her parents had no legal standing in the courts, so they became the legal guardians of their daughter. They petitioned a Missouri trial court to have the feeding tube removed. The court gave Cruzan's parents the right to terminate ANH. However, the state and the court-appointed guardian ad litem appealed to the Missouri Supreme Court. Although the guardian ad litem believed it was in Cruzan's best interests to have the artificial feeding tube removed, he considered it his duty as her attorney to take the case to the state supreme court because it was a case of first impression (without a precedent) in the state of Missouri.

THE RIGHT TO PRIVACY. In *Nancy Beth Cruzan, by Co-guardians, Lester L. Cruzan Jr. and Joyce Cruzan v. Robert Harmon* (760 S.W.2d 408 [Mo.banc 1988]), the Missouri Supreme Court stressed that the state constitution did not expressly provide for the right of privacy, which would support an individual's right to refuse medical treatment. Although the U.S. Supreme Court had recognized the right of privacy in cases such as *Griswold v. Connecticut* (381 U.S. 479 [1965]) and *Roe v. Wade* (410 U.S. 113 [1973]), this right did not extend to the withdrawal of food and water. In fact, the U.S. Supreme Court, in *Roe v. Wade*, stressed that it "has refused to recognize an unlimited right of this kind in the past."

THE STATE'S INTEREST IN LIFE. In Cruzan's case the Missouri Supreme Court majority confirmed that the state's interest in life encompassed the sanctity of life and the prolongation of life. The state's interest in the prolongation of life was especially valid in Cruzan's case. She was not terminally ill and, based on medical evidence, would "continue a life of relatively normal duration if allowed basic sustenance." Furthermore, the state was not interested in the quality of life. The court was mindful that its decision would apply not only to Cruzan but also to others and feared treading a slippery slope. "Were the quality of life at issue, persons with all manner of handicaps might find the state seeking to terminate their lives. Instead, the state's interest is in life; that interest is unqualified."

THE GUARDIANS' RIGHTS. The Missouri Supreme Court ruled that Cruzan had no constitutional right to die and that there was no clear and convincing evidence that she would not wish to continue her vegetative existence. The majority further found that her parents, or guardians, had no right to exercise substituted judgment on their daughter's behalf. The court concluded, "We find no principled legal basis which permits the co-guardians in this case to choose the death of their ward. In the absence of such a legal basis for that decision and in the face of this State's strongly stated policy in favor of life, we choose to err on the side of life, respecting the rights of incompetent persons who may wish to live despite a severely diminished quality of life."

Therefore, the Missouri Supreme Court reversed the judgment of the Missouri trial court that had allowed discontinuance of Cruzan's artificial feeding.

THE STATE DOES NOT HAVE AN OVERRIDING INTEREST. In his dissent, Judge Charles B. Blackmar (1922–2007) indicated that the state should not be involved in cases such as Cruzan's. He was not convinced that the state had spoken better for Cruzan's interests than did her parents. He also questioned the state's interest in life in the context of espousing capital punishment, which clearly establishes "the proposition that some lives are not worth preserving."

Judge Blackmar did not share the majority's opinion that yielding to the guardians' request would lead to the mass euthanasia of handicapped people whose conditions did not come close to Cruzan's. He stressed that a court ruling is precedent only for the facts of that specific case. Besides, one of the purposes of courts is to protect incompetent people against abuse. He claimed, "The principal opinion attempts to establish absolutes, but does so at the expense of human factors. In so doing it unnecessarily subjects Nancy and those close to her to continuous torture which no family should be forced to endure."

"ERRONEOUS DECLARATION OF LAW." Judge Andrew J. Higgins (1921–2011), also dissenting, mainly disagreed with the majority's premise that the more than 50 precedent-setting cases from 16 other states were based on an "erroneous declaration of law." Yet, he noted that all the cases cited by the majority upheld an individual's right to refuse life-sustaining treatment, either personally or through the substituted judgment of a guardian. He could not understand the majority's contradiction of its own argument.

Cruzan v. Director, Missouri Department of Health

Cruzan's father appealed the Missouri Supreme Court's decision, and in December 1989 the U.S. Supreme Court heard arguments in *Cruzan v. Director, Missouri Department of Health* (497 U.S. 261 [1990]). This was the first time the right-to-die issue had been brought before the U.S. Supreme Court, which chose not to rule on whether Cruzan's parents could have her feeding tube removed. Instead, it considered whether the U.S. Constitution prohibited the state of Missouri from requiring clear and convincing evidence that an incompetent person desires withdrawal of life-sustaining treatment. In a 5–4 decision the court held that the Constitution did not prohibit the state of Missouri from requiring convincing evidence that an incompetent person wants life-sustaining treatment withdrawn.

Chief Justice William H. Rehnquist (1924–2005) wrote the opinion, with Justices Byron R. White (1917–2002), Sandra Day O'Connor (1930–), Antonin Scalia (1936–), and Anthony M. Kennedy (1936–) joining. The court majority believed that the Missouri Supreme Court's rigorous requirement of clear and convincing evidence that Cruzan had refused termination of life-sustaining treatment was justified. An erroneous decision not to withdraw the patient's feeding tube meant that the patient would continue to be sustained artificially. Possible medical advances or new evidence of the patient's intent could correct the error. An erroneous decision to terminate the artificial feeding could not be corrected, because the result of that decision (death) is irrevocable. The chief justice concluded, "No doubt is engendered by anything in this record but that Nancy Cruzan's mother and father are loving and caring parents. If the State were required by the United States Constitution to repose a right of 'substituted judgment' with anyone, the Cruzans would surely qualify. But we do not think the Due Process Clause requires the State to repose judgment on these matters with anyone but the patient herself." The due process clause of the 14th Amendment provides that no state shall "deprive any person of life, liberty, or property, without due process of law."

STATE INTEREST SHOULD NOT OUTWEIGH THE FREEDOM OF CHOICE. Dissenting, Justice William J. Brennan Jr. (1906–1997) pointed out that the state of Missouri's general interest in the preservation of Cruzan's life in no way outweighed her freedom of choice (in this case the choice to refuse medical treatment). He stated, "The regulation of constitutionally protected decisions ... must be predicated on legitimate state concerns other than disagreement with the choice the individual has made.... Otherwise, the interest in liberty protected by the Due Process Clause would be a nullity."

Justice Brennan believed the state of Missouri had imposed an uneven burden of proof. The state would accept only clear and convincing evidence that the patient had made explicit statements refusing ANH. It did not, however, require any proof that she had made specific statements desiring continuance of such treatment. Hence, it could not be said that the state had accurately determined Cruzan's wishes.

Justice Brennan disagreed that it is better to err on the side of life than death. He argued that, to the patient, erring from either side is "irrevocable." He explained, "An erroneous decision to terminate artificial nutrition and hydration, to be sure, will lead to failure of that last remnant of physiological life, the brain stem, and result in complete brain death. An erroneous decision not to terminate life-support, however, robs a patient of the very qualities protected by the right to avoid unwanted medical treatment. His own degraded existence is perpetuated; his family's suffering is protracted; the memory he leaves behind becomes more and more distorted."

STATE USES NANCY CRUZAN FOR "SYMBOLIC EFFECT." In a separate dissenting opinion, Justice John Paul Stevens (1920–) believed the state of Missouri was using Cruzan for the "symbolic effect" of defining life. The state sought to equate Cruzan's physical existence with life. Justice Stevens, however, pointed out that life is more than physiological functions. In fact, life connotes a person's experiences that make up his or her whole history, as well as "the practical manifestation of the human spirit."

Justice Stevens viewed the state's refusal to let Cruzan's guardians terminate her artificial feeding as ignoring their daughter's interests, and therefore, was "unconscionable":

> Insofar as Nancy Cruzan has an interest in being remembered for how she lived rather than how she died, the damage done to those memories by the prolongation of her death is irreversible. Insofar as Nancy Cruzan has an interest in the cessation of any pain, the continuation of her pain is irreversible. Insofar as Nancy Cruzan has an interest in a closure to her life consistent with her own beliefs rather than those of the Missouri legislature, the State's imposition of its contrary view is irreversible. To deny the importance of these consequences is in effect to deny that Nancy Cruzan has interests at all, and thereby to deny her personhood in the name of preserving the sanctity of her life.

***CRUZAN* CASE FINALLY RESOLVED.** On December 14, 1990, nearly eight years after Cruzan's car accident, a Missouri circuit court ruled that new evidence presented by three more friends constituted clear and convincing evidence that she would not want to continue existing in a PVS. The court allowed the removal of her artificial feeding. Within two hours of the ruling, Cruzan's doctor removed the tube. Cruzan's family kept a 24-hour vigil with her, until she died on December 26, 1990. Cruzan's family, however, believed she had left them many years earlier.

THE TERRI SCHIAVO CASE

Like Cruzan, the case of Terri Schiavo (1963–2005) involved a young woman in a PVS and the question of whether her nutrition and hydration could be discontinued.

In 1990 Schiavo suffered a loss of potassium in her body due to an eating disorder. This physiological imbalance caused her heart to stop beating, which deprived her brain of oxygen and resulted in a coma. She underwent surgery to implant a stimulator in her brain, an experimental treatment. The brain stimulator implant appeared to be a success, and the young woman appeared to be slowly emerging from her coma.

Nonetheless, even though Schiavo was continually provided with appropriate stimulation to recover, she remained in a PVS years later. Her husband, Michael Schiavo, believing that she would never recover and saying that his wife did not want to be kept alive by artificial means, petitioned a Florida court to remove her feeding tube. Her parents, however, believed that she could feel, understand, and respond. They opposed the idea of removing the feeding tube.

In 2000 a Florida trial court determined that Schiavo did not wish to be kept alive by artificial means based on her clear and direct statement to that effect to her husband. However, Schiavo's parents appealed the ruling, based on their belief that their daughter responded to their voices and could improve with therapy. They also contested the assertion that their daughter did not want to be kept alive by artificial means. Schiavo had left no living will to clarify her position, but under Florida's Health Care Advance Directives Law, a patient's spouse was second in line to decide about whether life support should be suspended (after a previously appointed guardian), adult children were third, and parents were fourth.

Constitutional Breach?

By October 2003 Schiavo's parents had exhausted their appeals, and the Florida appellate courts upheld the ruling of the trial court. At that time, a Florida judge ruled that removal of the tube take place. Schiavo's parents, however, requested that the Florida governor Jeb Bush (1953–) intervene. In response, the Florida legislature developed House Bill 35-E (Terri's Law) and passed this bill on October 21, 2003. The law gave Governor Bush the authority to order Schiavo's feeding tube reinserted, and he did that by issuing Executive Order No. 03-201 that same day, six days after the feeding tube had been removed.

Legal experts noted that the Florida legislature, in passing Terri's Law, appeared to have taken judicial powers away from the judicial branch of the Florida government and had given them to the executive branch. If this were the case, then the law was unconstitutional under article 2, section 3 of the Florida constitution, which states, "No person belonging to one branch shall exercise any powers appertaining to either of the other branches unless expressly provided herein." Thus, Michael Schiavo challenged the law's constitutionality in Pinellas County Circuit Court. Governor Bush requested that the Pinellas County Circuit Court judge dismiss Schiavo's lawsuit arguing against Terri's Law. On April 30, 2004, Judge Charles A. Davis Jr. (1948–) rejected the governor's technical challenges, thereby denying the governor's motion to dismiss. In May 2004 the law that allowed Governor Bush to intervene in the case was ruled unconstitutional by a Florida appeals court.

Continued Appeals

Schiavo's parents then appealed the case to the Florida Supreme Court, which heard the case in September 2004. The court upheld the ruling of the lower court, with the seven justices ruling unanimously and writing that Terri's Law was "an unconstitutional encroachment on the power that has been reserved for the independent judiciary." Nonetheless, Schiavo's parents continued their legal fight to keep her alive, so a stay on the tube's removal was put in place while their appeals were pending. In October 2004 Governor Bush asked the Florida Supreme Court to reconsider its decision. The court refused the request.

Attorneys for the Florida governor then asked the U.S. Supreme Court to hear the Schiavo case. The Supreme Court rejected the request, essentially affirming the lower court rulings that the governor had no legal right to intervene in the matter. In February 2005 a Florida judge ruled that Michael Schiavo could remove his wife's feeding tube in March of that year. On March 18, 2005, the tube was removed. Days later, in an unprecedented action, the U.S. House of Representatives and the U.S. Senate approved legislation, which was quickly signed by President George W. Bush (1946–), that granted Terri Schiavo's parents the right to sue in federal court. In effect, this legislation allowed the court to intervene in the case and restore Terri's feeding tube. Nonetheless, when Schiavo's parents appealed to the court, a federal judge refused to order the feeding tube reinserted. They then filed an appeal with the U.S. Supreme Court. Once again, the high court refused to hear the case.

The Effect of the Schiavo Situation on End-of-Life Decision Making

Terri Schiavo died on March 31, 2005. Her death and the events leading up to her death resulted in an intense debate among Americans over end-of-life decisions and brought new attention to the question of who should make the decision to stop life support.

Timothy Williams reports in "Schiavo's Brain Was Severely Deteriorated, Autopsy Says" (NYTimes.com, June 15, 2005) that the medical examiners who conducted Schiavo's autopsy found her brain "severely 'atrophied,'" weighing half the normal size, and noted that "no amount of therapy or treatment would have regenerated the massive loss of neurons." An autopsy cannot definitively establish a PVS, but the Schiavo findings were seen as "consistent" with a PVS.

THE CONSTITUTIONALITY OF ASSISTED SUICIDE

Washington v. Glucksberg

In January 1994 four doctors from Washington state, three terminally ill patients, and the organization Compassion in Dying filed a suit in the U.S. District Court. The plaintiffs sought to have the Washington Revised Code 9A.36.060(1) (1994) declared unconstitutional.

This law states, "A person is guilty of promoting a suicide attempt when he knowingly causes or aids another person to attempt suicide."

The plaintiffs argued that under the equal protection clause of the 14th Amendment mentally competent terminally ill adults have the right to a physician's assistance in determining the time and manner of their death. In *Compassion in Dying v. Washington* (850 F. Supp. 1454, 1456 n.2 [WD Wash. 1994]), the U.S. District Court agreed, stating that the Washington Revised Code violated the equal protection clause's provision that "all persons similarly situated ... be treated alike."

In its decision, the district court relied on *Planned Parenthood of Southeastern Pennsylvania v. Casey* (505 U.S. 833 [1992]; a reaffirmation of *Roe v. Wade*'s holding of the right to abortion) and *Cruzan v. Director, Missouri Department of Health* (the right to refuse unwanted life-sustaining treatment). The court found Washington's statute against assisted suicide "unconstitutional because it places an undue burden on the exercise of that constitutionally protected liberty interest."

In *Compassion in Dying v. State of Washington* (49 F. 3d 586, 591 [1995]), a panel (three or more judges but not the full court) of the Court of Appeals for the Ninth Circuit Court reversed the district court's decision, stressing that in over 200 years of U.S. history no court had ever recognized the right to assisted suicide. In *Compassion in Dying v. State of Washington* (79 F. 3d 790, 798 [1996]), however, the Ninth Circuit Court reheard the case en banc (by the full court), reversed the panel's decision, and affirmed the district court's ruling.

The en banc Court of Appeals for the Ninth Circuit Court did not mention the equal protection clause violation as indicated by the district court. Nevertheless, it referred to *Casey* and *Cruzan*, adding that the U.S. Constitution recognizes the right to die. Quoting from *Casey*, Judge Stephen R. Reinhardt (1931–) wrote, "Like the decision of whether or not to have an abortion, the decision how and when to die is one of 'the most intimate and personal choices a person may make in a lifetime, ... central to personal dignity and autonomy.'"

THE U.S. SUPREME COURT DECIDES. The state of Washington and its attorney general appealed the case *Washington v. Glucksberg* (521 U.S. 702 [1997]) to the U.S. Supreme Court. Instead of addressing the plaintiffs' initial question of whether mentally competent terminally ill adults have the right to physician-assisted suicide, Chief Justice Rehnquist reframed the issue by focusing on "whether Washington's prohibition against 'caus[ing]' or 'aid[ing]' a suicide offends the 14th Amendment to the United States Constitution."

Chief Justice Rehnquist recalled the more than 700 years of Anglo American common-law tradition disapproving of suicide and assisted suicide. He added that assisted suicide is considered to be a crime in almost every state, with no exceptions granted to mentally competent terminally ill adults.

PREVIOUS SUBSTANTIVE DUE-PROCESS CASES. The plaintiffs argued that in previous substantive due-process cases, such as *Cruzan*, the U.S. Supreme Court had acknowledged the principle of self-autonomy by ruling "that competent, dying persons have the right to direct the removal of life sustaining medical treatment and thus hasten death." Chief Justice Rehnquist claimed that, although committing suicide with another's help is just as personal as refusing life-sustaining treatment, it is not similar to refusing unwanted medical treatment. In fact, according to the chief justice, the *Cruzan* court specifically stressed that most states ban assisted suicide.

STATE'S INTEREST. The court pointed out that the state of Washington's interest in preserving human life includes the entire spectrum of that life, from birth to death, regardless of a person's physical or mental condition. The court agreed with the state that allowing assisted suicide might imperil the lives of vulnerable populations such as the poor, the elderly, and the disabled. The state included the terminally ill in this group.

Furthermore, the court agreed with the state of Washington that legalizing physician-assisted suicide would eventually lead to voluntary and involuntary euthanasia. Because a health care proxy's decision is legally accepted as an incompetent patient's decision, what if the patient cannot self-administer the lethal medication? In such a case a physician or a family member would have to administer the drug, thus committing euthanasia.

The court unanimously ruled that:

> [The Washington Revised] Code ... does not violate the 14th Amendment, either on its face or "as applied to competent, terminally ill adults who wish to hasten their deaths by obtaining medication prescribed by their doctors."
>
> Throughout the Nation, Americans are engaged in an earnest and profound debate about the morality, legality, and practicality of physician assisted suicide. Our holding permits this debate to continue, as it should in a democratic society. The decision of the en banc Court of Appeals is reversed, and the case is remanded [sent back] for further proceedings consistent with this opinion.

PROVISION OF PALLIATIVE CARE. Concurring, Justices O'Connor and Stephen G. Breyer (1938–) wrote that "dying patients in Washington and New York can obtain palliative care [care that relieves pain, but does not cure the illness], even when doing so would hasten their deaths." Hence, the justices did not see the need to address a dying person's constitutional right to obtain relief from pain. Justice O'Connor believed the court was justified in banning assisted suicide for two reasons, "The difficulty in defining terminal illness and the risk that a dying patient's request for assistance in ending his or her life might not be truly voluntary."

Vacco, Attorney General of New York et al. v. Quill et al.

REFUSING LIFE-SUSTAINING TREATMENT IS ESSENTIALLY THE SAME AS ASSISTED SUICIDE. In 1994 three New York physicians and three terminally ill patients sued the New York attorney general. In *Quill v. Koppell* (870 F. Supp. 78, 84 [SDNY 1994]), they claimed before the U.S. District Court that New York violated the equal protection clause by prohibiting physician-assisted suicide. The state permits a competent patient to refuse life-sustaining treatment, but not to obtain physician-assisted suicide. The plaintiffs claimed that these are "essentially the same thing." The court disagreed, stating that withdrawing life support to let nature run its course differs from intentionally using lethal drugs to cause death.

The plaintiffs brought their case *Quill v. Vacco* (80 F. 3d 716 [1996]) to the Court of Appeals for the Second Circuit (appellate court), which reversed the district court's ruling. The appellate court found that the New York statute does not treat equally all competent terminally ill patients wishing to hasten their death. The court stated, "The ending of life by [the withdrawal of life-support systems] is nothing more nor less than assisted suicide."

REFUSING LIFE-SUSTAINING TREATMENT DIFFERS FROM ASSISTED SUICIDE. New York's attorney general appealed the case to the U.S. Supreme Court. In *Vacco, Attorney General of New York et al. v. Quill et al.* (521 U.S. 793 [1997]), the court distinguished between withdrawing life-sustaining medical treatment and assisted suicide. The court contended that when a patient refuses life support, he or she dies because the disease has run its natural course. By contrast, if a patient self-administers lethal drugs, death results from that medication.

The court also distinguished between the physician's role in both scenarios. A physician who complies with a patient's request to withdraw life support does so to honor a patient's wish because the treatment no longer benefits the patient. Likewise, when a physician prescribes painkilling drugs, the needed drug dosage might hasten death, although the physician's only intent is to ease pain. However, when a physician assists in suicide, his or her prime intention is to hasten death. Therefore, the court reversed the ruling made by the Court of Appeals for the Second Circuit.

Gonzales v. Oregon

In their *Quill* opinions, Justices Stevens and David H. Souter (1939–) let it be known that they thought there might be legal grounds for permitting physician-assisted suicide in certain cases. Oregon legislators had by that time already passed the Oregon Death with Dignity Act, and the act survived a number of challenges in state court. Voters reaffirmed the act via a 1997 referendum, and the act was implemented in 1998. In late 2001 the U.S. attorney general John D. Ashcroft (1942–) took aim at the Oregon law, reversing a decision made by his predecessor, Janet Reno (1938–), and asserting that the Controlled Substances Act of 1970 could be used against Oregon physicians who helped patients commit suicide by prescribing lethal drugs. The U.S. Drug Enforcement Administration could thereby revoke the prescription-writing privileges of any Oregon physician who prescribed drugs commonly used for assisted suicide, and those physicians would be subject to criminal prosecution. In response, the state of Oregon filed in November 2001 a lawsuit against Ashcroft's decision, claiming that he was acting unconstitutionally.

In April 2002, in *State of Oregon and Peter A. Rasmussen et al. v. John Ashcroft* (Civil No. 01-1647-JO), Judge Robert E. Jones (1927–) of the U.S. District Court for the District of Oregon ruled in favor of the Oregon Death with Dignity Act. The U.S. Department of Justice appealed the ruling to the U.S. Court of Appeals for the Ninth Circuit in San Francisco. In May 2004 the court upheld the Oregon Death with Dignity Act. The decision, by a divided three-judge panel, said the Department of Justice did not have the power to punish physicians for prescribing medication for the purpose of assisted suicide. The majority opinion stated that Ashcroft overstepped his authority in trying to block enforcement of Oregon's law.

In February 2005 the U.S. Supreme Court agreed to hear the Bush administration's challenge of Oregon's physician-assisted suicide law. On January 17, 2006, the court let stand in *Gonzales v. Oregon* (546 U.S. 243) Oregon's physician-assisted suicide law. The high court held that the Controlled Substances Act "does not allow the Attorney General to prohibit doctors from prescribing regulated drugs for use in physician-assisted suicide under state law permitting the procedure." Writing for the majority, Justice Kennedy explained that both Ashcroft and Alberto Gonzales (1955–), who succeeded Ashcroft as the U.S. attorney general, did not have the power to override the Oregon physician-assisted suicide law. Furthermore, Justice Kennedy added that the attorney general does not have the authority to make health and medical policy.

Baxter v. Montana

Physician-assisted suicide technically became legal in the state of Montana in 2009 via a court case rather than a legislative act, as in the other three states (Oregon,

Washington, and Vermont) allowing the practice. The Montana court case was originally initiated at the district level by Robert Baxter, a 76-year-old Montana truck driver with terminal cancer. Four physicians and the organization Compassion & Choices joined Baxter in the case *Baxter v. State of Montana* (Case No. ADV-2007-787). Baxter had been battling leukemia for over a decade and wished to end his life with prescribed medication. On December 5, 2008, Judge Dorothy McCarter ruled that the Montana constitution protected a mentally competent terminally ill patient's right to die with the help of medication prescribed by a physician. The ruling, which Baxter never heard, came the same day he died of his underlying disease.

The state of Montana appealed the ruling to the Montana Supreme Court in *Baxter v. State of Montana* (DA 09-0051 [2009 MT 449]). On December 31, 2009, the high court ruled 5–2 that physician-assisted suicide was not criminalized by either the Montana constitution or public policy. Although the court ruling protected physicians from prosecution in physician-assisted suicide, it did not declare that physician-assisted suicide is a right allowed to Montana residents. The high court left that debate to be settled in the state legislature.

OTHER HIGH-PROFILE CASES

Besides the many precedent-setting cases discussed above, there have been numerous high-profile cases centering on end-of-life and right-to-die issues that do not set legal precedent. Often, these cases make their way into the media based on the poignancy of the situations or the advocacy of individuals or organizations who believe the cases support right-to-die or pro-life stances.

For example, in December 2013, Jahi McMath, a 13-year-old girl who was in an Oakland, California, hospital undergoing a tonsillectomy, suffered cardiac arrest while on the operating table and was declared brain dead. McMath's family members were devout Christians, however, and they insisted that she was still alive as long as her heart was beating. The family thus pressed for the right to have McMath remain on a ventilator and receiving ANH despite the fact that she was dead according to California law. McMath was kept on life support during the weeks-long court case before a judge finally ruled, in early January 2014, that the hospital could not be required to keep her alive by artificial means. The family ultimately won the right to keep McMath on life support while she was transported from the hospital to an undisclosed facility, where her body was being kept alive as of March 2014.

The McMath case neither raised new legal issues nor involved any controversial interpretation of existing issues. Instead, it created a media sensation in which McMath's family's claims that the young girl was still alive were frequently repeated uncritically by newscasters and journalists, and in which comparisons were drawn to such cases as that of Terri Schiavo. Schiavo, however, had not been brain dead but in a PVS, a condition raising very different and more contentious legal and ethical issues. Bioethicists lamented the media coverage of the McMath case, noting that it wrongly obscured the relevant ethical and legal issues. "The ability to get clear about brain death has been a real obstacle," Arthur Caplan, a bioethicist at New York University's Langone Medical Center, told Lee Romney in "Jahi McMath Case Muddies an Already Agonizing Subject" (LATimes.com, January 6, 2014). "This hasn't helped at all."

CHAPTER 10
THE COST OF HEALTH CARE

Advances in health care have revolutionized life in the developed world, eradicating or controlling once-fatal diseases, making infant and child mortality a rarity rather than a nearly universal occurrence, and extending average life spans dramatically. The elderly population in wealthy countries has accordingly grown, both in raw numerical terms and as a share of total population.

Although the health advances that have led to increased life expectancies represent one of humankind's greatest achievements, it is an achievement that has given rise to many new problems. In the United States, one of the largest unsolved problems relating to end-of-life care (and to health care in general), is cost. An aging population is a population with an ever-expanding need for medical care, and new technological and pharmaceutical advances are expensive, more so in the United States than in any other country.

THE HIGH COST OF HEALTH CARE IN THE UNITED STATES

Most developed countries other than the United States manage their health care systems for the benefit of the public rather than as an ordinary part of the market economy. The United States, by contrast, has a predominantly private and market-based health care system, in which health care companies and caregivers are allowed to price their goods and services according to their interests as for-profit businesses or nonprofit foundations tasked with maximizing their efficiency. In the United States most people pay for their health care with private insurance policies that they obtain through their employers (who typically share costs with employees) or on their own, although a substantial proportion receive care subsidized through government programs. In other developed countries the government typically provides a base level of free or subsidized health care coverage to the entire population. Although other countries' systems may offer much of the same technology and pharmaceuticals as in the United States, and although their physicians and nurses receive the same level of training, their governments are able to exert greater influence on the market for health care and keep prices down. In the United States, by contrast, the government exerts less downward pressure on the price of health care.

Many advocates for the market-based health care system maintain that high health costs in the United States are a function not of insufficient government participation in the system but of insufficiently free markets. In this view, one main problem with the U.S. system is that consumers, accustomed to paying only part of the fees for the medical goods and services they obtain (while employers share the costs of insurance and insurers pay medical bills in full), do not make well-reasoned economic decisions in the realm of health care. In other words, when people know that they will get considerably more health care than they pay for on their own, they consent to more medical care than they need. If, according to this theory, Americans were more often forced to pay for service directly and in full, they would reason more efficiently and spend their money more wisely, and prices would fall system-wide as health care providers begin to compete for customers on the basis of price.

Another frequently cited reason for the high cost of health care in the United States is the burden placed on hospitals and physicians by frivolous lawsuits. Doctors and facilities pay a great deal of money to insure themselves against malpractice claims, and they pass these costs along to consumers.

As Figure 10.1 shows, in 2010 average annual health care spending per person in the United States was $8,233, compared with $4,445 in Canada, $3,758 in Sweden, $3,433 in the United Kingdom, and $3,035 in Japan. The much higher spending on American health care did not translate into better health outcomes across the

FIGURE 10.1

Health care spending per person and life span, U.S. and other developed countries, 2010

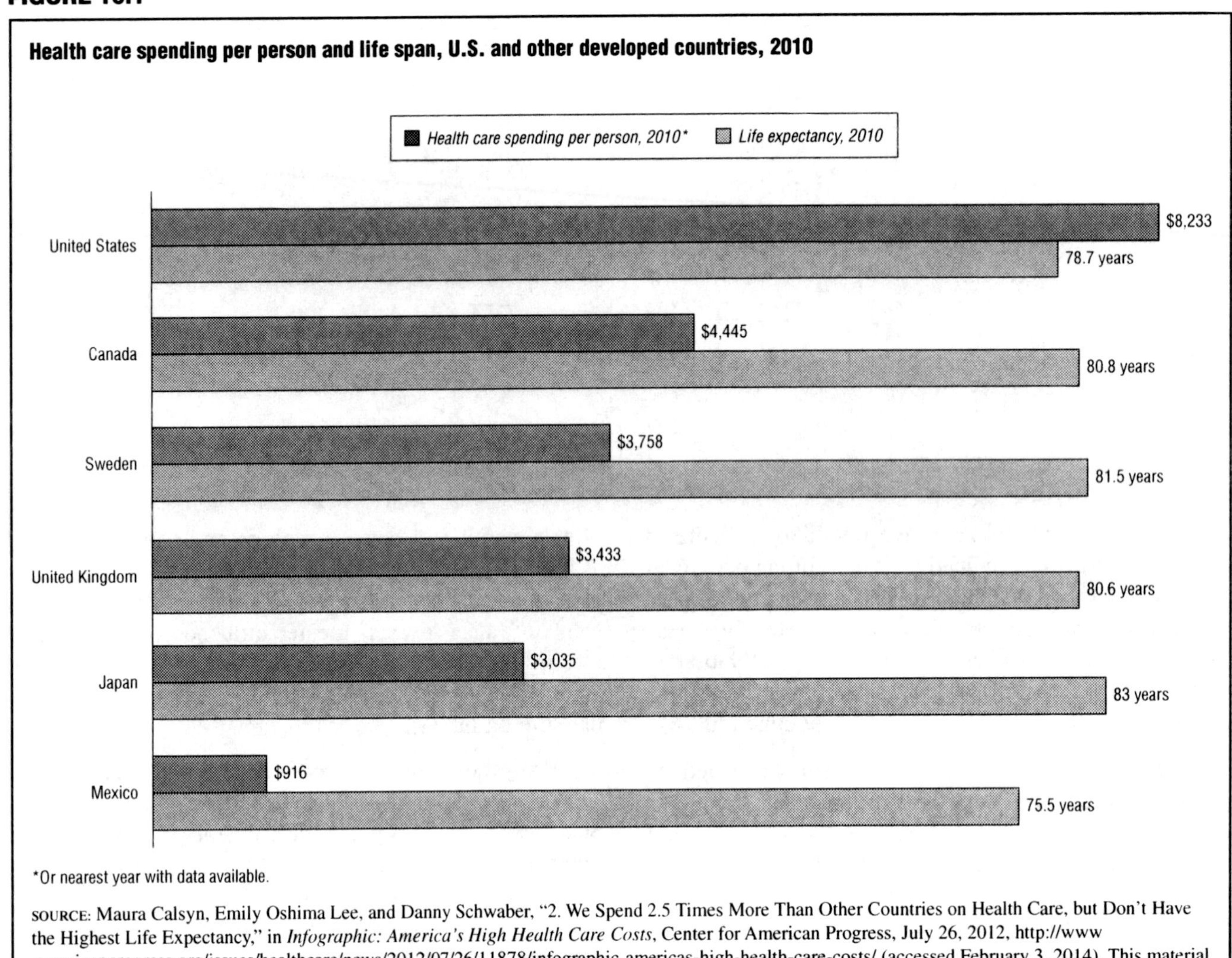

*Or nearest year with data available.

SOURCE: Maura Calsyn, Emily Oshima Lee, and Danny Schwaber, "2. We Spend 2.5 Times More Than Other Countries on Health Care, but Don't Have the Highest Life Expectancy," in *Infographic: America's High Health Care Costs*, Center for American Progress, July 26, 2012, http://www.americanprogress.org/issues/healthcare/news/2012/07/26/11878/infographic-americas-high-health-care-costs/ (accessed February 3, 2014). This material was created by the Center for American Progress (www.americanprogress.org).

population, however. Life expectancy in the United States was 78.7 years in 2010, compared with 80.8 in Canada, 81.5 in Sweden, 80.6 in the United Kingdom, and 83 in Japan. Life expectancy in Mexico was 75.5 years, only three years lower than in the United States, although Mexico's health care spending per person was $916, or approximately eight times lower.

The International Federation of Health Plans, the global health insurance industry's leading trade group, conducts an annual survey of health care costs worldwide. In *International Federation of Health Plans 2012 Comparative Price Report: Variation in Medical and Hospital Prices by Country* (2013, https://static.squarespace.com/), the group notes that the average price that insurers pay to health care providers for virtually every variety of medical service and treatment, from routine office visits to major surgery, was significantly higher in the United States in 2012 than in other developed countries. For example, a routine office visit cost an average of $95 in the United States, compared with $30 in both Canada and France, and only $11 in Spain. Lipitor, a drug commonly prescribed to treat high cholesterol, cost an average of $124 per month in the United States, compared with $43 in the United Kingdom, $13 in Spain, and $6 in New Zealand. An angiogram (an X-ray of the blood vessels used to diagnose various heart conditions) cost $914, on average, in the United States, compared with $264 in France, $218 in Switzerland, and $35 in Canada. The average cost of one day in the hospital was $4,287, compared with $1,472 in Australia, $853 in France, and $476 in Spain. The cost of bypass surgery (commonly used to reduce the risk of death from heart disease) averaged $73,420 in the United States, $43,230 in Australia, $22,844 in France, and $14,117 in the United Kingdom. (The International Federation of Health Plans notes that although its figures for the United States are based on averages from over 100 million claims paid by multiple insurers, its numbers for other countries are based on one plan per country and thus may not reflect the overall average in those countries.)

These prices represent costs paid by insurers (including government insurance programs). In the United States and elsewhere, however, insurers may pay only part of the total cost of health care. Depending on the type of health plan someone is enrolled in, they may be expected to pay a premium (a set fee) on a regular schedule in order to be covered by insurance at all. Some insurance plans feature co-payments, meaning that their members must pay a portion of the total cost of whatever services they do use. Deductibles, which are also a feature of many health plans, require plan members to pay a certain amount of health care costs themselves each year before the insurer will step in to cover any remaining expenses. Premiums, co-payments, and deductibles are not exclusive to the U.S. health care system, but they are very common features of health insurance plans there. This means that the relatively high cost of care borne by insurers in the United States is also being passed on to consumers to some degree.

Additionally, many in the United States have no insurance coverage at all. Such individuals must pay their medical fees in full when they receive care. Payment in full of health care expenses is beyond the means of many Americans, however, so many people without health insurance forgo health care except in emergency situations. Emergency medical care is much more expensive than the routine preventive care, which can often treat illnesses before a patient's condition becomes critical. Unlike nonemergency physicians' offices, however, in the United States most emergency medical facilities are legally obliged to care for anyone in need, whether or not they can pay for the care that they receive. State and federal funds are typically used to reimburse hospitals for the emergency treatment of uninsured people. The cost of such treatment, which is passed on to taxpayers, is another significant driver of overall health care spending in the United States.

As Table 10.1 shows, health care spending in the United States has risen much faster than the population has grown. Total national health expenditures stood at $27.4 billion in 1960, when the population was 186 million. By 2011 the population had grown by a factor of nearly 1.7, reaching 311 million, but health expenditures had risen by a factor of nearly 100, to $2.7 trillion. In 1960 health care spending represented 5.2% of the gross domestic product (GDP; the total value of all goods and services produced in the country in a given year); by 2011 health care spending represented 17.9% of GDP.

The cost of health care has been increasing, over this period, not only relative to previous eras but relative to the costs of other goods and services. As measured by the consumer price index (CPI), a numerical value meant to quantify the cost of an average "basket of goods" for the purposes of measuring changes in prices, the cost of health care has risen more rapidly since the late 20th century than all other basic goods and services Americans typically purchase. (See Table 10.2.) Between 1960 and 2011 the cost of medical care as measured by the CPI rose by a factor of nearly 18, from 22.3 to 400.3. By contrast, the price of the next-most costly set of goods ordinarily purchased—energy (including both fuel for automobiles and electricity and gas for the home)—rose by a factor of just less than 11 during the same period. The prices of other goods, such as food and housing, while substantially more expensive in 2011 than in 1960, likewise rose much more slowly than the price of medical care.

By 2012 health care spending was a major financial burden for many families. As Figure 10.2 shows, 16.5% of American families had trouble paying medical bills at some point in 2012 and 8.9% had medical bills that they were completely unable to pay at the time they were surveyed. More than one in four families (26.8%) reported that medical care represented a financial burden for their households, including 21.4% of families that had made arrangements to pay medical debts over time. This burden was, understandably, most pressing for those families with the least amount of income. Figure 10.3 shows the prevalence of financial burdens related to medical care according to income level. Those families making below 250% of the federal poverty level (the poverty level is an income threshold below which a household is considered officially poor, according to the federal government) were substantially more likely to have trouble paying their medical bills than those who made more than that amount. Sizable percentages of families making between 250% and 400% struggled to pay their medical bills as well. Even among those making more than 400% of poverty (400% of poverty for a family of four was $92,200 in 2012), 16.6% considered themselves financially burdened due to medical care and 14.9% were paying medical bills in installments.

The Affordable Care Act

It was in large part to relieve some of these financial burdens that President Barack Obama (1961–) made it a legislative priority to reform the U.S. health care system during his first term in office. The resulting Patient Protection and Affordable Care Act (commonly called the Affordable Care Act, or the ACA), which Obama signed into law in 2010, had provisions outlawing the insurance industry practice of denying coverage to those who were ill or otherwise in need of care, offering subsidized insurance policies to households making less than 400% of poverty, and expanding Medicaid, the federally funded, state-administered program of health care coverage for low-income Americans. The Medicaid expansion was designed to offer coverage to all adults and children

TABLE 10.1

National health expenditures, selected years 1960–2011

Item	1960	1970	1980	1990	2000	2001	2002	2003	2004	2005	2006	2007	2008	2009	2010	2011
	Amount in billions															
National health expenditures	$27.4	$74.9	$255.8	$724.3	$1,377.2	$1,493.3	$1,638.0	$1,775.4	$1,901.6	$2,030.5	$2,163.3	$2,298.3	$2,406.6	$2,501.2	$2,600.0	$2,700.7
Health consumption expenditures	24.8	67.1	235.7	675.6	1,289.6	1,402.1	1,535.9	1,665.5	1,784.2	1,904.0	2,032.4	2,154.6	2,252.8	2,355.1	2,450.8	2,547.2
Personal health care	23.4	63.1	217.2	616.8	1,165.4	1,265.3	1,371.9	1,480.2	1,589.4	1,697.1	1,804.4	1,914.1	2,010.4	2,111.6	2,190.0	2,279.3
Government administration and net cost of health insurance	1.1	2.6	12.0	38.8	81.2	90.0	111.9	131.8	141.0	150.9	165.7	171.8	169.8	167.9	181.5	188.9
Government public health activities	0.4	1.4	6.4	20.0	43.0	46.8	52.0	53.5	53.8	56.0	62.3	68.7	72.6	75.6	79.3	79.0
Investment	2.6	7.8	20.1	48.7	87.5	91.3	102.0	110.0	117.4	126.5	130.9	143.7	153.8	146.1	149.1	153.5
	Millions															
U.S. population[a]	186	210	230	254	282	285	288	290	293	295	298	301	304	306	309	311
	Amount in billions															
Gross domestic product[b]	$526	$1,038	$2,788	$5,801	$9,952	$10,286	$10,642	$11,142	$11,853	$12,623	$13,377	$14,029	$14,292	$13,974	$14,499	$15,076
	Per capita amount															
National health expenditures	$147	$356	$1,110	$2,854	$4,878	$5,240	$5,695	$6,121	$6,497	$6,875	$7,255	$7,636	$7,922	$8,163	$8,417	$8,680
Health consumption expenditures	133	319	1,023	2,662	4,568	4,919	5,340	5,742	6,096	6,447	6,816	7,158	7,416	7,686	7,934	8,187
Personal health care	125	300	943	2,430	4,128	4,439	4,770	5,103	5,430	5,746	6,051	6,360	6,618	6,891	7,090	7,326
Government administration and net cost of health insurance	6	12	52	153	288	316	389	454	482	511	556	571	559	548	588	607
Government public health activities	2	6	28	79	152	164	181	185	184	190	209	228	239	247	257	254
Investment	14	37	87	192	310	320	355	379	401	428	439	477	506	477	483	493
	Average annual percent change from previous year shown															
National health expenditures		10.6%	13.1%	11.0%	6.6%	8.4%	9.7%	8.4%	7.1%	6.8%	6.5%	6.2%	4.7%	3.9%	3.9%	3.9%
Health consumption expenditures		10.5	13.4	11.1	6.7	8.7	9.5	8.4	7.1	6.7	6.7	6.0	4.6	4.5	4.1	3.9
Personal health care		10.4	13.2	11.0	6.6	8.6	8.4	7.9	7.4	6.8	6.3	6.1	5.0	5.0	3.7	4.1
Government administration and net cost of health insurance		9.4	16.4	12.4	7.7	10.8	24.4	17.7	7.0	7.0	9.8	3.7	−1.2	−1.1	8.1	4.1
Government public health activities		13.8	16.9	12.0	8.0	8.7	11.2	2.8	0.5	4.1	11.2	10.3	5.8	4.1	4.9	−0.5
Investment		11.7	10.0	9.2	6.0	4.3	11.8	7.8	6.8	7.8	3.5	9.7	7.1	−5.0	2.1	2.9
U.S. population[a]		1.2	0.9	1.0	1.1	1.0	0.9	0.8	0.9	0.9	1.0	0.9	0.9	0.9	0.8	0.7
Gross domestic product[b]		7.0	10.4	7.6	5.5	3.4	3.5	4.7	6.4	6.5	6.0	4.9	1.9	−2.2	3.8	4.0
	Percent distribution															
National health expenditures	100.0%	100.0%	100.0%	100.0%	100.0%	100.0%	100.0%	100.0%	100.0%	100.0%	100.0%	100.0%	100.0%	100.0%	100.0%	100.0%
Health consumption expenditures	90.6	89.6	92.1	93.3	93.6	93.9	93.8	93.8	93.8	93.8	93.9	93.7	93.6	94.2	94.3	94.3
Personal health care	85.4	84.3	84.9	85.2	84.6	84.7	83.8	83.4	83.6	83.6	83.4	83.3	83.5	84.4	84.2	84.4
Government administration and net cost of health insurance	3.9	3.5	4.7	5.4	5.9	6.0	6.8	7.4	7.4	7.4	7.7	7.5	7.1	6.7	7.0	7.0
Government public health activities	1.4	1.8	2.5	2.8	3.1	3.1	3.2	3.0	2.8	2.8	2.9	3.0	3.0	3.0	3.1	2.9
Investment	9.4	10.4	7.9	6.7	6.4	6.1	6.2	6.2	6.2	6.2	6.1	6.3	6.4	5.8	5.7	5.7
	Percent															
National health expenditures as a percent of gross domestic product	5.2%	7.2%	9.2%	12.5%	13.8%	14.5%	15.4%	15.9%	16.0%	16.1%	16.2%	16.4%	16.8%	17.9%	17.9%	17.9%

[a]Census resident-based population less armed forces overseas and population of outlying areas.
[b]U.S. Department of Commerce, Bureau of Economic Analysis.

SOURCE: "Table 1. National Health Expenditures; Aggregate and Per Capita Amounts, Annual Percent Change and Percent Distribution: Selected Calendar Years 1960–2011," in *National Health Expenditure Data: Historical—NHE Tables*, Centers for Medicare and Medicaid Services, 2012, http://www.cms.gov/Research-Statistics-Data-and-Systems/Statistics-Trends-and-Reports/NationalHealthExpendData/Downloads/tables.pdf (accessed December 28, 2013)

TABLE 10.2

Consumer price index and average annual percentage change for all items, selected items, and medical care components, selected years 1960–2011

[Data are based on reporting by samples of providers and other retail outlets]

Items and medical care components	1960	1970	1980	1990	1995	2000	2005	2010	2011
				Consumer Price Index (CPI)					
All items	29.6	38.8	82.4	130.7	152.4	172.2	195.3	218.1	224.9
All items less medical care	30.2	39.2	82.8	128.8	148.6	167.3	188.7	209.7	216.3
Services	24.1	35.0	77.9	139.2	168.7	195.3	230.1	261.3	265.8
Food	30.0	39.2	86.8	132.4	148.4	167.8	190.7	219.6	227.8
Apparel	45.7	59.2	90.9	124.1	132.0	129.6	119.5	119.5	122.1
Housing	—	36.4	81.1	128.5	148.5	169.6	195.7	216.3	219.1
Energy	22.4	25.5	86.0	102.1	105.2	124.6	177.1	211.4	243.9
Medical care	22.3	34.0	74.9	162.8	220.5	260.8	323.2	388.4	400.3
Components of medical care									
Medical care services	19.5	32.3	74.8	162.7	224.2	266.0	336.7	411.2	423.8
Professional services	—	37.0	77.9	156.1	201.0	237.7	281.7	328.2	335.7
Physician services	21.9	34.5	76.5	160.8	208.8	244.7	287.5	331.3	340.3
Dental services	27.0	39.2	78.9	155.8	206.8	258.5	324.0	398.8	408.0
Eyeglasses and eye care[a]	—	—	—	117.3	137.0	149.7	163.2	176.7	178.3
Services by other medical professionals[a]	—	—	—	120.2	143.9	161.9	186.8	214.4	217.4
Hospital and related services	—	—	69.2	178.0	257.8	317.3	439.9	607.7	641.5
Hospital services[b]	—	—	—	—	—	115.9	161.6	227.2	241.2
Inpatient hospital services[b, c]	—	—	—	—	—	113.8	156.6	221.5	236.6
Outpatient hospital services[a, c]	—	—	—	138.7	204.6	263.8	373.0	520.6	546.9
Hospital rooms	9.3	23.6	68.0	175.4	251.2	—	—	—	—
Other inpatient services[a]	—	—	—	142.7	206.8	—	—	—	—
Nursing homes and adult day care[b]	—	—	—	—	—	117.0	145.0	177.0	182.2
Health insurance[d]	—	—	—	—	—	—	—	106.6	105.5
Medical care commodities	46.9	46.5	75.4	163.4	204.5	238.1	276.0	314.7	324.1
Medicinal drugs[e]	—	—	—	—	—	—	—	102.3	105.5
Prescription drugs[f]	54.0	47.4	72.5	181.7	235.0	285.4	349.0	407.8	425.0
Nonprescription drugs[e]	—	—	—	—	—	—	—	100.0	98.6
Medical equipment and supplies[e]	—	—	—	—	—	—	—	99.1	99.3
Nonprescription drugs and medical supplies[a, g]	—	—	—	120.6	140.5	149.5	151.7	—	—
Internal and respiratory over-the-counter drugs[h]	—	42.3	74.9	145.9	167.0	176.9	179.7	—	—
Nonprescription medical equipment and supplies[i]	—	—	79.2	138.0	166.3	178.1	180.6	—	—
			Average annual percent change from previous year shown						
All items	. . .	2.7	7.8	4.7	3.1	2.5	2.5	1.6	3.2
All items less medical care	. . .	2.6	7.8	4.5	2.9	2.4	2.4	1.5	3.2
Services	. . .	3.8	8.3	6.0	3.9	3.0	3.3	0.8	1.7
Food	. . .	2.7	8.3	4.3	2.3	2.5	2.6	0.8	3.7
Apparel	. . .	2.6	4.4	3.2	1.2	−0.4	−1.6	−0.5	2.2
Housing	. . .	—	8.3	4.7	2.9	2.7	2.9	−0.4	1.3
Energy	. . .	1.3	12.9	1.7	0.6	3.4	7.3	9.5	15.4
Medical care	. . .	4.3	8.2	8.1	6.3	3.4	4.4	3.4	3.0
Components of medical care									
Medical care services	. . .	5.2	8.8	8.1	6.6	3.5	4.8	3.5	3.1
Professional services	. . .	—	7.7	7.2	5.2	3.4	3.5	2.8	2.3
Physician services	. . .	4.6	8.3	7.7	5.4	3.2	3.3	3.3	2.7
Dental services	. . .	3.8	7.2	7.0	5.8	4.6	4.6	2.7	2.3
Eyeglasses and eye care[a]	. . .	—	—	—	3.2	1.8	1.7	0.7	0.9
Services by other medical professionals[a]	. . .	—	—	—	3.7	2.4	2.9	2.2	1.4
Hospital and related services	. . .	—	—	9.9	7.7	4.2	6.8	7.0	5.6
Hospital services[b]	. . .	—	—	—	—	—	6.9	7.8	6.2
Inpatient hospital services[b, c]	. . .	—	—	—	—	—	6.6	8.8	6.8
Outpatient hospital services[a, c]	. . .	—	—	—	8.1	5.2	7.2	6.1	5.1
Hospital rooms	. . .	9.8	11.2	9.9	7.4	—	—	—	—
Other inpatient services[a]	. . .	—	—	—	7.7	—	—	—	—
Nursing homes and adult day care[b]	. . .	—	—	—	—	—	4.4	3.1	2.9
Health insurance[d]	. . .	—	—	—	—	—	—	−3.5	−1.1
Medical care commodities	. . .	−0.1	5.0	8.0	4.6	3.1	3.0	3.1	3.0
Medicinal drugs[e]	. . .	—	—	—	—	—	—	. . .	3.1
Prescription drugs[f]	. . .	−1.3	4.3	9.6	5.3	4.0	4.1	4.3	4.2
Nonprescription drugs[e]	. . .	—	—	—	—	—	—	. . .	−1.3
Medical equipment and supplies[e]	. . .	—	—	—	—	—	—	. . .	0.3
Nonprescription drugs and medical supplies[a, g]	. . .	—	—	—	3.1	1.2	0.3	—	—
Internal and respiratory over-the-counter drugs[f]	. . .	—	5.9	6.9	2.7	1.2	0.3	—	—
Nonprescription medical equipment and supplies[g]	. . .	—	—	5.7	3.8	1.4	0.3	—	—

TABLE 10.2

Consumer price index and average annual percentage change for all items, selected items, and medical care components, selected years 1960–2011 [CONTINUED]

[Data are based on reporting by samples of providers and other retail outlets]

—Data not available.
. . .Category not applicable.
[a]December 1986 = 100.
[b]December 1996 = 100.
[c]Special index based on a substantially smaller sample.
[d]December 2005 = 100.
[e]December 2009 = 100.
[f]Prior to 2006, this category included medical supplies.
[g]Starting with 2010 updates, this index series will no longer be published.
[h]Starting with 2010 updates, replaced by the series, Nonprescription drugs.
[i]Starting with 2010 updates, replaced by the series, Medical equipment and supplies.
Notes: CPI for all urban consumers (CPI-U) U.S. city average, detailed expenditure categories. 1982–1984 = 100, except where noted. Data are not seasonally adjusted. Data for additional years are available.

SOURCE: "Table 112. Consumer Price Index and Average Annual Percent Change for All Items, Selected Items, and Medical Care Components: United States, Selected Years 1960–2011," in *Health, United States, 2012: With Special Feature on Emergency Care*, Centers for Disease Control and Prevention, National Center for Health Statistics, 2013, http://www.cdc.gov/nchs/data/hus/hus12.pdf (accessed December 27, 2013)

FIGURE 10.2

Percentage of families with selected financial burdens related to medical care, 2012

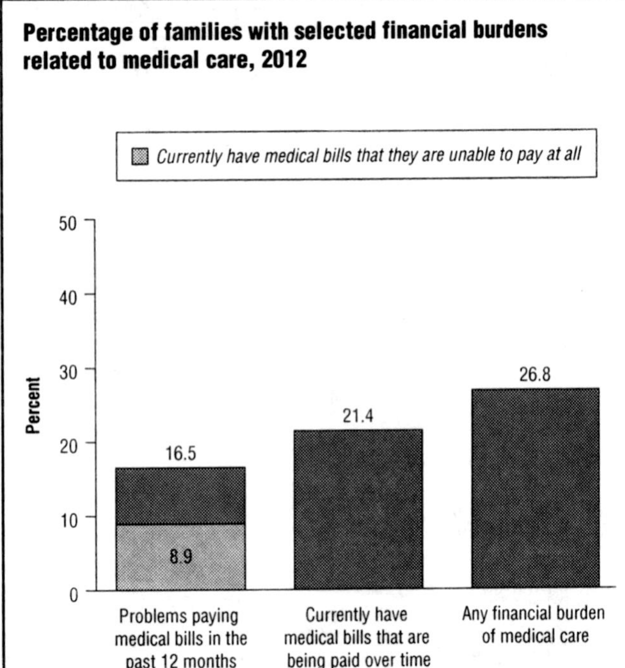

Notes: Data are based on household interviews of a sample of the civilian noninstitutionalized population. Any financial burden of medical care is based on a positive response to a question asking whether anyone in the family experienced "problems paying medical bills in the past 12 months" or a positive response to a question asking whether anyone in the family currently had "medical bills that are being paid over time." Only those who responded positively to the former question were asked if they currently had medical bills that they were unable to pay at all.

SOURCE: Robin A. Cohen and Whitney K. Kirzinger, "Figure 1. Percentage of Families with Selected Financial Burdens of Medical Care: United States, 2012," in "Financial Burden of Medical Care: A Family Perspective," *NCHS Data Brief*, no. 142, Centers for Disease Control and Prevention, National Center for Health Statistics, January 2014, http://www.cdc.gov/nchs/data/databriefs/db142.pdf (accessed February 3, 2014)

making less than 138% of poverty, building on Medicaid's traditional mission of serving needy families with dependent children, pregnant women, the disabled, and other selected groups of low-income people (with variations in eligibility occurring at the state level).

The ACA reached full implementation in January 2014, but its success at expanding health care coverage to those in need was uncertain in the months that followed. One limit on the expansion of coverage came in the form of state opposition to the Medicaid expansion. As of early 2014 at least 23 states had chosen not to expand Medicaid. Additionally, unrelenting opposition from Republicans and other opponents of the law had a significant effect on public perceptions of the ACA, possibly depressing the numbers of enrollees. Furthermore, the federal website created to allow consumers a means of purchasing subsidized insurance experienced major technical difficulties, setting back the enrollment process even further. In an April 1, 2014, news conference, however, Obama stated that 7.1 million Americans had enrolled in health plans under the ACA. The high level of political polarization surrounding the law meant that a clear view of its successes and failures was likely to be obscured for years after the reforms took effect.

Although government subsidies and coverage expansions under the ACA were likely to relieve some of the financial burden felt by a number of poor and middle-class families, it was unclear what effect the law would have on overall health care costs at the national level. In spite of representing a significant enhancement of the government's role in the health care system, the ACA's reforms did not bring about a centralized system such as those that were in place in other wealthy countries. Private health care businesses—such as hospitals, insurance companies, and physicians' offices—were subject to new government regulations, but they remained central players in the health care marketplace.

FIGURE 10.3

Percentage of families with selected financial burdens related to medical care, by poverty level, 2012

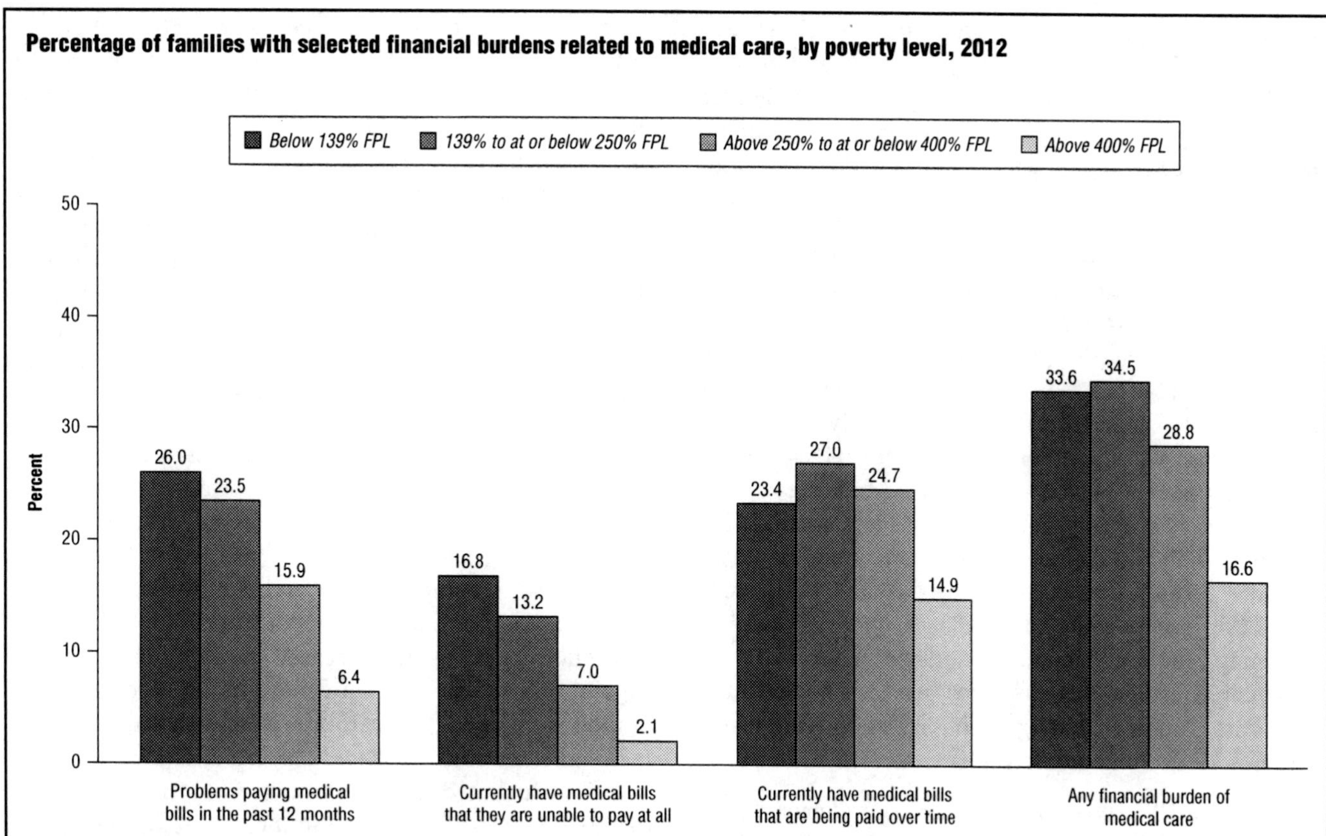

Notes: Data are based on household interviews of a sample of the civilian noninstitutionalized population. Any financial burden of medical care is based on a positive response to a question asking whether anyone in the family experienced "problems paying medical bills in the past 12 months" or a positive response to a question asking whether anyone in the family currently had "medical bills that are being paid over time." Only those who responded positively to the former question were asked if they currently had medical bills that they were unable to pay at all. FPL = federal poverty level.

SOURCE: Robin A. Cohen and Whitney K. Kirzinger, "Figure 2. Percentage of Families with Selected Financial Burdens of Medical Care, by Poverty Level: United States, 2012," in "Financial Burden of Medical Care: A Family Perspective," *NCHS Data Brief*, no. 142, Centers for Disease Control and Prevention, National Center for Health Statistics, January 2014, http://www.cdc.gov/nchs/data/databriefs/db142.pdf (accessed February 3, 2014)

MEETING THE END-OF-LIFE HEALTH CARE NEEDS OF THE ELDERLY

As Donna L. Hoyer and Jiaquan Xu of the National Center for Health Statistics note in "Deaths: Preliminary Data for 2011" (*National Vital Statistics Reports*, vol. 61, no. 6, October 10, 2012), 1.8 million (72.8%) of the 2.5 million people who died in 2011 were aged 65 years and older. Most of these people were covered by Medicare, the federal government program offering universal health care coverage to those aged 65 years and older. As a major source of health care funding for the impoverished and disabled, Medicaid also plays a significant role in end-of-life care for Americans of all ages. Health programs under the U.S. Department of Veterans Affairs and the U.S. Department of Defense also pay for terminal care for some Americans. Many older Americans also make substantial out-of-pocket payments toward their medical expenses.

Medicare

Although not centrally affected by the health care reform effort, which was focused on the insurance market for nonelderly adults and children, Medicare is a major player in the overall medical marketplace. A primary source of funding for most end-of-life care, Medicare consists of a base program that is free for all eligible individuals as well as supplemental forms of fee-based coverage. Medicare's viability as a program has been brought into question as a result of rising health care costs and the rapid growth of the elderly population.

Enacted in 1965 as part of an amendment to the Social Security Act of 1935, Medicare went into effect in 1966 and has been subject to numerous additions and amendments since that time. Today Medicare is divided into two primary components: part A, or hospital insurance; and part B, or supplementary medical insurance. Part A covers costs related to hospital stays, temporary stays in skilled nursing facilities, home health care, and hospice care. Part A is free for all eligible individuals, although there are coverage limits beyond which participants may be required to share costs. Part B covers a range of preventive medical services and other medically necessary care not covered under Part A; most of these services and forms of care, by contrast with Part A, are delivered on an outpatient basis. Part B is optional for as long as participants have other health coverage through an employer or a spouse's employer, but thereafter individuals are subject to penalties if they do not participate in a Part B plan. Participants must reach a deductible under Part B coverage, beyond which Medicare pays for 80% of costs.

There is also a Medicare Part D, introduced in 2003 by the George W. Bush administration and implemented in 2006, which covers prescription drugs. Part D is significantly smaller, as a percentage of total costs, than Parts A and B, but it has rapidly become a major element of the overall Medicare effort. Additionally, there is a Medicare Part C, which consists of health plans offered by private insurers but managed under Medicare regulations. Part C is not truly separate from Parts A and B but represents, rather, a different way of accessing the benefits other people access under Parts A and B. Besides these basic components of Medicare, program participants may purchase Medigap insurance, a form of supplemental coverage that pays for services not covered under Parts A and B. Medigap policies are private insurance, not a government program.

As Table 10.3 shows, the number of Medicare enrollees more than doubled between 1970 and 2011, from 20.4 million to 48.7 million. Medicare's board of trustees, who provide an annual report to Congress on the financial status of the program, predict that the number of Medicare enrollees will again more than double between 2011 and 2080, rising to 112.1 million. (See Figure 10.4.)

The combination of rapidly rising prices for health care and a growing elderly population has resulted in massive increases in overall Medicare spending. In 1970 the total cost of providing seniors with health care coverage under Medicare was $7.5 billion; by 2011 the cost was $549.1 billion. (See Table 10.3.) The elderly have a disproportionate need for medical care, relative to the population as a whole. Those aged 65 years and older accounted for a little over 13% of the U.S. population as of 2010. (See Figure 1.4 in Chapter 1.) Just a year later, in 2011, Medicare accounted for 23% of total health care spending in the United States. (See Figure 10.5.)

Medicare spending, like health care spending in general, has risen more rapidly than GDP since the 1970s. Between 1970 and 2000 Medicare spending grew from 0.7% of GDP to 2.3% of GDP. (See Figure 10.6.) By 2010 continued growth of the elderly population together with the addition of the Part D prescription drug benefit drove accelerated spending, and Medicare spending stood at 3.6% of GDP. Medicare's trustees project that by 2080 Medicare spending will grow to 6.5% of GDP.

The total amount of Medicare spending in 2011 was split almost evenly between Part A ($256.7 billion) and Part B ($225.3 billion). (See Table 10.3.) Part D, the prescription drug benefit, accounted for the remaining $67.1 billion in spending. As Figure 10.7 shows, the components of Medicare spending have shifted over time. In 2006 inpatient hospital stays accounted for 31% of spending, and outpatient managed care accounted for 16% of spending; by 2012 spending on managed care had grown relative to overall spending, accounting for 24% of spending, while spending on inpatient hospital stays had fallen relative to the whole, accounting for 25% of spending. Spending on prescription drugs, physicians' fees, medical equipment, skilled nursing facilities, home health care, and hospice care remained steadier during this period.

Although most Medicare beneficiaries are aged 65 years and older, some nonelderly disabled people and nonelderly people with end-stage renal disease qualify for benefits. (End-stage renal disease is the final phase of irreversible kidney disease and requires either kidney transplantation or dialysis, a medical procedure in which a machine performs the diseased organ's functions.) As Figure 10.8 shows, 83.5% of those in the Medicare population were aged, while 15.5% were disabled and 0.9% had end-stage renal disease. The beneficiaries with disabilities accounted for a slightly disproportionate amount of spending (16.1%) relative to their share of the overall Medicare population, and those beneficiaries with end-stage renal disease accounted for a significantly disproportionate amount of spending, at 6.4% of the total. By age, the costliest groups to cover under Medicare were those under the age of 65 years (who were either disabled or had end-stage renal disease) and those aged 75 years and older. (See Figure 10.9.) Those aged 65 to 74 years accounted for 43.7% of the Medicare population but only 33.1% of total spending.

ELDERLY MEDICAID BENEFICIARIES. Medicaid is not primarily a program for the elderly, but some impoverished people aged 65 years and older are covered by both Medicare and Medicaid. These beneficiaries tend to be unable to afford supplemental Medicare coverage, and they are among the most expensive of Medicaid patients to insure. As Table 10.4 shows, those aged 65 years and older accounted for 6.7% of Medicaid's 62.6 million beneficiaries in 2009. Although the average yearly payment per Medicaid beneficiary was $5,209, the average payment per elderly Medicaid beneficiary was $15,337.

Hospice Care

In 1982 Congress created a Medicare hospice benefit program, via the Tax Equity and Fiscal Responsibility Act, to provide services to terminally ill patients with an anticipated six months or less to live. In 1989 the U.S. General Accounting Office (GAO; now called the U.S. Government Accountability Office) reported that only 35% of eligible hospices were Medicare certified, in part due to the Health

TABLE 10.3

Medicare enrollees and expenditures, by Medicare program and type of service, selected years 1970–2011

[Data are compiled from various sources by the Centers for Medicare & Medicaid Services]

Medicare program and type of service	1970	1980	1990	1995	2000	2005	2008	2009	2010	2011[a]
Enrollees					Number, in millions					
Total Medicare[b]	20.4	28.4	34.3	37.6	39.7	42.6	45.5	46.6	47.7	48.7
Hospital insurance	20.1	28.0	33.7	37.2	39.3	42.2	45.1	46.3	47.3	48.3
Supplementary medical insurance (SMI)[c]	19.5	27.3	32.6	35.6	37.3	—	—	—	—	—
Part B	19.5	27.3	32.6	35.6	37.3	39.8	42.0	42.9	43.9	44.9
Part D[d]	—	—	—	—	—	1.8	32.6	33.6	34.8	35.7
Expenditures					Amount, in billions					
Total Medicare	$7.5	$36.8	$111.0	$184.2	$221.8	$336.4	$468.2	$509.0	$522.9	$549.1
Total hospital insurance (HI)	5.3	25.6	67.0	117.6	131.1	182.9	235.6	242.5	247.9	256.7
HI payments to managed care organizations[e]	—	0.0	2.7	6.7	21.4	24.9	50.6	59.4	60.7	64.6
HI payments for fee-for-service utilization	5.1	25.0	63.4	109.5	105.1	156.6	172.8	179.5	183.3	186.9
Inpatient hospital	4.8	24.1	56.9	82.3	87.1	123.3	130.3	133.9	136.1	132.7
Skilled nursing facility	0.2	0.4	2.5	9.1	11.1	19.3	24.4	26.2	27.0	32.9
Home health agency	0.1	0.5	3.7	16.2	4.0	6.0	6.7	7.1	7.2	7.3
Hospice	—	—	0.3	1.9	2.9	8.0	11.4	12.3	13.1	14.0
Incentive payments[f]	—	—	—	—	—	—	—	—	0.0	0.9
Home health agency transfer[g]	—	—	—	—	1.7	—	—	—	—	—
Medicare Advantage premiums[h]	—	—	—	—	—	—	0.1	0.1	0.2	0.2
Accounting error (CY 2005–2008)[i]	—	—	—	—	—	−1.9	8.5	—	—	—
Administrative expenses[j]	0.2	0.5	0.9	1.4	2.9	3.3	3.6	3.5	3.8	4.1
Total supplementary medical insurance (SMI)[c]	2.2	11.2	44.0	66.6	90.7	153.5	232.6	266.5	274.9	292.5
Total Part B	2.2	11.2	44.0	66.6	90.7	152.4	183.3	205.7	212.9	225.3
Part B payments to managed care organizations[e]	0.0	0.2	2.8	6.6	18.4	22.0	48.1	53.4	55.2	59.1
Part B payments for fee-for-service utilization[k]	1.9	10.4	39.6	58.4	72.2	125.0	140.5	149.0	154.3	162.3
Physician/supplies[l]	1.8	8.2	29.6	—	—	—	—	—	—	—
Outpatient hospital[m]	0.1	1.9	8.5	—	—	—	—	—	—	—
Independent laboratory[n]	0.0	0.1	1.5	—	—	—	—	—	—	—
Physician fee schedule	—	—	—	31.7	37.0	57.7	60.6	61.8	63.9	67.5
Durable medical equipment	—	—	—	3.7	4.7	8.0	8.6	8.2	8.3	8.2
Laboratory[o]	—	—	—	4.3	4.4	6.9	7.9	8.7	8.9	8.9
Other[p]	—	—	—	9.9	13.6	26.7	29.6	32.4	33.3	34.7
Hospital[q]	—	—	—	8.7	8.1	18.7	23.6	26.3	28.1	30.7
Home health agency	0.0	0.2	0.1	0.2	4.5	7.1	10.3	11.6	11.8	12.4
Home health agency transfer[g]	—	—	—	—	−1.7	—	—	—	—	—
Medicare Advantage premiums[h]	—	—	—	—	—	—	0.1	0.1	0.2	0.2
Accounting error (CY 2005–2008)[i]	—	—	—	—	—	1.9	−8.5	—	—	—
Administrative expenses[j]	0.2	0.6	1.5	1.6	1.8	2.8	3.1	3.2	3.2	3.7
Part D start-up costs[r]	—	—	—	—	—	0.7	0.0	—	—	—
Total Part D[d]	—	—	—	—	—	1.1	49.3	60.8	62.1	67.1
					Percent distribution of expenditures					
Total hospital insurance (HI)	100.0	100.0	100.0	100.0	100.0	100.0	100.0	100.0	100.0	100.0
HI payments to managed care organizations[e]	—	0.0	4.0	5.7	16.3	13.6	21.5	24.5	24.5	25.2
HI payments for fee-for-service utilization	97.0	97.9	94.6	93.1	80.2	85.6	73.4	74.0	73.9	72.8
Inpatient hospital	91.4	94.3	85.0	70.0	66.4	67.4	55.3	55.2	54.9	51.7
Skilled nursing facility	4.7	1.5	3.7	7.8	8.5	10.6	10.4	10.8	10.9	12.8
Home health agency	1.0	2.1	5.5	13.8	3.1	3.3	2.8	2.9	2.9	2.8
Hospice	—	—	0.5	1.6	2.2	4.4	4.8	5.1	5.3	5.5
Incentive payments[f]	—	—	—	—	—	—	—	—	0.0	0.3
Home health agency transfer[g]	—	—	—	—	1.3	—	—	—	—	—
Medicare Advantage premiums[h]	—	—	—	—	—	—	0.0	0.1	0.1	0.1
Accounting error (CY 2005–2008)[i]	—	—	—	—	—	−1.0	3.6	—	—	—
Administrative expenses[j]	3.0	2.1	1.4	1.2	2.2	1.8	1.5	1.4	1.5	1.6
Total supplementary medical insurance (SMI)[c]	100.0	100.0	100.0	100.0	100.0	100.0	100.0	100.0	100.0	100.0
Total Part B	100.0	100.0	100.0	100.0	100.0	99.3	78.8	77.2	77.4	77.1
Part B payments to managed care organizations[e]	1.2	1.8	6.4	9.9	20.2	14.3	20.7	20.0	20.1	20.2
Part B payments for fee-for-service utilization[k]	88.1	92.8	90.1	87.6	79.6	81.5	60.4	55.9	56.1	55.5
Physician/supplies[l]	80.9	72.8	67.3	—	—	—	—	—	—	—
Outpatient hospital[m]	5.2	16.9	19.3	—	—	—	—	—	—	—
Independent laboratory[n]	0.5	1.0	3.4	—	—	—	—	—	—	—
Physician fee schedule	—	—	—	47.5	40.8	37.6	26.0	23.2	23.2	23.1
Durable medical equipment	—	—	—	5.5	5.2	5.2	3.7	3.1	3.0	2.8
Laboratory[o]	—	—	—	6.4	4.8	4.5	3.4	3.3	3.3	3.1
Other[p]	—	—	—	14.8	15.0	17.4	12.7	12.2	12.1	11.9
Hospital[q]	—	—	—	13.0	8.9	12.2	10.1	9.9	10.2	10.5
Home health agency	1.5	2.1	0.2	0.3	4.9	4.6	4.4	4.3	4.3	4.2

TABLE 10.3

Medicare enrollees and expenditures, by Medicare program and type of service, selected years 1970–2011 [CONTINUED]

[Data are compiled from various sources by the Centers for Medicare & Medicaid Services]

Medicare program and type of service	1970	1980	1990	1995	2000	2005	2008	2009	2010	2011[a]
Home health agency transfer[g]	—	—	—	—	−1.9	—	—	—	—	—
Medicare advantage premiums[h]	—	—	—	—	—	—	0.0	0.0	0.1	0.1
Accounting error (CY 2005–2008)[i]	—	—	—	—	—	1.2	−3.6	—	—	—
Administrative expenses[j]	10.7	5.4	3.5	2.4	2.0	1.8	1.3	1.2	1.2	1.3
Part D start-up costs[r]	—	—	—	—	—	0.4	0.0	—	—	—
Total Part D[d]	—	—	—	—	—	**0.7**	**21.2**	**22.8**	**22.6**	**22.9**

—Category not applicable or data not available.
0.0 Quantity more than zero but less than 0.05.
[a]Preliminary estimates.
[b]Average number enrolled in the hospital insurance (HI) and/or supplementary medical insurance (SMI) programs for the period.
[c]Starting with 2004 data, the SMI trust fund consists of two separate accounts: Part B (which pays for a portion of the costs of physicians' services, outpatient hospital services, and other related medical and health services for voluntarily enrolled individuals) and Part D (Medicare Prescription Drug Account, which pays private plans to provide prescription drug coverage).
[d]The Medicare Modernization Act, enacted December 8, 2003, established within SMI two Part D accounts related to prescription drug benefits: the Medicare Prescription Drug Account and the Transitional Assistance Account. The Medicare Prescription Drug Account is used in conjunction with the broad, voluntary prescription drug benefits that began in 2006. The Transitional Assistance Account was used to provide transitional assistance benefits, beginning in 2004 and extending through 2005, for certain low-income beneficiaries prior to the start of the new prescription drug benefit. The amounts shown for Total Part D expenditures—and thus for total SMI expenditures and total Medicare expenditures—for 2006 and later years include estimated amounts for premiums paid directly from Part D beneficiaries to Part D prescription drug plans.
[e]Medicare-approved managed care organizations.
[f]Includes Community-Based Care Transitions Program ($125 million in 2011) and Electronic Health Records Incentive Program ($739 million in 2011).
[g]For 1998 to 2003 data, reflects annual home health HI to SMI transfer amounts.
[h]When a beneficiary chooses a Medicare Advantage plan whose monthly premium exceeds the benchmark amount, the additional premiums (that is, amounts beyond those paid by Medicare to the plan) are the responsibility of the beneficiary. Beneficiaries subject to such premiums may choose to either reimburse the plans directly or have the additional premiums deducted from their Social Security checks. The amounts shown here are only those additional premiums deducted from Social Security checks. These amounts are transferred to the HI trust and SMI trust funds and then transferred from the trust funds to the plans.
[i]Represents misallocation of benefit payments between the HI trust fund and the Part B account of the SMI trust fund from May 2005 to September 2007, and the transfer made in June 2008 to correct the misallocation.
[j]Includes expenditures for research, experiments and demonstration projects, peer review activity (performed by Peer Review Organizations from 1983 to 2001 and by Quality Review Organizations from 2002 to present), and to combat and prevent fraud and abuse.
[k]Type-of-service reporting categories for fee-for-service reimbursement differ before and after 1991.
[l]Includes payment for physicians, practitioners, durable medical equipment, and all suppliers other than independent laboratory through 1990. Starting with 1991 data, physician services subject to the physician fee schedule are shown. Payments for laboratory services paid under the laboratory fee schedule and performed in a physician office are included under Laboratory beginning in 1991. Payments for durable medical equipment are shown separately beginning in 1991. The remaining services from the Physician/supplies category are included in other.
[m]Includes payments for hospital outpatient department services, skilled nursing facility outpatient services, Part B services received as an inpatient in a hospital or skilled nursing facility setting, and other types of outpatient facilities. Starting with 1991 data, payments for hospital outpatient department services, except for laboratory services, are listed under Hospital. Hospital outpatient laboratory services are included in the Laboratory line.
[n]Starting with 1991 data, those independent laboratory services that were paid under the laboratory fee schedule (most of the independent laboratory category) are included in the Laboratory line; the remaining services are included in the Physician fee schedule and other lines.
[o]Payments for laboratory services paid under the laboratory fee schedule performed in a physician office, independent laboratory, or in a hospital outpatient department.
[p]Includes payments for physician-administered drugs; freestanding ambulatory surgical center facility services; ambulance services; supplies; freestanding end-stage renal disease (ESRD) dialysis facility services; rural health clinics; outpatient rehabilitation facilities; psychiatric hospitals; and federally qualified health centers.
[q]Includes the hospital facility costs for Medicare Part B services that are predominantly in the outpatient department, with the exception of hospital outpatient laboratory services, which are included on the Laboratory line. Physician reimbursement is included on the Physician fee schedule line.
[r]Part D start-up costs were funded through the SMI Part B account in 2004–2008.
Notes: Estimates are subject to change as more recent data become available. Totals may not equal the sum of the components because of rounding. Estimates are for Medicare-covered services furnished to Medicare enrollees residing in the United States, Puerto Rico, Virgin Islands, Guam, other outlying areas, foreign countries, and unknown residence. Estimates in this table have been revised and differ from previous editions of *Health, United States*.

SOURCE: "Table 126. Medicare Enrollees and Expenditures and Percent Distribution, by Medicare Program and Type of Service: United States and Other Areas, Selected Years 1970–2011," in *Health, United States, 2012: With Special Feature on Emergency Care*, Centers for Disease Control and Prevention, National Center for Health Statistics, 2013, http://www.cdc.gov/nchs/data/hus/hus12.pdf (accessed December 27, 2013)

Care Financing Administration's low rates of reimbursement to hospices. That same year Congress gave hospices a 20% increase in reimbursement rates through a provision in the Omnibus Budget Reconciliation Act.

Under the Balanced Budget Act (BBA) of 1997, Medicare hospice benefits are divided into three benefit periods:

- An initial 90-day period
- A subsequent 90-day period
- An unlimited number of subsequent 60-day periods, but only if a patient continues to satisfy the program eligibility requirements

At the start of each period the Medicare patient must be recertified as terminally ill. After the patient's death, the patient's family receives up to 13 months of bereavement counseling.

The National Association for Home Care and Hospice (NAHCH; http://www.nahc.org/assets/1/7/2011hhas.pdf) reports that as of April 2011 there were 3,533 Medicare-certified hospices. At that time Medicare paid most of the cost of hospice care. Terminally ill patients who stay in a hospice incur lower Medicare costs than those who stay in a hospital or skilled nursing facility. In 2009 a one-day stay in a hospice cost Medicare $153, compared with $622 for a skilled nursing facility and $6,200 for a hospital. (See Table 10.5.)

FIGURE 10.4

Historic and projected Medicare enrollment, 1970–2080

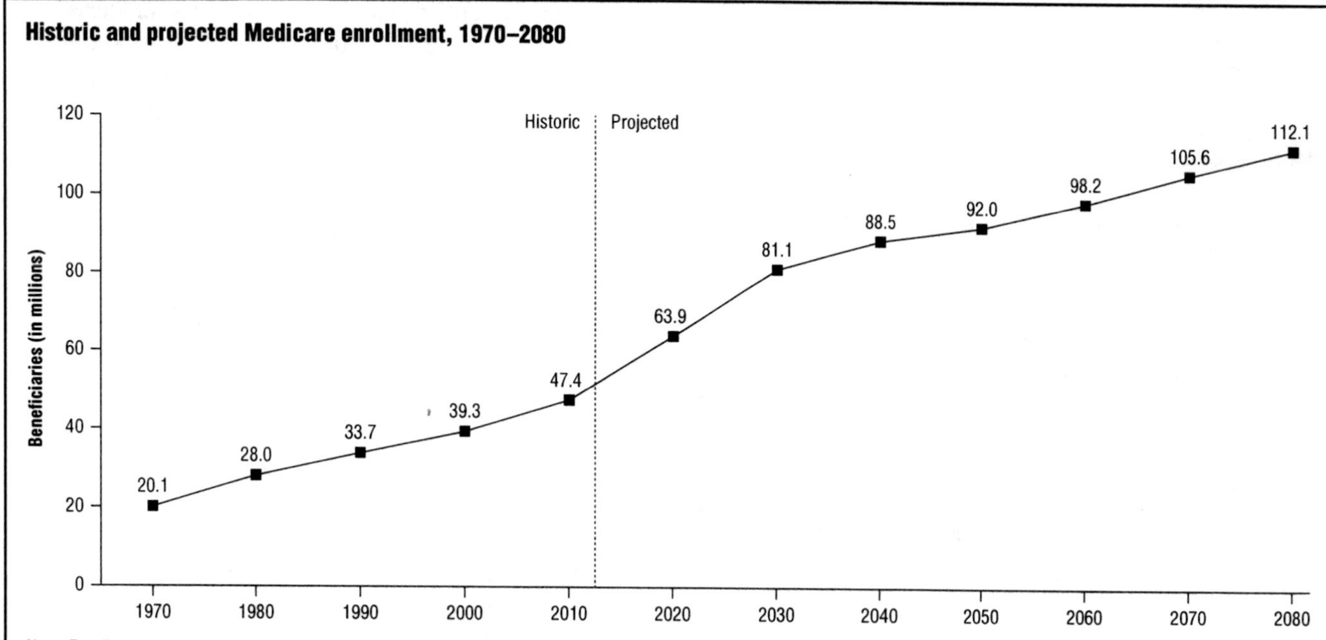

Note: Enrollment numbers are based on Part A enrollment only. Beneficiaries enrolled only in Part B are not included.

SOURCE: "Chart 2-4. Enrollment in the Medicare Program Is Projected to Grow Rapidly in the Next 20 Years," in *A Data Book: Health Care Spending and the Medicare Program*, Medicare Payment Advisory Commission (MedPAC), June 2013, http://www.medpac.gov/documents/Jun13DataBookEntireReport.pdf (accessed December 29, 2013)

Home Health Care

The concept of home health care began as postacute care after hospitalization, an alternative to longer, costlier hospital stays. The Centers for Medicare and Medicaid Services explains in *Medicare and Home Health Care* (June 2010, http://www.medicare.gov/Publications/Pubs/pdf/10969.pdf) that in the 21st century Medicare's home health care services provide medical help, prescribed by a doctor, to home-bound people who are covered by Medicare. Having been hospitalized is not a prerequisite. There are no limits to the number of professional visits or to the length of coverage. As long as the patient's condition warrants it, the following services are provided:

- Part-time or intermittent skilled nursing and home health aide services
- Speech-language pathology services
- Physical and occupational therapy
- Medical social services
- Medical supplies
- Durable medical equipment (such as walkers and hospital beds, with a 20% co-pay)

According to the NAHCH, as of April 21, 2011, there were 11,633 Medicare-certified home health agencies. However, Medicare coverage of home health needs tends to be temporary. Those patients who have a protracted need for constant medical attention in the home must typically find other funding sources.

Long-Term Care

Longer life spans and improved life-sustaining technologies have created an increasing need for long-term care, usually defined as care that is continuously ongoing for an average of three years. The Kaiser Family Foundation (KFF) notes in "A Short Look at Long-Term Care for Seniors" (*Journal of the American Medical Association*, vol. 301, no. 8, August 28, 2013) that 70% of all adults aged 65 years and older will need long-term care before their deaths, and 20% will require long-term care that lasts for five years or more. Of the 12 million Americans who needed long-term care in 2010, 87% received it from family members on an unpaid basis. The KFF estimates the annual value of unpaid labor devoted to long-term care at $450 billion as of 2009, and it projects that the number of Americans requiring long-term care will more than double by 2050, increasing from 12 million to 27 million.

Although Medicare covers postacute home health care and temporary care in skilled nursing facilities (which are similar to nursing homes), it typically does not cover long-term care, whether that care is delivered in the home or in an institution such as a nursing home. Medicaid, however, does cover long-term care for those impoverished elderly adults who meet the program's eligibility criteria. Among long-term care recipients who were paying for that care in 2011, Medicaid was the single largest source of funding, accounting for 40% of the total $357 billion spent on long-term care that year. (See Figure 10.10.) Another 21% of

FIGURE 10.5

Percentage of total health care spending funded by public and private payers, 2011

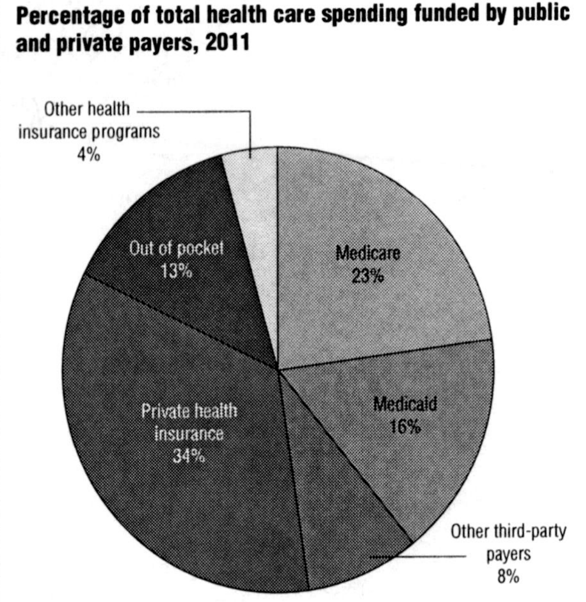

Total = $2.28 trillion

Note: All data are for calendar year 2011. Out-of-pocket spending includes cost sharing for both privately and publicly insured individuals. Personal health care is a subset of national health expenditures. It includes spending for all medical goods and services that are provided to treat or prevent a specific disease or condition in a specific person and excludes other spending, such as government administration, the net cost of health insurance, public health, and investment. Premiums are included with each program (e.g., Medicare, private insurance) rather than in the out-of-pocket category. Other health insurance programs include the Children's Health Insurance Program, Department of Defense, and Department of Veterans' Affairs. Other third-party payers include worksite health care, other private revenues, Indian Health Service, workers' compensation, general assistance, maternal and child health, vocational rehabilitation, other federal programs, Substance Abuse and Mental Health Services Administration, other state and local programs, and school health. Numbers do not add to 100 percent due to rounding.

SOURCE: "Chart 1-3. Medicare Made up over One-Fifth of Spending on Personal Health Care in 2011," in *A Data Book: Health Care Spending and the Medicare Program*, Medicare Payment Advisory Commission (MedPAC), June 2013, http://www.medpac.gov/documents/Jun13DataBookEntireReport.pdf (accessed December 29, 2013)

total long-term care expenditures were paid for under Medicare's postacute care coverage, 15% was paid out-of-pocket by patients and their families, 7% was paid for by private insurers, and 18% was paid for by other private and public sources.

As Medicare does not cover long-term care and Medicaid covers only people who are poor, Americans who are not impoverished must either have private insurance that covers long-term care, the assets to pay for long-term care out-of-pocket, or family members who are able and willing to provide them with long-term care. Otherwise, the costs of such care will exhaust whatever funds they do have, driving them into poverty and the Medicaid program. In spite of the fact that most people will require long-term care at the end of life, only 35% of people aged 40 years and older have set aside money to pay for such care, according to the KFF.

NURSING HOMES. Among long-term care options, nursing homes are by far the most costly. For those who require labor-intensive, round-the-clock care, however, nursing homes may be the only viable option. Nursing homes provide terminally ill residents with end-of-life services in a variety of ways:

- Caring for patients in the nursing home
- Transferring patients who request it to hospitals or hospices
- Contracting with hospices to provide palliative care (care that relieves the pain but does not cure the illness) within the nursing home

Since the 1990s the number of people being cared for in nursing homes has declined at the national level, with some variations at the state level. (See Table 10.6.) Growth of the home health care industry is likely partly responsible for the decline in nursing home populations, as home health care is a less costly option for those needing long-term care. Another factor is likely the increased popularity of assisted-living and continuing-care retirement communities, which offer alternatives to nursing home care for those people who need less than round-the-clock assistance, and which cost less on average than nursing home care. There is also a trend toward healthy aging—more older adults are living longer with fewer disabilities. Finally, the high cost of nursing home care is a prohibitive factor for many older Americans.

In 2011 there were 15,702 nursing homes in the United States with a combined occupancy of just over 1.7 million beds, down from 16,389 nursing homes and 1.75 million beds in 1995. (See Table 10.6.) Slightly fewer than 1.4 million adults were nursing home residents in 2011, for an overall occupancy rate of 81.6%. The lowest occupancy rates were in Oregon (61.3%), Utah (65%), and Indiana (66.3%). The highest occupancy rates were in the District of Columbia (94.2%), Alaska (91.7%), New York (91.6%), and Rhode Island (91.6%). According to the *Genworth 2013 Cost of Care Survey* (2013, https://www.genworth.com/dam/Americas/US/PDFs/Consumer/corporate/130568_032213_Cost%20of%20Care_Final_nonsecure.pdf), a comprehensive annual survey of long-term care costs produced by Genworth Financial (a public company that offers long-term care insurance), the median rate paid by nursing home residents in 2012 was $207 per day (or $75,555 per year) for a semiprivate room and $230 per day (or $83,950 per year) for a private room.

PATIENTS WITH TERMINAL DISEASES

Acquired Immunodeficiency Syndrome

The acquired immunodeficiency syndrome (AIDS) is a set of signs, symptoms, and diseases that occur together when the immune system of a person who is infected with the human immunodeficiency virus (HIV) becomes

FIGURE 10.6

Projected increases in Medicare spending as a percentage of GDP, 1970–2080

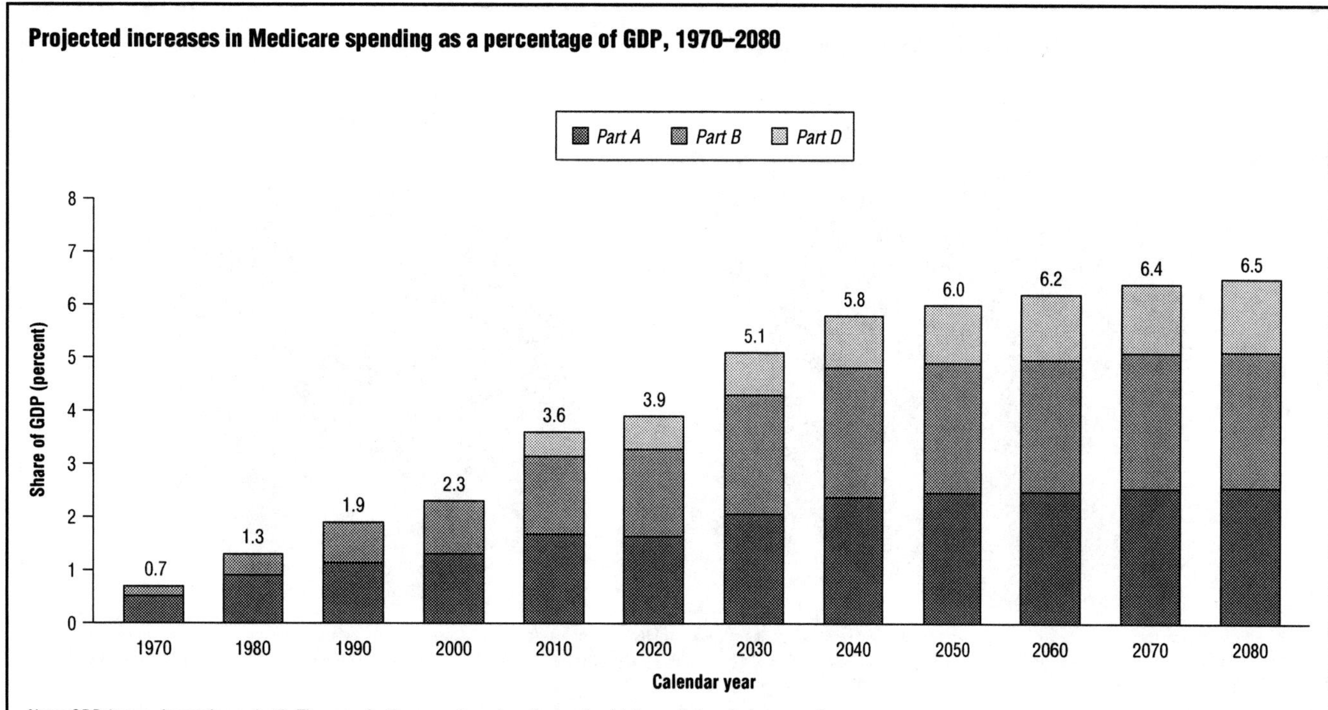

Note: GDP (gross domestic product). These projections are based on the trustees' intermediate set of assumptions.

SOURCE: "Chart 1-6. Trustees Project Medicare Spending to Increase As a Share of GDP," in *A Data Book: Health Care Spending and the Medicare Program*, Medicare Payment Advisory Commission (MedPAC), June 2013, http://www.medpac.gov/documents/Jun13DataBookEntireReport.pdf (accessed December 29, 2013)

FIGURE 10.7

Medicare spending by type of service, 2006 and 2012

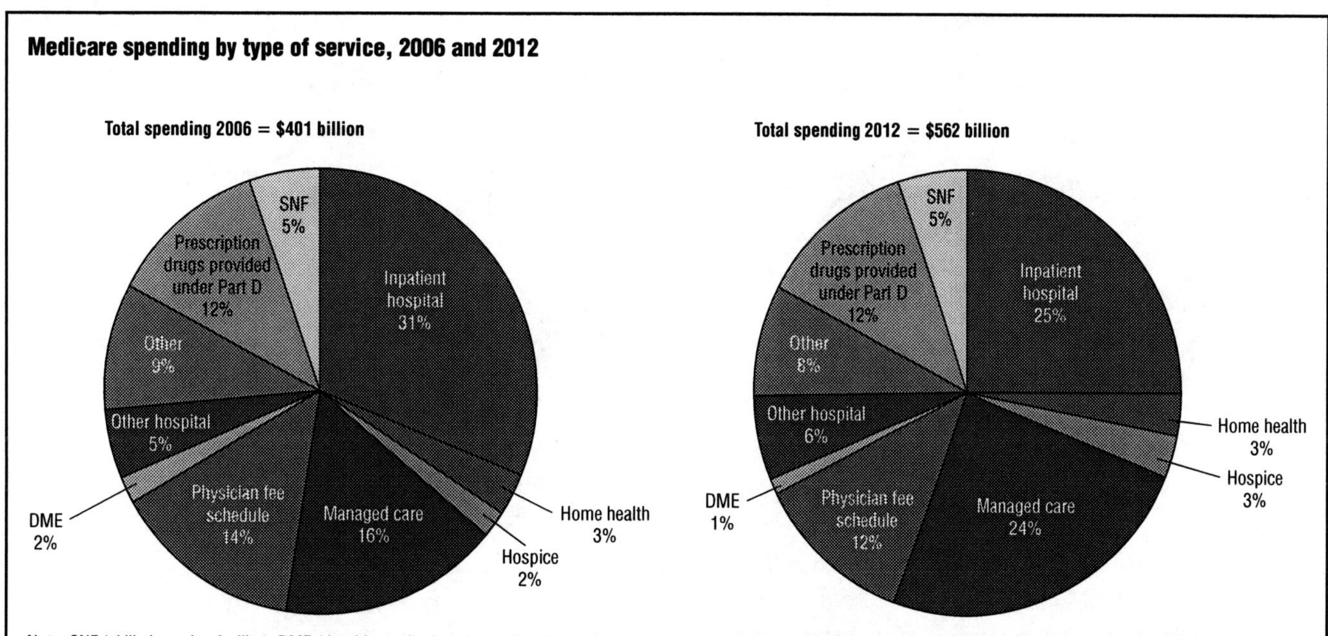

Note: SNF (skilled nursing facility), DME (durable medical equipment). All data are by calendar year. Dollars are Medicare spending only and do not include beneficiary cost sharing. "Other" includes carrier lab, other carrier, intermediary lab, and other intermediary. Totals may not sum to 100 percent due to rounding.

SOURCE: "Chart 1-9. Medicare Spending Is Concentrated in Certain Services and Has Shifted over Time," in *A Data Book: Health Care Spending and the Medicare Program*, Medicare Payment Advisory Commission (MedPAC), June 2013, http://www.medpac.gov/documents/Jun13DataBookEntireReport.pdf (accessed December 29, 2013)

extremely weakened. Advances in treatment during the mid- to late 1990s made it possible to slow the progression of HIV infection to AIDS, which led to dramatic decreases in AIDS deaths. Whereas an HIV diagnosis represented a death sentence in the 1980s, by the early 21st century HIV-infected individuals were able to

FIGURE 10.8

Medicare enrollment and spending, by type of beneficiary, 2009

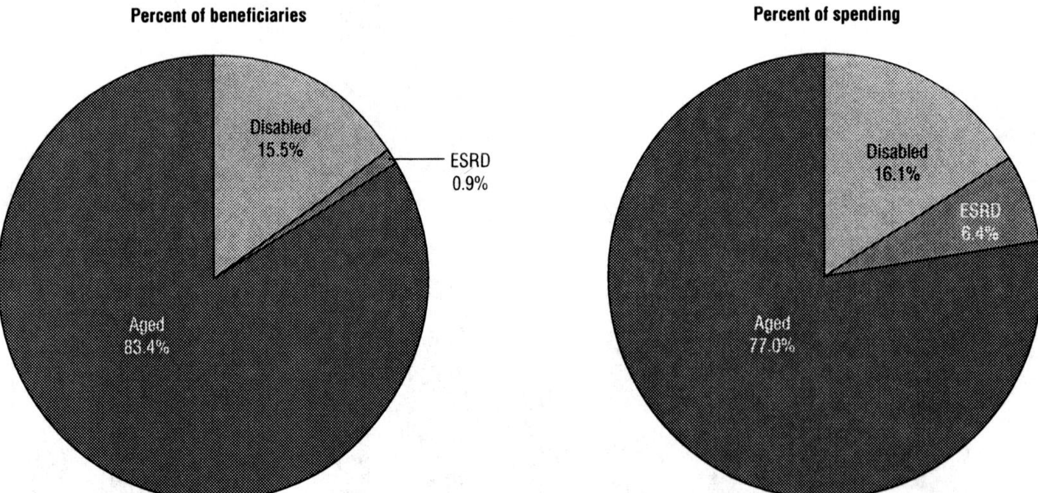

Note: ESRD (end-stage renal disease). The aged category refers to beneficiaries age 65 or older without ESRD. The disabled category refers to beneficiaries under age 65 without ESRD. The ESRD category refers to beneficiaries with ESRD, regardless of age. Results include fee-for-service. Medicare Advantage, community dwelling, and institutionalized beneficiaries. Totals may not sum to 100 percent due to missing data or to rounding.

SOURCE: "Chart 2-1. Aged Beneficiaries Account for the Greatest Share of the Medicare Population and Program Spending, 2009," in *A Data Book: Health Care Spending and the Medicare Program*, Medicare Payment Advisory Commission (MedPAC), June 2013, http://www.medpac.gov/documents/Jun13DataBookEntireReport.pdf (accessed December 29, 2013)

FIGURE 10.9

Medicare enrollment and spending, by age group, 2009

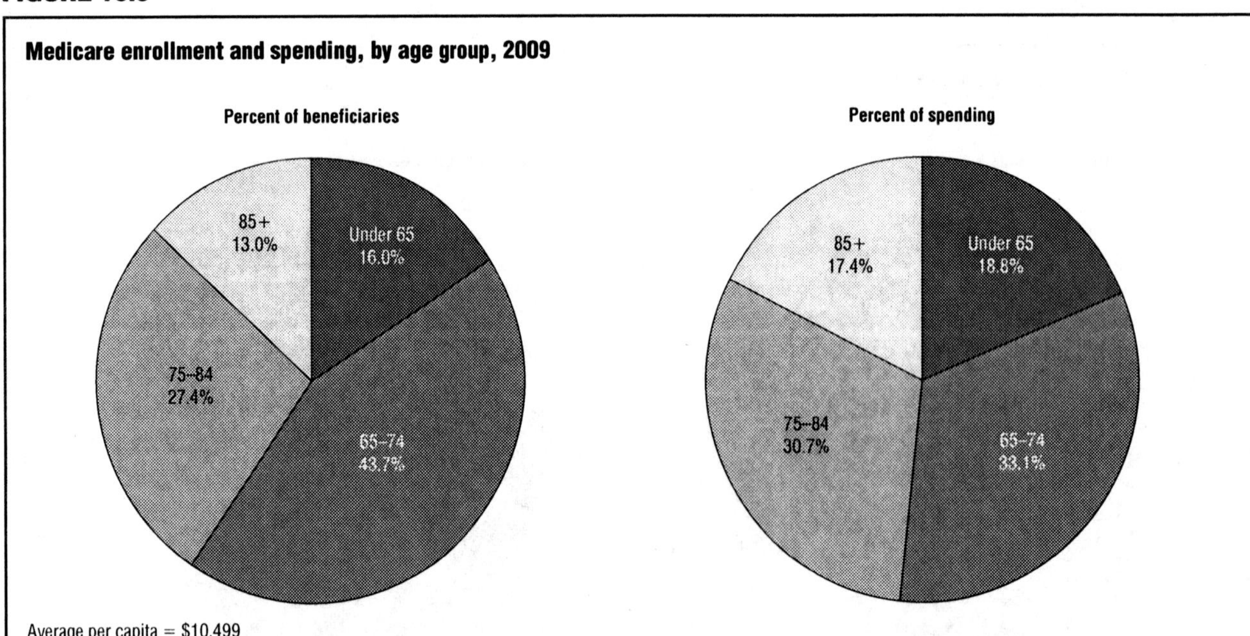

Average per capita = $10,499

Note: Results include fee-for-service, Medicare Advantage, community dwelling, and institutionalized beneficiaries. Totals may not sum to 100 percent due to rounding.

SOURCE: "Chart 2-2. Medicare Enrollment and Spending by Age Group, 2009," in *A Data Book: Health Care Spending and the Medicare Program*, Medicare Payment Advisory Commission (MedPAC), June 2013, http://www.medpac.gov/documents/Jun13DataBookEntireReport.pdf (accessed December 29, 2013)

manage their conditions and live relatively normal lives, provided that they had access to high-quality health care and drug treatments.

Among the poor, however, HIV infection retains much of its deadly force. The disease is more common, more likely to develop into AIDS, and more likely to lead to

TABLE 10.4

Medicaid recipients and payments, by basis of eligibility, and by race and Hispanic origin, selected fiscal years 1999–2009

[Data are compiled by the Centers for Medicare & Medicaid Services from the Medicaid Data System]

Basis of eligibility and race and Hispanic origin	1999	2000	2003	2004	2005	2006	2007	2008	2009
Beneficiaries[a]					Number, in millions				
All beneficiaries	40.1	42.8	52.0	55.6	57.7	57.8	56.8	58.8	62.6
Basis of eligibility:					Percent of beneficiaries				
Aged (65 years and over)	9.4	8.7	7.8	7.8	7.6	7.6	7.1	7.1	6.7
Blind and disabled	16.7	16.1	14.8	14.6	14.2	14.4	14.8	14.8	14.4
Adults in families with dependent children[b]	18.7	20.5	22.5	22.5	21.5	21.9	21.8	21.8	22.7
Children under age 21[c]	46.9	46.1	47.8	47.8	47.5	48.0	48.4	48.0	47.7
Other Title XIX[d]	8.4	8.6	7.2	7.3	9.1	8.1	7.8	8.4	8.4
Race and Hispanic origin:[e]									
White	—	—	41.2	41.1	39.3	39.1	38.6	38.1	38.2
Black or African American	—	—	22.4	22.1	21.5	21.8	21.6	21.1	20.7
American Indian or Alaska Native	—	—	1.4	1.3	1.2	1.2	1.2	1.3	1.2
Asian or Pacific Islander	—	—	3.3	3.3	3.5	3.5	3.5	3.5	3.6
Asian	—	—	2.4	2.4	2.5	2.6	2.6	2.6	2.7
Pacific Islander	—	—	0.9	0.9	0.9	0.9	0.9	0.9	0.9
Hispanic or Latino	—	—	19.3	19.4	20.6	21.0	21.6	21.7	22.3
Multiple race or unknown	—	—	12.5	12.7	13.9	13.3	13.5	14.3	14.0
Payments[f]					Amount, in billions				
All payments	$153.5	$168.3	$233.2	$257.7	$274.9	$269.0	$276.2	$294.2	$326.0
					Percent distribution				
Total	**100.0**	**100.0**	**100.0**	**100.0**	**100.0**	**100.0**	**100.0**	**100.0**	**100.0**
Basis of eligibility:									
Aged (65 years and over)	27.7	26.4	23.7	23.1	23.1	21.6	20.7	20.6	19.7
Blind and disabled	42.9	43.2	43.7	43.3	43.4	43.3	43.3	43.5	43.4
Adults in families with dependent children[b]	10.3	10.6	11.5	12.0	11.7	12.3	12.4	12.6	13.8
Children under age 21[c]	15.7	15.9	17.1	17.2	17.3	18.8	19.4	19.4	19.6
Other Title XIX[d]	3.4	3.9	4.0	4.5	4.6	3.9	4.2	4.0	3.4
Race and Hispanic origin:[e]									
White	—	—	53.8	53.4	53.0	52.1	50.7	50.2	50.0
Black or African American	—	—	19.7	19.8	19.8	20.4	20.8	20.6	20.7
American Indian or Alaska Native	—	—	1.2	1.2	1.2	1.2	1.2	1.3	1.2
Asian or Pacific Islander	—	—	2.4	2.5	2.7	2.8	2.8	2.9	3.1
Asian	—	—	1.6	1.7	1.9	2.0	2.0	2.1	2.3
Pacific Islander	—	—	0.8	0.8	0.8	0.8	0.8	0.8	0.8
Hispanic or Latino	—	—	10.6	10.7	12.2	12.8	13.1	13.7	14.2
Multiple race or unknown	—	—	12.2	12.3	11.1	10.8	11.4	11.4	10.8
Payments per beneficiary[f]					Amount				
All beneficiaries	$3,819	$3,936	$4,487	$4,639	$4,768	$4,657	$4,862	$5,051	$5,209
Basis of eligibility:									
Aged (65 years and over)	11,268	11,929	13,677	13,687	14,427	13,276	14,141	14,742	15,337
Blind and disabled	9,832	10,559	13,303	13,714	14,531	13,982	14,194	14,843	15,670
Adults in families with dependent children[b]	2,104	2,030	2,292	2,471	2,587	2,622	2,753	2,917	3,152
Children under age 21[c]	1,282	1,358	1,606	1,664	1,735	1,825	1,951	2,038	2,145
Other Title XIX[d]	1,532	1,778	2,474	2,896	2,380	2,255	2,622	2,407	2,125
Race and Hispanic origin:[e]									
White	—	—	5,870	6,026	6,422	6,199	6,390	6,657	6,809
Black or African American	—	—	3,944	4,158	4,397	4,358	4,669	4,928	5,216
American Indian or Alaska Native	—	—	4,001	4,320	4,626	4,489	4,826	5,218	5,382
Asian or Pacific Islander	—	—	3,327	3,513	3,710	3,696	3,863	4,133	4,402
Asian	—	—	2,993	3,198	3,624	3,657	3,847	4,123	4,386
Pacific Islander	—	—	4,223	4,366	3,947	3,799	3,907	4,161	4,448
Hispanic or Latino	—	—	2,463	2,563	2,822	2,831	2,960	3,175	3,322
Multiple race or unknown	—	—	4,396	4,493	3,816	3,770	4,106	4,014	4,025

premature death among those who live in poverty or who do not have reliable access to health care. Medicaid has historically played a major role in providing for the care of the HIV-positive population in the United States. Even before the ACA expanded Medicaid eligibility, many HIV patients qualified for coverage because the disease had permanently disabled them. Besides those who are poor at the time that they contract HIV, many patients become impoverished because of the condition, and Medicaid then becomes their primary recourse for health care coverage. For example, people in whom the disease progresses are often forced to discontinue working. If these people have private health insurance through their employers, they lose their coverage when they become too ill to work.

TABLE 10.4

Medicaid recipients and payments, by basis of eligibility, and by race and Hispanic origin, selected fiscal years 1999–2009 [CONTINUED]

[Data are compiled by the Centers for Medicare & Medicaid Services from the Medicaid Data System]

—Data not available.
[a]Beneficiaries include those who received services through Medicaid.
[b]Includes adults who meet the requirements for the Aid to Families with Dependent Children (AFDC) program that were in effect in their state on July 16, 1996, or, at state option, more liberal criteria (with some exceptions). Includes adults in the Temporary Assistance for Needy Families (TANF) program. Starting with 2001 data, includes women in the Breast and Cervical Cancer Prevention and Treatment Program and unemployed adults.
[c]Includes children (including those in the foster care system) in the TANF program.
[d]Includes some participants in the Supplemental Security Income program and other people deemed medically needy in participating states. Prior to 2001, includes unemployed adults. Excludes foster care children and includes unknown eligibility.
[e]Race and Hispanic origin are as determined on initial Medicaid application. Categories are mutually exclusive. Starting with 2001 data, the Hispanic category included Hispanic persons, are gardless of race. Persons indicating more than one race were included in the multiple race category.
[f]Medicaid payments exclude disproportionate share hospital (DSH) payments ($14.7 billion in fiscal year 2009) and DSH mental health facility payments ($3.1 billion in fiscal year 2009).
Notes: Data are for fiscal year ending September 30. Some data have been revised and differ from previous editions of *Health, United States*. Data for additional years are available.

SOURCE: "Table 129. Medicaid Beneficiaries and Payments, by Basis of Eligibility, and Race and Hispanic Origin: United States, Selected Fiscal Years 1999–2009," in *Health, United States, 2012: With Special Feature on Emergency Care*, Centers for Disease Control and Prevention, National Center for Health Statistics, 2013, http://www.cdc.gov/nchs/data/hus/hus12.pdf (accessed December 27, 2013)

TABLE 10.5

Comparison of hospital, skilled nursing facility, and hospice Medicare charges, 1999–2009

	1999	2000	2001	2002	2003	2004	2005	2006	2007	2008	2009
Hospital inpatient charges per day	$2,583	$2,762	$3,069	$3,574	$4,117	$4,559	$4,999	$5,475	$5,895	$6,196	$6,200
Skilled nursing facility charges per day	424	413	422	475	487	493	504	519	558	590	622
Hospice charges per covered day of care	113	112	119	125	129	132	138	141	146	150	153

Notes: Hospital data for 2008 & 2009 are updated using the Bureau of Labor Statistics' (BLS) General medical and surgical hospitals Producer Price Index (PPI). SNF data for 2006–2009 are updated using the BLS Nursing care facilities PPI. Hospice data for 2008 & 2009 are updated using the BLS Home health care services PPI. SNF = Skilled nursing facility-based.

SOURCE: "Table 24. Comparison of Hospital, SNF, and Hospice Medicare Charges, 1999–2009," in *Hospice Facts and Statistics*, Hospice Association of America, November 2010, http://www.nahc.org/assets/1/7/HospiceStats10.pdf (accessed March 3, 2012). Reproduced with the express and limited permission from the National Association for Home Care & Hospice.

It was uncertain, as of 2014, how the ACA would affect the HIV-positive population, but the Medicaid expansion was certain to provide coverage to many more low-income Americans with the infection. Additionally, the ACA prohibits insurers from denying people coverage based on preexisting medical conditions. This makes it less likely that people living well above the poverty line will be financially devastated by a disease such as HIV. In the event that a middle- or high-income person with HIV is forced to stop working, that person no longer becomes immediately uninsurable.

THE RYAN WHITE COMPREHENSIVE AIDS RESOURCES EMERGENCY ACT. The Ryan White Comprehensive AIDS Resources Emergency (CARE) Act is a federal program that provides funds for the care, treatment, and support of low-income, uninsured or underinsured people with AIDS. It is the largest federally funded program for helping people with AIDS. The act is named after an Indiana teenager who had AIDS and worked against AIDS-related discrimination. The act was initially passed in 1990 and has since been reauthorized numerous times, including in 2009. According to the U.S. Department of Health and Human Services, in the fact sheet "Ryan White HIV/AIDS Program Overview" (January 2013, http://hab.hrsa.gov/abouthab/files/programoverviewfacts2012.pdf), "For Program clients, the Program is the payor of last resort, because they are un- or underinsured and no other source of payment for services—public or private—is available." As of 2008, according to the fact sheet, over 70% of program clients were members of racial or ethnic minority groups, 67% were male, and 33% were female. Most of the funds for the program are used to pay for primary medical care and support services for clients. As of 2013, the program was funded at $2.4 billion.

Cancer

Cancer, in all its forms, is expensive to treat. Compared with other diseases, there are more options for cancer treatment, more adverse side effects that require additional treatment, and a greater potential for unrelieved pain. In *Cancer Facts and Figures 2013* (2013, http://www.cancer.org/acs/groups/content/@epidemiologysurveilance/documents/document/acspc-036845.pdf), the American Cancer Society (ACS) reports that the overall

FIGURE 10.10

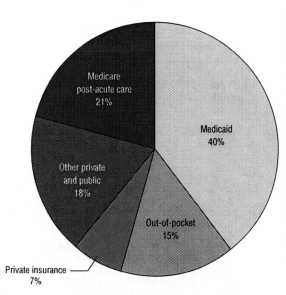

Sources of funding for long-term care, 2011

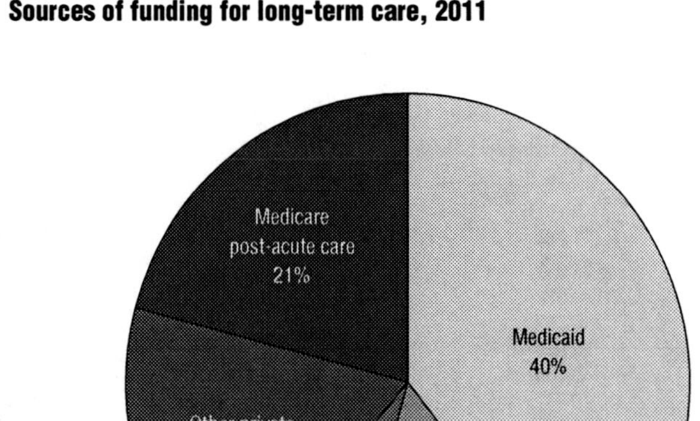

Total long-term care spending, 2011 = $357 billion.

Note: Total LTSS expenditures include spending on residential care facilities, nursing homes, home health services, and home and community-based waiver services. Expenditures also include spending on ambulance providers. All home and community-based waiver services are attributed to Medicaid. LTSS = Long-term services and support.

SOURCE: "Medicaid Is the Primary Payer of Long-Term Care," in "A Short Look at Long-Term Care for Seniors, JAMA, August 27, 2013," The Henry J. Kaiser Family Foundation, August 27, 2013, http://kff.org/slideshow/a-short-look-at-long-term-care-for-seniors-jama-august-27-2013/ (accessed February 5, 2014). Data from Kaiser Commission on Medicaid and the Uninsured estimates based on Centers for Medicare & Medicaid Services National Health Expenditure Accounts data for 2011.

estimated cost of cancer to the nation was $201.5 billion in 2008. Of this amount, $77.4 billion was spent on medical care and $124 billion was the cost of lost productivity due to premature death.

The ACS further notes that cancer costs are generally higher for those who are uninsured: "Uninsured patients and those from ethnic minorities are substantially more likely to be diagnosed with cancer at a later stage, when treatment can be more extensive and more costly." This more extensive and costly treatment is, moreover, less likely to be successful than treatments begun in the early stages of cancer. Cancer is also, like AIDS, likely to leave individuals unable to continue with their careers as the disease progresses. Thus, those who have health insurance through their employers may end up losing coverage. The ACA's prohibition of coverage denials based on preexisting conditions was expected to be helpful to cancer patients who were able to afford private insurance coverage. The expansion of coverage through Medicaid and subsidies was also potentially helpful in enabling previously uninsured Americans to access preventive care that would allow for earlier diagnoses of cancer, bringing down costs and increasing the chances of survival.

Alzheimer's Disease

Alzheimer's disease is a form of dementia that is characterized by memory loss, behavior and personality changes, and decreasing capacity for clear thought. The disease is terminal, and it worsens over time. The chances of developing Alzheimer's increase with age. Thus, it is a particularly pressing concern in countries with rapidly expanding populations of people who live longer into old age.

The Alzheimer's Association reports in *2013 Alzheimer's Disease Facts and Figures* (2013, http://www.alz.org/downloads/facts_figures_2013.pdf) that an estimated 5.2 million people in the United States had Alzheimer's disease in 2013, 5 million of whom were aged 65 years and older and 200,000 of whom were younger people suffering from a specific subset of the disease known as younger-onset Alzheimer's. The organization went on to state that one in nine adults aged 65 years and older had Alzheimer's and that 32% of adults aged 85 years and older had the disease. Of the 5 million elderly adults with Alzheimer's in 2013, 3.2 million (64%) were women. This is not a result of a higher susceptibility to the disease, however, but a consequence of the fact that women live longer, on average, than men.

Because of the deterioration of their mental faculties, Alzheimer's patients require round-the-clock supervision and can be extremely demanding. Compared with other older people who require daily care, Alzheimer's patients are more likely to need help getting in and out of bed, dressing, using the toilet, bathing, and eating. Likewise, the progression of the disease is slow compared with other terminal conditions, so caregivers often must provide for the needs of patients for longer than caregivers of other older patients. Most care of Alzheimer's patients falls to family members. According to the Alzheimer's Association, 15.4 million family and other unpaid caregivers provided an estimated 17.5 billion hours of care to U.S. Alzheimer's patients in 2012. The association estimates the value of this care (using a pay rate of $12.33 per hour, which is significantly lower than the hourly pay of most home health workers) at $216.4 billion.

Besides unpaid care, Alzheimer's patients received paid care costing $203 billion in 2013, according to the Alzheimer's Association. Medicare and Medicaid covered approximately 70% of this total. An average Alzheimer's patient who was cared for in the home received $26,869 worth of paid care in 2012, $18,380 of which was paid for by Medicare. An average Alzheimer's patient who was cared for in a residential

TABLE 10.6

Nursing homes, beds, residents, and occupancy rates, by state, selected years 1995–2011

[Data are based on a census of certified nursing facilities]

State	Nursing homes				Beds			
	1995	2000	2010	2011	1995	2000	2010	2011
	Number							
United States	**16,389**	**16,886**	**15,690**	**15,702**	**1,751,302**	**1,795,388**	**1,703,398**	**1,703,486**
Alabama	221	225	227	228	23,353	25,248	26,656	26,692
Alaska	15	15	15	15	814	821	682	662
Arizona	152	150	139	141	16,162	17,458	16,460	16,401
Arkansas	256	255	232	234	29,952	25,715	24,548	24,600
California	1,382	1,369	1,239	1,235	140,203	131,762	121,167	120,833
Colorado	219	225	213	212	19,912	20,240	20,259	20,115
Connecticut	267	259	239	238	32,827	32,433	29,255	29,045
Delaware	42	43	47	47	4,739	4,906	4,990	4,990
District of Columbia	19	20	19	19	3,206	3,078	2,775	2,772
Florida	627	732	678	681	72,656	83,365	82,226	82,567
Georgia	352	363	360	359	38,097	39,817	39,960	39,857
Hawaii	34	45	48	48	2,513	4,006	4,303	4,315
Idaho	76	84	79	79	5,747	6,181	6,153	6,131
Illinois	827	869	787	781	103,230	110,766	101,061	100,346
Indiana	556	564	506	510	59,538	56,762	57,721	58,782
Iowa	419	467	443	442	39,959	37,034	32,842	32,548
Kansas	429	392	340	341	30,016	27,067	25,598	25,683
Kentucky	288	307	285	282	23,221	25,341	26,063	25,934
Louisiana	337	337	281	281	37,769	39,430	36,098	35,990
Maine	132	126	109	109	9,243	8,248	7,127	7,121
Maryland	218	255	231	231	28,394	31,495	29,004	28,763
Massachusetts	550	526	427	426	54,532	56,030	49,175	49,095
Michigan	432	439	428	425	49,473	50,696	47,054	46,903
Minnesota	432	433	385	384	43,865	42,149	32,339	31,620
Mississippi	183	190	203	203	16,059	17,068	18,589	18,632
Missouri	546	551	514	514	52,679	54,829	55,393	55,114
Montana	100	104	88	85	7,210	7,667	6,991	6,927
Nebraska	231	236	222	222	18,169	17,877	16,065	16,141
Nevada	42	51	50	51	3,998	5,547	5,856	5,984
New Hampshire	74	83	79	78	7,412	7,837	7,692	7,710
New Jersey	300	361	360	362	43,967	52,195	51,101	51,681
New Mexico	83	80	70	71	6,969	7,289	6,769	6,789
New York	624	665	635	634	107,750	120,514	117,984	117,931
North Carolina	391	410	424	422	38,322	41,376	44,392	44,421
North Dakota	87	88	85	84	7,125	6,954	6,438	6,370
Ohio	943	1,009	960	962	106,884	105,038	93,043	92,584
Oklahoma	405	392	314	312	33,918	33,903	28,932	29,073
Oregon	161	150	137	137	13,885	13,500	12,218	12,232
Pennsylvania	726	770	710	710	92,625	95,063	88,829	88,927
Rhode Island	94	99	86	85	9,612	10,271	8,802	8,792
South Carolina	166	178	184	188	16,682	18,102	19,474	19,605
South Dakota	114	114	110	111	8,296	7,844	7,932	6,892
Tennessee	322	349	318	319	37,074	38,593	37,279	37,235
Texas	1,266	1,215	1,173	1,194	123,056	125,052	130,665	133,268
Utah	91	93	99	100	7,101	7,651	8,255	8,377
Vermont	23	44	40	40	1,862	3,743	3,276	3,250
Virginia	271	278	286	286	30,070	30,595	32,152	32,358
Washington	285	277	229	228	28,464	25,905	21,837	21,811
West Virginia	129	139	127	125	10,903	11,413	10,840	10,789
Wisconsin	413	420	392	393	48,754	46,395	36,113	35,859
Wyoming	37	40	38	38	3,035	3,119	2,965	2,969

facility received $71,917 worth of paid care, $23,792 of which was paid for by Medicare, $24,942 of which was paid for by Medicaid, and $18,780 of which was paid for out of pocket. By comparison, the average Medicare beneficiary without Alzheimer's or other forms of dementia received an annual total of $14,452 of paid care. Alzheimer's patients with other coexisting medical conditions—such as kidney disease, heart disease, stroke, diabetes, and cancer—were also more likely to require hospitalization in a given year than other older people who had those other conditions but did not have Alzheimer's.

The Alzheimer's Association expected these costs, and the number of older people requiring treatment for the disease, to grow rapidly through the middle of the 21st century. The organization projected that the cost of paid care for Alzheimer's patients would reach $1.2 trillion by 2050.

TABLE 10.6

Nursing homes, beds, residents, and occupancy rates, by state, selected years 1995–2011 [CONTINUED]

[Data are based on a census of certified nursing facilities]

State	Residents				Occupancy rate*			
	1995	2000	2010	2011	1995	2000	2010	2011
				Number				
United States	**1,479,550**	**1,480,076**	**1,396,473**	**1,389,241**	**84.5**	**82.4**	**82.0**	**81.6**
Alabama	21,691	23,089	22,968	22,855	92.9	91.4	86.2	85.6
Alaska	634	595	641	607	77.9	72.5	94.0	91.7
Arizona	12,382	13,253	11,878	11,472	76.6	75.9	72.2	69.9
Arkansas	20,823	19,317	17,864	18,071	69.5	75.1	72.8	73.5
California	109,805	106,460	102,591	102,377	78.3	80.8	84.7	84.7
Colorado	17,055	17,045	16,302	16,099	85.7	84.2	80.5	80.0
Connecticut	29,948	29,657	25,972	25,748	91.2	91.4	88.8	88.6
Delaware	3,819	3,900	4,145	4,195	80.6	79.5	83.1	84.1
District of Columbia	2,576	2,858	2,595	2,610	80.3	92.9	93.5	94.2
Florida	61,845	69,050	71,907	72,068	85.1	82.8	87.5	87.3
Georgia	35,933	36,559	34,704	34,272	94.3	91.8	86.8	86.0
Hawaii	2,413	3,558	3,880	3,800	96.0	88.8	90.2	88.1
Idaho	4,697	4,640	4,388	4,315	81.7	75.1	71.3	70.4
Illinois	83,696	83,604	75,224	74,580	81.1	75.5	74.4	74.3
Indiana	44,328	42,328	39,167	38,994	74.5	74.6	67.9	66.3
Iowa	27,506	29,204	25,463	25,121	68.8	78.9	77.5	77.2
Kansas	25,140	22,230	18,985	18,877	83.8	82.1	74.2	73.5
Kentucky	20,696	22,730	23,252	23,242	89.1	89.7	89.2	89.6
Louisiana	32,493	30,735	25,198	25,586	86.0	77.9	69.8	71.1
Maine	8,587	7,298	6,417	6,391	92.9	88.5	90.0	89.7
Maryland	24,716	25,629	24,816	24,683	87.0	81.4	85.6	85.8
Massachusetts	49,765	49,805	42,880	42,801	91.3	88.9	87.2	87.2
Michigan	43,271	42,615	39,894	39,545	87.5	84.1	84.8	84.3
Minnesota	41,163	38,813	29,434	28,529	93.8	92.1	91.0	90.2
Mississippi	15,247	15,815	16,489	16,447	94.9	92.7	88.7	88.3
Missouri	39,891	38,586	37,839	37,519	75.7	70.4	68.3	68.1
Montana	6,415	5,973	4,943	4,799	89.0	77.9	70.7	69.3
Nebraska	16,166	14,989	12,630	12,522	89.0	83.8	78.6	77.6
Nevada	3,645	3,657	4,735	4,717	91.2	65.9	80.9	78.8
New Hampshire	6,877	7,158	6,932	6,906	92.8	91.3	90.1	89.6
New Jersey	40,397	45,837	45,917	45,486	91.9	87.8	89.9	88.0
New Mexico	6,051	6,503	5,555	5,645	86.8	89.2	82.1	83.1
New York	103,409	112,957	109,044	108,077	96.0	93.7	92.4	91.6
North Carolina	35,511	36,658	37,199	37,486	92.7	88.6	83.8	84.4
North Dakota	6,868	6,343	5,629	5,733	96.4	91.2	87.4	90.0
Ohio	79,026	81,946	79,234	78,673	73.9	78.0	85.2	85.0
Oklahoma	26,377	23,833	19,227	19,491	77.8	70.3	66.5	67.0
Oregon	11,673	9,990	7,549	7,498	84.1	74.0	61.8	61.3
Pennsylvania	84,843	83,880	81,014	80,253	91.6	88.2	91.2	90.2
Rhode Island	8,823	9,041	8,043	8,053	91.8	88.0	91.4	91.6
South Carolina	14,568	15,739	17,133	17,240	87.3	86.9	88.0	87.9
South Dakota	7,926	7,059	6,497	6,471	95.5	90.0	81.9	93.9
Tennessee	33,929	34,714	31,927	31,437	91.5	89.9	85.6	84.4
Texas	89,354	85,275	91,099	92,133	72.6	68.2	69.7	69.1
Utah	5,832	5,703	5,361	5,448	82.1	74.5	64.9	65.0
Vermont	1,792	3,349	2,931	2,833	96.2	89.5	89.5	87.2
Virginia	28,119	27,091	28,314	28,308	93.5	88.5	88.1	87.5
Washington	24,954	21,158	18,065	17,578	87.7	81.7	82.7	80.6
West Virginia	10,216	10,334	9,557	9,448	93.7	90.5	88.2	87.6
Wisconsin	43,998	38,911	30,618	29,801	90.2	83.9	84.8	83.1
Wyoming	2,661	2,605	2,427	2,401	87.7	83.5	81.9	80.9

*Percentage of beds occupied (number of nursing home residents per 100 nursing home beds).
Notes: Annual numbers of nursing homes, beds, and residents are based on the Online Survey Certification and Reporting Database reporting cycle. Data for additional years are available.

SOURCE: "Table 109. Nursing Homes, Beds, Residents, and Occupancy Rates, by State: United States, Selected Years 1995–2011," in *Health, United States, 2012: With Special Feature on Emergency Care*, Centers for Disease Control and Prevention, National Center for Health Statistics, 2013, http://www.cdc.gov/nchs/data/hus/hus12.pdf (accessed December 27, 2013)

IMPORTANT NAMES AND ADDRESSES

AARP
601 E St. NW
Washington, DC 20049
1-888-687-2277
E-mail: member@aarp.org
URL: http://www.aarp.org/

Aging with Dignity
3050 Highland Oaks Terrace
Tallahassee, FL 32301-3841
(850) 681-2010
1-888-594-7437
FAX: (850) 681-2481
E-mail: fivewishes@agingwithdignity.org
URL: http://www.agingwithdignity.org/

Alzheimer's Association
225 N. Michigan Ave., 17th Floor
Chicago, IL 60601-7633
(312) 335-8700
1-800-272-3900
FAX: 1-866-699-1246
E-mail: info@alz.org
URL: http://www.alz.org/

American Association of Suicidology
5221 Wisconsin Ave. NW
Washington, DC 20015
(202) 237-2280
FAX: (202) 237-2282
URL: http://www.suicidology.org/

American Cancer Society
250 Williams St. NW
Atlanta, GA 30303
1-800-227-2345
URL: http://www.cancer.org/

American Foundation for Suicide Prevention
120 Wall St., 29th Floor
New York, NY 10005
(212) 363-3500
1-888-333-2377
FAX: (212) 363-6237
E-mail: info@afsp.org
URL: http://www.afsp.org/

Centers for Disease Control and Prevention
1600 Clifton Rd.
Atlanta, GA 30333
1-800-232-4636
URL: http://www.cdc.gov/

Children's Hospice International
1101 King St., Ste. 360
Alexandria, VA 22314
(703) 684-0330
E-mail: Info@CHIonline.org
URL: http://www.chionline.org/

Compassion & Choices
PO Box 101810
Denver, CO 80250
1-800-247-7421
FAX: 1-866-312-2690
URL: http://
www.compassionandchoices.org/

Hastings Center
21 Malcolm Gordon Rd.
Garrison, NY 10524-4125
(845) 424-4040
FAX: (845) 424-4545
E-mail: mail@thehastingscenter.org
URL: http://www.thehastingscenter.org/

Health Resources and Services Administration Information Center
5600 Fishers Ln.
Rockville, MD 20857
1-888-275-4772
E-mail: ask@hrsa.gov
URL: http://www.hrsa.gov/

March of Dimes
1275 Mamaroneck Ave.
White Plains, NY 10605
(914) 997-4488
URL: http://www.marchofdimes.com/

National Association for Home Care and Hospice
228 Seventh St. SE
Washington, DC 20003
(202) 547-7424
FAX: (202) 547-3540
URL: http://www.nahc.org/

National Council on Aging
1901 L St. NW, Fourth Floor
Washington, DC 20036
(202) 479-1200
URL: http://www.ncoa.org/

National Hospice and Palliative Care Organization
1731 King St.
Alexandria, VA 22314
(703) 837-1500
FAX: (703) 837-1233
URL: http://www.nhpco.org/

National Institute on Aging
Bldg. 31, Rm. 5C27
31 Center Dr., MSC 2292
Bethesda, MD 20892
(301) 496-1752
1-800-222-2225
FAX: (301) 496-1072
E-mail: niaic@nia.nih.gov
URL: http://www.nia.nih.gov/

National Right to Life Committee
512 10th St. NW
Washington, DC 20004
(202) 626-8800
URL: http://www.nrlc.org/

Older Women's League
1625 K St. NW, Ste. 1275
Washington, DC 20006
(202) 567-2606
E-mail: info@owl-national.org
URL: http://www.owl-national.org/

United Network for Organ Sharing
700 N. Fourth St.
Richmond, VA 23219
(804) 782-4800
1-888-894-6361
FAX: (804) 782-4817
URL: http://www.unos.org/

RESOURCES

Many of the most authoritative sources of data and information on end-of-life issues are published by various agencies of the U.S. government.

The National Center for Health Statistics (NCHS), which is affiliated with the Centers for Disease Control and Prevention (CDC), provides a number of annual publications on health-related matters. Among the most useful sources for the topics covered in this book were *Health, United States, 2012: With Special Feature on Emergency Care*, as well as several reports published as part of the *National Vital Statistics Reports* series, including "Deaths: Preliminary Data for 2011" (October 2012, Donna L. Hoyer and Jiaquan Xu), "Births: Final Data for 2011" (June 2013, Joyce A. Martin et al.), and "Deaths: Final Data for 2010" (May 2013, Sherry L. Murphy, Jiaquan Xu, and Kenneth D. Kochanek). A number of papers issued as part of the *NCHS Data Brief* series were also helpful, including "75 Years of Mortality in the United States, 1935–2010" (March 2012, Donna L. Hoyert), "Death in the United States, 2011" (March 2013, Arialdi M. Miniño), "Use of Advance Directives in Long-Term Care Populations" (January 2011, Adrienne L. Jones, Abigail J. Moss, and Lauren D. Harris-Kojetin), and "Financial Burden of Medical Care: A Family Perspective" (January 2014, Robin A. Cohen and Whitney K. Kirzinger). Other important CDC sources include the series *Morbidity and Mortality Weekly Report*, in particular the data release "Youth Risk Behavior Surveillance—United States, 2011" (June 2012).

Numerous data sources from the U.S. Department of Health and Human Services and its subordinate agencies were also instrumental in compiling this book. These include the Organ Procurement and Transplantation Network's (OPTN) online database (http://optn.transplant.hrsa.gov/data/default.asp), as well as the OPTN's *United States Organ Transplantation: OPTN & SRTR Annual Data Report 2011* (December 2012); the Maternal and Child Health Bureau's *Child Mortality in the United States, 1935–2007: Large Racial and Socioeconomic Disparities Have Persisted over Time* (2010, Gopal K. Singh); and the Administration on Aging's *A Profile of Older Americans: 2012* (April 2013).

The U.S. Census Bureau provides a wealth of data on the U.S. population in the form of reports as well as freely accessible online data tables. Census Bureau reports used in compiling this book include *Income, Poverty, and Health Insurance Coverage in the United States: 2012* (September 2013, Carmen DeNavas-Walt, Bernadette D. Proctor, and Jessica C. Smith) and *The Older Population: 2010* (November 2011, Carrie A. Werner). The bureau's *2012 National Population Projections: Summary Tables* provided a useful collection of online data tables.

Other important government data sources were *Older Americans 2012: Key Indicators of Well-Being* (June 2012) by the Federal Interagency Forum on Aging Related Statistics, *National Health Expenditure Data: Historical—NHE Tables* (2012) by the Centers for Medicare and Medicaid Services, and *A Data Book: Health Care Spending and the Medicare Program* (June 2013) by the Medicare Payment Advisory Commission.

The mission of the National Hospice and Palliative Care Organization (NHPCO) is "improving end of life care and expanding access to hospice care with the goal of profoundly enhancing quality of life for people dying in America and their loved ones." The Hospice Association of America represents hospices, caregivers, and volunteers who serve terminally ill patients and their families. The NHPCO and the Hospice Association of America both collect data about hospice care that were helpful in addressing this topic.

Journals that frequently publish studies dealing with life-sustaining treatment, medical ethics, and medical costs include *American Family Physician, American Journal of Hospice and Palliative Medicine, American Journal of Nursing, Annals of Internal Medicine, Archives of Disease in Childhood, BMC Medicine, Current Opinion in Critical Care, Journal of the American Medical Association, Journal of Medical Ethics, Journal of Neurology, Journal of Palliative Medicine, Mayo Clinic Proceedings, Neurology, New England Journal of Medicine, Pediatrics, Psychological Science*, and *Trends in Cognitive Sciences*.

The Gallup Organization, Harris Interactive, the Pew Research Center, and the Roper Center for Public Opinion Research have all conducted opinion polls on topics that are related to death and dying; a number of such polls and the reports accompanying them were used to provide perspective on public opinions about controversial end-of-life issues.

The Henry J. Kaiser Family Foundation provides a wealth of information on health-related topics, including most of the issues raised in this book.

INDEX

Page references in italics refer to photographs. References with the letter t *following them indicate the presence of a table. The letter* f *indicates a figure. If more than one table or figure appears on a particular page, the exact item number for the table or figure being referenced is provided.*

A

D

E

F

G

H

I

J

K

L

M

N

Q

R

T

U

V

W

X

Y

Advance praise for *Teenagers and Their Babies*

I love this manual. It respects the very important role of the home visitor and acknowledges the need for preparation for this role, likewise it respects adolescence and the importance of training care providers to understand this very dynamic developmental stage. It provides concrete, helpful, hopeful, and respectful tools for these very special workers, enabling them to build the developmental scaffolding that promotes strong and successful young families. This is a really wonderful resource for anyone working with young families.

Patricia Flanagan, MD
Director "Teens with Tots Program," Hasbro Children's Hospital, Associate Professor of Pediatrics, Brown University

Teenagers and Their Babies: A Perinatal Home Visitor's Guide is a "user-friendly" creative guide that elaborates not only on what knowledge a home visitor needs for her/his work, but, also is unique for including a description of feelings that may emerge. The *Guide* is designed to assist the home visitor at several different and important levels and to integrate knowledge and feelings in her/his work. I believe that this perspective is unique, but may be the key to success in being sensitive to and supporting young mothers. *Teenagers and TheirBabies: A Perinatal Home Visitor's Guide* should be recommended for all professionals and paraprofessionals working in this area.

Joy D. Osofsky, PhD
Professor of Pediatrics and Psychiatry
LSU Health Sciences Center, New Orleans

This book is an outstanding guide for all home visitors and doulas who care for teenage parents during pregnancy and after birth. It focuses on sensitive and helpful methods to engage the young parents at their own pace to understand and express their own feelings and needs as well as become aware of the fetus' vast array of sensory and motor responses. This method of support illustrates a model of care that parents can internalize. We highly recommend this excellent book.

Marshall Klaus, MD, and Phyllis Klaus, MFT, LCSW
Authors: *Your Amazing Newborn*, *Bonding*, *The Doula Book*

Teenagers and Their Babies: A Perinatal Home Visitor's Guide

Ida Cardone, Linda Gilkerson, and Nick Wechsler
Ounce of Prevention Fund

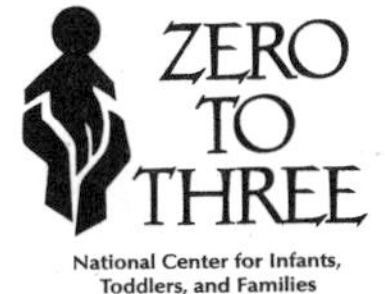

Washington, DC

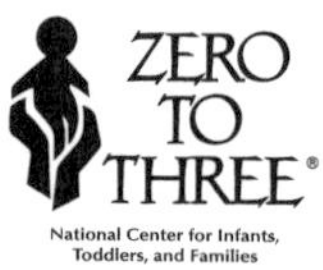

ZERO TO THREE
2000 M St., NW, Suite 200, Washington, DC 20036-3307
(202) 638-1144; Toll-free orders (800) 899-4301
Fax: (202) 638-0851
Web: www.zerotothree.org

The mission of the ZERO TO THREE Press is to publish authoritative research, practical resources, and new ideas for those who work with and care about infants, toddlers, and their families. Books are selected for publication by an independent Editorial Board.

Cover and text design: Design Consultants, Inc.

Library of Congress Cataloging-in-Publication Data
Cardone, Ida.
Teenagers and their babies: a perinatal home visitor's guide / Ida Cardone, Linda Gilkerson and Nick Wechsler.
p. cm.
"For the Ounce of Prevention Fund."
ISBN 978-1-934019-16-0
1. Teenage pregnancy. 2. Teenage mothers--Counselling of. 3. Teenage parents--Counselling of. 4. Prenatal care. 5. Home-based family services. I. Gilkerson, Linda, 1947- II. Wechsler, Nick, 1947- III. Title
RG556.5.C38 2007
618.200835--dc22

2007025459

10 9 8 7 6 5 4 3 2 1
ISBN 978-1-934019-16-0
Printed in the United States of America

Suggested citation: Cardone, I., Gilkerson, L., & Wechsler, N. (2008). *Teenagers and their babies: A perinatal home visitor's guide.* Washington, DC: ZERO TO THREE.

Table of Contents

ACKNOWLEDGMENTS

The authors are deeply grateful for the generous and gracious assistance of preeminent clinicians, research scientists, and administrators in the areas of infant mental health. The Community-Based FANA (Family Administered Neonatal Activities) was willed into being by two very strong forces: Harriet Meyer, executive director of the Ounce of Prevention Fund, and the staff of the Ounce's Parents Too Soon Programs throughout Illinois. Thank you, Harriet, for your persistence and enthusiastic motivation. Thank you, staff, for encouraging us to take FANA into the community.

Transforming the perinatal intervention, the Community-Based FANA, into *Teenagers and Their Babies: A Perinatal Home Visitor's Guide* was driven by the inspiration of a giant in our field, the late Emily Fenichel. After hearing about this intervention, each time Emily encountered one of the authors she would greet us with, "So, when will you turn it into a guide that we can publish?" Although Emily is irreplaceable, her inspiration continues to carry us all to more meaningful places. Now, every parent and newborn who benefits from *Teenagers and Their Babies* will be embraced by Emily as they begin their new lives as a family.

The Community-Based FANA is a modification and extension of the Family Administered Neonatal Activities (FANA), developed in 1986 by Cardone and Gilkerson and their colleagues at the Perinatal Family Support Center of Evanston Northwestern Healthcare/Evanston Hospital. The FANA continues to be available at the hospital to families at the time of birth or at discharge from the neonatal intensive care unit. The FANA, itself, is an adaptation of the Brazelton Neonatal Behavioral Assessment Scale developed by T. Berry Brazelton, MD, and Kevin Nugent, PhD (1995). The FANA was kept alive in the Parents Too Soon Programs by Victor Bernstein, PhD. The authors are indebted to and have benefited enormously from this rich heritage.

Very special thanks to those who have been generous with their time and expertise in reviewing the draft of the Community-Based FANA: Jeannie Beck, Lynn Bos, Mimi Graham, Alicia Lieberman, Polly Malory, Joy Osofsky, Jolene Pearson,

Nancy Sinclair, and Barbara White. They have provided invaluable suggestions and revisions.

We thank all of the home visitors, doulas, and directors who have so generously contributed to this work: Maria Espejel, Ana Martinez, Bonnie Matty, and Mary Dru Anderson, all of whom spent hours sharing their experience and insights.

The collaboration between The Ounce of Prevention Fund and the Chicago Health Connection that resulted in the Chicago Doula Project inspired and informed our work. Thanks to the doulas, Lovie Griffin, Loretha Weisinger, Anita Moss, Peggy Brewer, and Wandy Hernandez, and thanks to Judy Tiebloom-Mishkin and Rachel Abrahamson. We appreciate the support and direction offered by the staff of Alivio Medical Center, Christopher House, and Marillac Social Center during the pilot training. The thoughts of Darnesha Lucas, Monique Strickland, and Ethel Washington from the Center for Successful Child Development added considerably to our understanding.

This work was developed with the generous support of the Illinois Department of Human Services.

We appreciate David Wilson, who helped our work progress from computer disc to the printed page. This final version of the guide has benefited from the mighty growth spurt brought to the manuscript by our editor, Mary McGonigel.

We are grateful to our colleagues who continue to guide and inspire us at our three institutions: Erikson Institute, Evanston Northwestern Healthcare/Evanston Hospital, and the Ounce of Prevention Fund. We are the beneficiaries of their wisdom and support.

Ida Cardone, Linda Gilkerson, and Nick Wechsler, August 2007

Reference

Brazelton, T., & Nugent, K. (1995). *Neonatal Behavioral Assessment Scale* (3rd ed.). London: MacKeith Press.

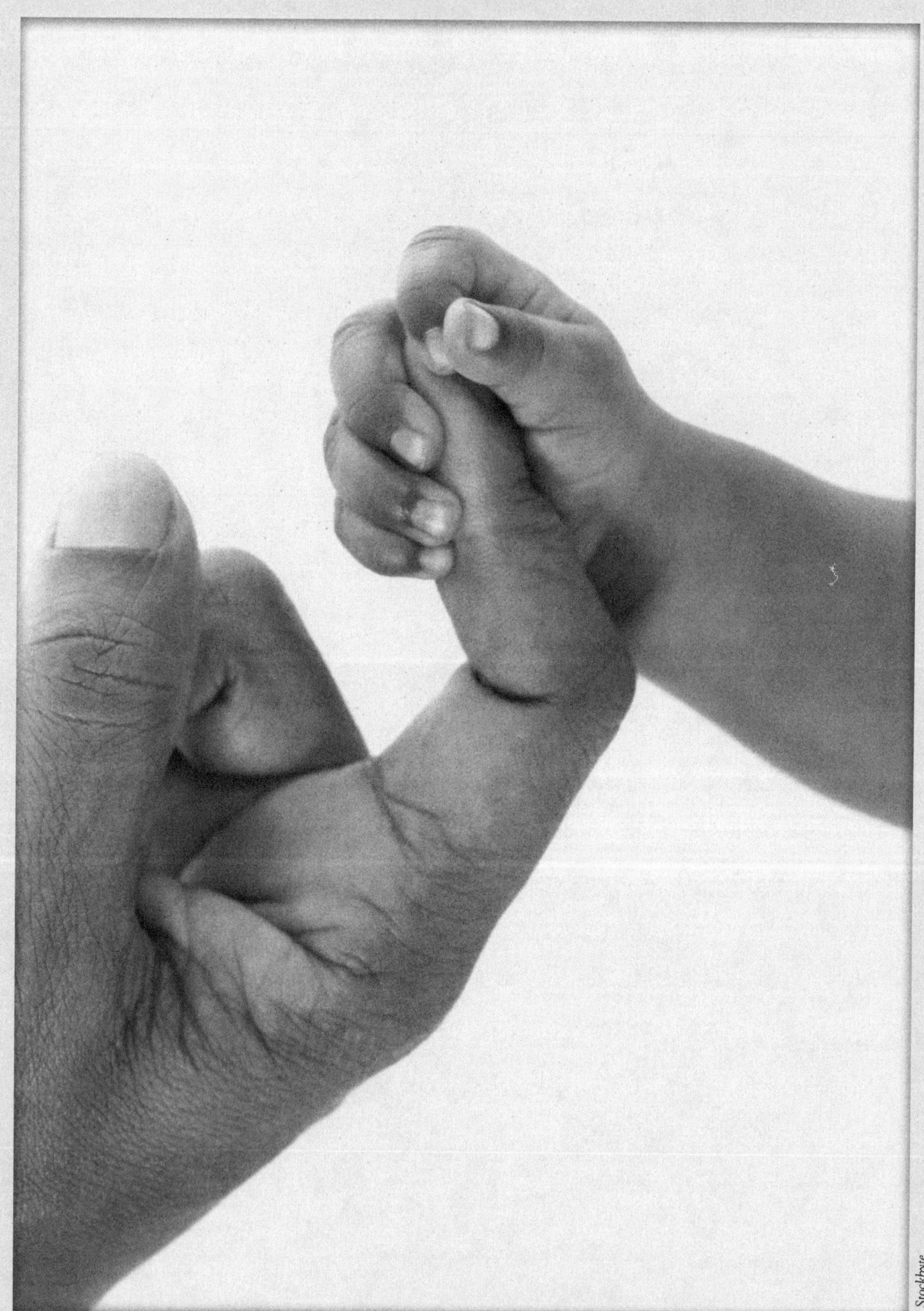

Stockbyte

CHAPTER 1

Know the Community-Based Family Administered Neonatal Activities

As a home-based infant–parent worker, you are continuing a long and fruitful tradition of caring for our most precious resource—infants and their families. Caring for teens during their pregnancies and after they have become mothers presents you with a double challenge. You must be constantly aware of the dramatic growth and changes in the fetus[1]—and, later, the baby—and must be equally aware of the growth and changes in the young mother, who is going through the breathtaking spurts in development common to all adolescents. We hope that *Teenagers and Their Babies: A Perinatal Home Visitor's Guide* will help you meet this challenge.

Working with adolescent parents brings you to a door that opens into a complex and rapidly changing environment that sizzles with change and growth—the teenager's solar system of relationships. These include relationships with her own sense of self, with her developing child, with the father, with her family, with her peers and social group, and, now, with you. To be effective you must work in five worlds simultaneously, in a manner that helps both you and the young parent feel grounded by the sense of gravity that holds you and her together.

You work in the world of your own feelings, experiences, wishes, and beliefs. You work in the world of the unborn and newborn child, a responsibility that requires care and attention in the present for the hope and promise of the future. You work in the world of the teenager, a world that swings from chaos to calm and challenges both her and you in your shared efforts to transform her new life as a parent from a "*me* thing" into a "*we* thing." You work in the world of the parent–child relationship, which encompasses both the teen's individual need for nurturing and the challenge of helping parent and child find in each other exactly what each requires in order to feel competent and secure with the other. And you work in the world of your unique relationship with the teenager, as she seeks your understanding and approval even as you build the trust that paves the way for your work with her.

---

[1]Although *fetus* is the medically correct term, always say *baby* in your work with expectant parents when referring to their unborn child. The Community-Based FANA models this usage, with the pronouns "*he*" and "*she*" used to refer to the fetus rather than the pronoun "it."

The relationship you and the teen build allows her to use the wisdom and safety that she finds with you as a guide and point of reference in her journey into parenthood. It is no wonder that you experience your work as challenging and taxing, yet are buoyed by your belief in the future!

Long years of clinical and life experience, as well as research, have taught us that a mother who is aware of and attaches to the baby growing within her is more likely to attach to her newborn (Fonagy, Steele, & Steele, 1991). The driving force behind the work of the infant–parent specialist—you—is the idea that a strong relationship between mother and child is the very best buffer against child abuse and neglect (Benoit, Zeanah, & Barton, 1989; Zeanah et al., 1993) and the very best way to ensure the solid emotional, physical, and intellectual development of the baby.

We developed *Teenagers and Their Babies: A Perinatal Home Visitor's Guide* to help paraprofessional home-based visitors engage expectant and new parents in an exploration of their baby's development and their expectations for parenthood. It provides you with ideas culled from theory, research, and practice that can help inform what you know about and how you plan for your work with families. It also includes service interventions—strategies, techniques, and activities—for you to use in your work. The ideas you are about to encounter in this guide will be useful in aspects of your work with all families, not just those who are expecting a baby. It offers a way of bringing your own personal style of being into a professional way of being.

Teenagers and Their Babies is based on an adaptation of the FANA (Family Administered Neonatal Activities), which was developed by Ida Cardone and Linda Gilkerson (1989, 1990), for community-based use. The FANA itself is an adaptation of the Brazelton Neonatal Behavioral Assessment Scale, created by T. Berry Brazelton, MD, and Kevin Nugent, PhD (1995). Nurses, child development specialists, and any program offering prenatal groups also can use this guide to learn how to support young families using the Community-Based FANA.

In this chapter, we introduce and describe the Community-Based FANA as a foundation for engaging young parents, review the importance of the home visitor in promoting attachment, and provide a chapter-by-chapter overview of the guide.

The Community-Based FANA

The Community-Based FANA is a set of principles, methods, and activities that home visitors can use to promote emotional availability and engagement between parents and their unborn infant and, later, their newborn. It is designed as a structured intervention that home visitors facilitate with pregnant teenagers and their partners. Many programs also are using the Community-Based FANA in other settings and with different populations, such as with adult parents or in center-based programs.

The Community-Based FANA offers detailed information and instructions for activities for prenatal and postnatal home visits covering the period from 26

Figure 1.1

Community-Based FANA Home Visit Structure

Prenatal Visits	**Postnatal Visits**
Preparation	Preparation
Parent Time	Parent Time
Parent and Baby Time	Parent and Baby Time
Family Time	Family Time
Reflection and Writing to the Baby	Reflection and Writing to the Baby

weeks gestation to 4 weeks after birth. Each Community-Based FANA home visit has the same basic structure (see Figure 1.1):

- Preparation: Reviewing past visits and preparing for the current visit
- Parent Time: Greeting and reconnecting with parents and asking about and validating parental observations
- Parent and Baby Time: Exploring the baby's present behavior and guiding parental exploration of their baby's prenatal and postnatal development
- Family Time: Making a special time for the parents and baby to be together and enjoy one another prenatally, creating a pattern of behavior that can continue after the baby is born
- Reflection and Writing to the Baby: Reflecting on the visit and writing to the baby.

The Community-Based FANA is divided into prenatal and postnatal activities. The prenatal activities begin in the last trimester of pregnancy. Although these activities are designed to span six prenatal home visits, they can be easily adapted for use with prenatal groups or for use over a longer or shorter period of time. Each of the prenatal visits focuses on a different aspect of development, guiding you as you help parents explore their unborn baby's development in utero and preview their newborn's development. "Previewing the Newborn" helps parents wonder about and anticipate what their baby will be like once she is born.

The postnatal Community-Based FANA activities are designed for home or hospital visits. You can facilitate these activities with parents in the days after the baby is born, or even as soon as hours after delivery. Because the Community-Based FANA creates and promotes engaged behavior patterns, as a general rule, the sooner you begin to use the postnatal activities with new parents, the better. These activities also can be repeated as often as the parents desire.

This guide provides all the information you need to begin using the Community-Based FANA as part of your work with young families. You will learn how to get to know each teen mother you visit and how to understand yourself and your reactions as you undertake the rich and challenging task of being her partner as she enters motherhood. You also will learn how to support and engage fathers.[2]

We provide guiding principles and key practices throughout *Teenagers and Their Babies* to help you in critical aspects of your work with families. To support you as you learn how to facilitate the Community-Based FANA with young families, scripted comments and questions and answers are provided for your use as you are getting started. As you gain more confidence with the Community-Based FANA, questions and comments will emerge from your experience with the work and your understanding of individual parents.

All of your self-study and preparation is geared to getting you ready to provide a meaningful, enjoyable experience for parents. Each home visit boosts the self-confidence and competence of the young family as you help the parents prepare for their new life with their baby.

What Research Tells Us—Attachment and Home Visiting

What is attachment? Why is it so important? Because you have chosen the infant–parent field, you probably already know the answers to these questions on an instinctive level. There is also an enormous body of research to back you up. Zeanah and Boris (2000) summarized the key features of attachment:

[2]Because most prenatal programs serve women and are staffed by women, this guide primarily uses *mother* and feminine pronouns, but the Community-Based FANA is used successfully with expectant and new fathers, too. A father experiences the same closer sense of awareness, comfort, and mastery, and he benefits from the powerful feelings of being connected and warmly attached to his newborn.

> *Emotional availability, nurturance and warmth, protection and provision of comfort are the most salient caregiver behaviors for the attachment relationship, corresponding to security and trust, balanced emotional regulation, vigilance and seeking comfort for distress in the young child.* (p. 356)

Sturdy mother–infant attachment is a product of a finely tuned and engaged interaction. Two of the many important factors that help a new mother stay attuned and engaged are (a) a strong social support network (Sequin, Potvin, St-Denis, & Loiselle, 1999) and (b) a mother's understanding of her child's signals (Wakschlag & Hans, 2000).

Where do you fit in as an infant–parent home visitor? The relationship you develop with the teens you work with is a critical part of that social support network. You not only provide a young mother with nurturant support but you also model the kind of warm, engaged relationship that you hope she will experience with her baby. All of this has a terrific effect on a teen's self-esteem and her capacity to mother (Osofsky, Hann, & Peebles, 1993). Through the Community-Based FANA, you also provide the teen with an exciting, interactive way of learning about her baby's competencies and the ways he has of signaling comfort, joy, discomfort, and frustration.

What happens when babies feel secure in their attachments? They grow into toddlers who are more likely to show empathy toward others, engage in enjoyable, back-and-forth play, and show resilience in the face of failure (Arend, Gove, & Sroufe, 1979; Waters, Wippman, & Sroufe, 1979). These children enjoy life more than children who do not feel cared for, thought about, or safe!

You have a remarkable opportunity to enter the life of a newly developing family. What you do now will have an effect for years to come (Coley & Chase-Landale, 1998; Furstenberg, Brooks-Gunn, & Morgan 1987). Does home visiting matter? You bet it does! A study found that even 15 years after home visits stopped, mothers who had been involved in a home-visiting program had fewer subsequent pregnancies and were more active participants in the labor force than mothers who had not had such visits (Kitzman et al., 2000; Olds et al., 1997).

Our challenge is to translate these research findings into good clinical practice. How do you as a home visitor make use of this information? This guide and the Community-Based FANA will help you learn the following:

- Promote the teen mother's recognition of her baby in utero
- Explore her perception of her baby in utero
- Explore her life as it unfolds in relation to her baby in utero and her newborn
- Promote her growing attachment to her unborn baby and, ultimately, her attachment and interest in her newborn.

Overview of the Guide

Teenagers and Their Babies contains everything you need to know to help expectant and new parents explore their baby's development and their expectations for parenthood. The first eight chapters offer a broad array of essential information and guidance; the actual Community-Based FANA activities are not introduced until chapter 9. If you skip ahead to take a look, be sure to come back to the beginning and you will be rewarded!

Chapter 2, "Know Yourself," provides general guidelines for exploring your own thoughts and feelings in relation to the young parents with whom you work. Your life experiences, from childhood until right now—your joys and struggles, defeats and victories—are all a part of what you bring to your relationship with young parents. Being aware of what has happened to you helps you connect with what a teen is living through. At the same time, it helps you maintain a healthy boundary and space between you and the teen parent (J. Osofsky, personal communication, October, 2000).

Chapter 3, "Know the Teen," is full of ideas for getting to know the teens with whom you are working. Because every teen is uniquely her own person, regardless of whether she is 13 or 19, it also offers guidelines for discovering where a teen is in terms of self-understanding, mood states, and the development of her unique identity.

Chapter 4, "Connecting With Fathers," discusses pregnancy, relating to the developing fetus, and meeting the newborn from the father's perspective. It provides guidance for working with a father while still following the mother's lead in involving him, as well as methods for including him in Community-Based FANA activities and experiences to solidify his growing relationship with his child.

Chapter 5, "Mutual Growth: The Trimesters of Pregnancy," explores the dynamic physical and emotional changes that a pregnant adolescent experiences in her new role as an expectant mother as she transforms her life from a *me* thing into a *we* thing. It describes by trimester and developmental area how the baby is growing within the mother.

Chapter 6, "The Birth," highlights issues that are important for the teen to address as she prepares for labor and delivery, and it offers guidance for the home visitor on how to help make this happen.

Chapter 7, "When Things Don't Go as Planned," examines unexpected and sorrowful events such as the death of the baby, prenatally or at birth, and health or developmental problems that are apparent at birth.

Chapter 8, "Coming Through the Door," outlines the structure of the Community-Based FANA and discusses the five main components of each home visit—Preparation, Parent Time, Parent and Baby Time, Family Time, and Reflection and Writing to the Baby. A variety of tools are provided throughout the chapter to guide your work.

Chapter 9, "Welcome Parents: The Prenatal Home Visits," presents the Community-Based FANA activities for prenatal home visits, along with detailed information and tools for tailoring each home visit component to the prenatal period.

Chapter 10, "Welcome Baby: The Postnatal Home Visits," presents activities and discussions for supporting parents and baby in the newborn period, from birth through the first month of life.

Chapter 11, "Getting Started," is a final message to you, the home visitor. It acknowledges the challenge of digesting new ideas and strategies and provides support in the most critical next step—turning the authors' work into your work with families.

Appendix A is a resource list, and Appendix B is a tool kit comprising all of the tools and activities provided throughout the guide.

Now you have a better idea of what lies ahead for you. As you use the guide, you will develop a fuller awareness of what lies ahead for parents as they work with you and learn about their new relationship both with you and with their developing baby. You will have many opportunities throughout the guide to build your capacity to work with new parents to help them feel close to their baby. Working with families, especially young families, challenges home visitors to balance what families bring to the conversation with what you need to introduce. *Teenagers and Their Babies: A Perinatal Home Visitor's Guide* and the Community-Based FANA offer you and parents a meaningful and enjoyable place to begin.

Now that you have this overview of the manual, you are in exactly the right place to roll up your sleeves and begin your preparation!

References

Arend, R., Gove, F. L., & Sroufe, L. A. (1979). Continuity of individual adaptation from infancy to kindergarten: A predictive study of eco-resiliency and curiosity in preschoolers. *Child Development*, 50, 950–959.

Benoit, D., Zeanah, C., & Barton, M. (1989). Maternal attachment disturbances in failure to thrive. *Infant Mental Health Journal, 10*, 185–202.

Brazelton, T. B., Nugent, K. (1995) *Neonatal Behavior Assessment Scale* (3rd ed.). London: MacKeith Press.

Cardone, I., & Gilkerson, L. (1989). Family administered neonatal activities: An innovative component of family-centered care. *Zero to Three, 10*(1), 23–28.

Cardone, I., &. Gilkerson, L. (1990). Family administered neonatal activities: An exploratory method for the integration of parental perceptions and newborn behavior. *Infant Mental Health Journal, 11*(2), 127–141.

Coley, R. L., & Chase-Landale, P. L. (1998). Adolescent pregnancy and parenthood: Recent evidence and future directions. *American Psychologist, 53*, 152–166.

Fonagy, P., Steele, H., & Steele, M. (1991). Maternal representations of attachment during pregnancy predict the organization of infant–mother attachment at one year of age. *Child Development, 62*, 891–905.

Furstenberg, F. F., Brooks-Gunn, J., & Morgan, P. (1987). *Adolescent mothers in later life*. New York: Cambridge University Press.

Kitzman, H., Olds, D., Sidora, K., Henderson, C., Hanks, C., Cole, R., et al. (2000). Enduring effects of nurse home visitation on maternal life course: A 3-year follow-up of a randomized trial. *Journal of the American Medical Association, 283*, 1983–1989.

Olds, D. L., Eckenrode, J., Henderson, Jr., C. R., Kitzman, H., Powers, J., Cole, R., et al. (1997). Long-term effects of home visitation on maternal life course and child abuse and neglect: 15-year follow-up of a randomized trial. *The Journal of the American Medical Association, 278*, 637–643.

Osofsky, J. D., Hann, D. M., & Peebles, C. (1993). Adolescent parenthood: Risks and opportunities for parents and infants. In C. Zeanah (Ed.), *Handbook of infant mental health* (2nd ed., pp. 106–119). New York: Guilford.

Sequin, L., Potvin, L., St-Denis, M., & Loiselle, J. (1999). Socio-environmental factors and postnatal depressive symptomatology: A longitudinal study. *Women and Health, 29*(1), 57–72.

Wakschlag, L. S., & Hans, S. L. (2000). Early parenthood in context: Implications for development and intervention. In C. Zeanah (Ed.), *Handbook of infant mental health* (2nd ed., pp. 129–144). New York: Guilford Press.

Waters, E., Wippman, J., & Sroufe, L. A. (1979). Attachment, positive affect, and competence in the peer group: Two studies in construct validation. *Child Development, 50*, 821–829.

Zeanah, C. H., Benoit, D., Barton, M., Regan, M., Hirshberg, L., & Lipsitt, L. (1993). Representations of attachment in mothers and their one-year-old infants. *Journal of the American Academy of Child and Adolescent Psychiatry, 32*(2), 278–286.

Zeanah, C. H., & Boris, N. W. (2000). Disturbances and disorders of attachment in early childhood. In
C. H. Zeanah (Ed.), *Handbook of infant mental health* (2nd ed., pp. 353–368). New York: Guilford Press.

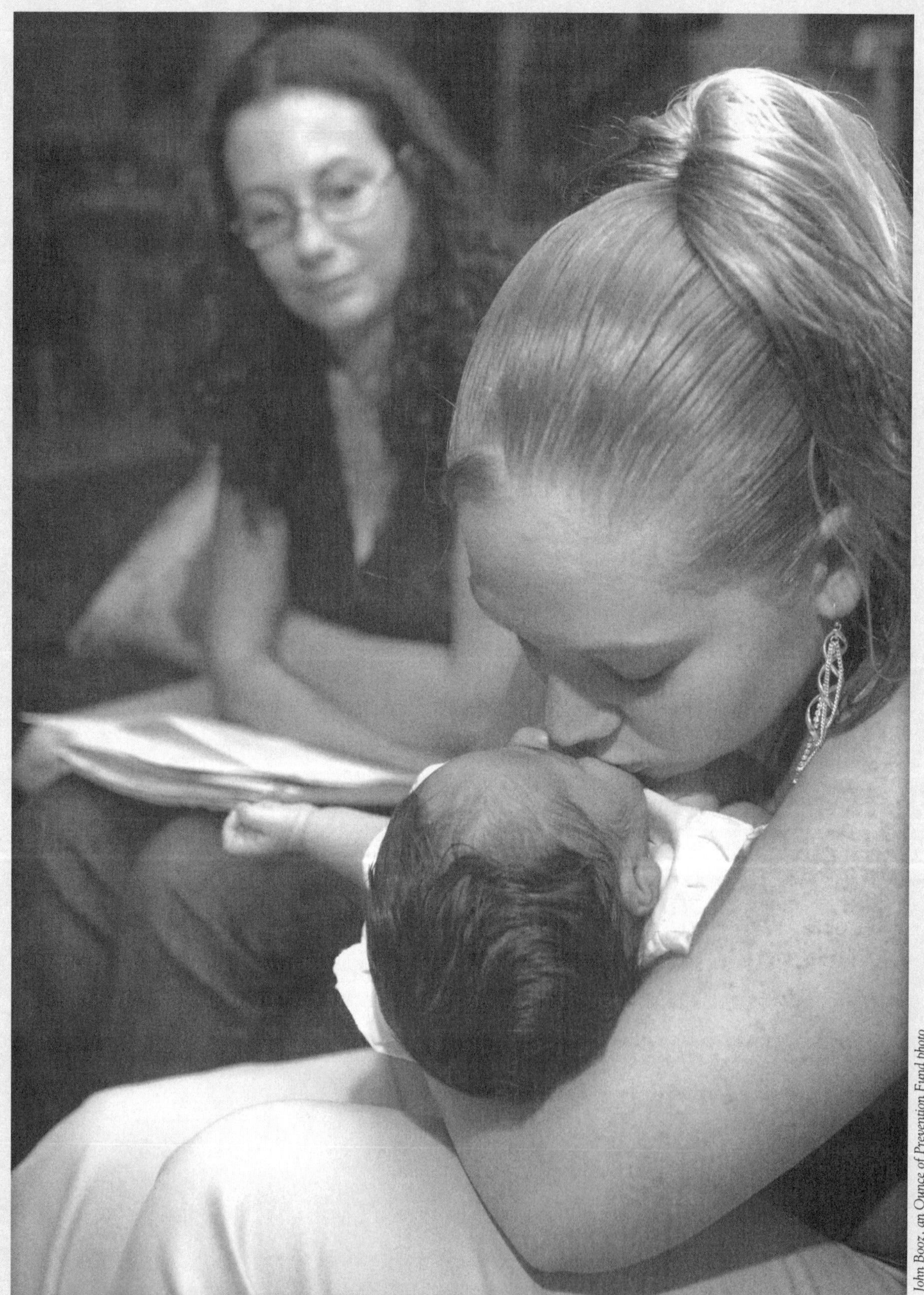

John Booz, an Ounce of Prevention Fund photo

Chapter 2

Know Yourself

In so many ways you are doing for the teen mother what you want her to do for her baby. No matter how happy or sad her life has been, you are entering it at a magical, momentous time when she is carrying new life. You have an unparalleled opportunity to be helpful at this special time in her life. You are eager to learn about the teen mom and help her identify and frame her strengths so that she can do the sometimes daunting job before her, but you also must identify and frame your own strengths.

This chapter is a guide to knowing yourself and being comfortable working in the distance that separates you and the parents with whom you work, while at the same time being close and connected to them. That distance and connection both create the ideal environment for the Community-Based Family Administered Neonatal Activities (FANA). It is an environment that invites the parent to see herself as the star of her story and to take her place as the one who knows her baby best.

Know Your Strengths

Your work as a home visitor is strength based. You attempt always to draw on the strengths of the young people you are working with, rather than focus on the deficits, but what about your own strengths? Do you know them? Take a good look at the strengths and resources you bring to your work.

When you are in a room with a mother, father, and infant, or a mother, father, and yet-to-be-born baby, there are at least four key players in that room—mother, father, baby, and you. All are important, and all have strengths, as well as equal but different kinds of knowledge. Your presence is powerful in that room, and the things that you want to learn about that young family are the very same things you need to know about yourself.

To help you learn about your strengths, ask yourself the questions in Figure 2.1.

Allow your strengths to be revealed to you during the course of your work. This is your own private space. What you learn about yourself, as a general rule, should not be shared with the young families with whom you are working. Remember that strengths are a two-way street. Allow your strengths to develop at the same time that you encourage the teens' developing strengths.

Figure 2.1

Ask Yourself These Questions . . .

About Your Age

- How does my age influence how I am viewed by the teen or family?
- Who is it that they see?
- What will they be able to hear from me?

How old or young you are is important because each age has its own magic. A 24-year-old home visitor may be able to say something to a teen mom about her purple hair that a 60-year-old visitor cannot. And a 60-year-old may be able to offer words of wisdom that would never be accepted from a 24-year-old. Thinking about these things is essential as you prepare for your work.

About Your Life Story

- Do I have children of my own?
- Am I a grandparent, aunt, or uncle, or are there other children in my life?

Your own life story profoundly affects how you approach your work. If, for example, you have a daughter the same age as the teen you are working with, consider what this means. Does your relationship with your daughter make you overly sympathetic with the teen's mother? Or, does it give you such a strong sense of why the youngster is so angry that you really understand where she's coming from?

About the People in Your Life

- How do my family, friends, and colleagues help me define myself?
- Who or what are the special strengths in my life—my supervisors, fellow workers, or people at my place of worship?

Examining these things about the people in your life will help you understand how the teen is defining herself. Does she have anything comparable in her life? Understanding what helps you feel good and whole will help you assess her special strengths as well as understand what may be missing from her life.

The Receptive Posture

An important part of knowing yourself is defining the attitude of mind that you bring to each and every encounter with teens and families—how you settle yourself in to listen and interact in each of your home-based sessions. Underlying all of our interactions with young parents is our commitment that we are wholly present, engaged, and attuned.

How do we turn this commitment into action? It requires a certain stillness, an internal sense of quietness and receptivity, an awareness that silence on the part of the skilled home-based visitor is powerful. Parents tend to fill gentle silences with their most profound hopes and fears. They do their best learning with an accepting, observing "other"—you—present. Our goal is a cascade of quiet, shared attention. If the teens you are working with are not in that place yet, know that part of the magic is that you will help them get there.

The receptive posture is an active, deliberate process of engagement. Receptive does not mean passive. We must be actively, wholly present and release ourselves from private concerns. We must be liberated in that moment, in that place.

Figure 2.2

Guiding Principles and Key Practices for Knowing Yourself

Guiding principle. We are all—and always—in a process of growth.

Key practice. Seek to understand the special magic of your age, no matter what age that is, and connect to the teen with this understanding in mind.

Guiding principle. We change through our work with teens, and they change as they work with us. We are both in a process of becoming.

Key practice. Create a space to coexist with the new you that you are becoming and the new person that the teen is becoming. Build your relationship and structure your interactions with a young parent to foster the strengths of each of you as you codevelop and coemerge.

Figure 2.3

The Receptive Posture

- Receptive, but not passive.
- Fully involved, but not instructional.
- Attuned, but not an echo.
- Still and centered, but not soundless.

We must be fully involved, but not instructional. We are guides to new learning with families. Just as strengths co-develop, so, too, does learning.

We must be attuned, but not an echo. We must bring the conversation to the next level of engagement. We've all seen mothers do this with their toddlers. The toddler says, "ball," and the mother, in a slightly higher tone with slightly different feeling, says, "Oh yes. A red ball." She brings the conversation to the next level of engagement.

We must be still and centered, but not soundless. We must enter a peaceful place. How do we do that? What are your strategies for making that happen? Is there a physical place in your body where you experience a tranquil sense? Your head, chest, stomach? Practice getting there, so that when you speak with families, you speak with gentle tranquility. What happens when we see the Grand Canyon—or our very own baby—for the first time? We say a whispered, "Wow!" Your voice can be a supportive embrace.

Receptive Posture Skills

You have all the skills in you right now to use the receptive posture! What are these skills? They are your voice, eyes, body, touch, and mind. (See Figure 2.4)

These are the same skills the teen mother has. You hope that she will use these things to encourage brain and body growth, trust, and a sense of being well with the world and her baby. And you can use your own voice, eyes, body, touch, and

Figure 2.4

Receptive Posture Skills and Ways to Use Them

Use:	*To:*
Your voice	Invite
Your touch	Encourage
Your eyes	Elaborate
Your mind	Discuss
Your body	Model
	Guide

mind to encourage growth, trust, and a sense of internal organization in her. Only the content will be different.

There are six important ways, adapted from Bromwich (1978), that you can use these specific skills: inviting, elaborating, modeling, encouraging, discussing, and guiding. How can you use your voice, eyes, body, touch, and mind in these ways?

Inviting. To invite, the home visitor actively solicits the teen's interest, perhaps by directing her attention to particular activities of her unborn baby or infant: "Let's see, Maggie, if you feel the baby moving." Or, "Let's see what the baby is doing right now."

Elaborating. To elaborate, the home visitor adds detail or new information to a recently presented observation: "Yes, Tamika, your baby is sound asleep right now. There are many ways a baby can be asleep . . . ."

Modeling. To model, the home visitor acts in a way that she hopes the teen will imitate: "Let's pretend, Chanel, that your baby is kicking really hard inside you. I wonder what would happen if you put your hands on your tummy like this (the home visitor puts her hands on either side of her own stomach) and spoke softly?" (The home visitor speaks in a whisper toward her own stomach.) The purpose of modeling is to engage the teen with her unborn baby or infant, rather than to achieve precision with a given activity.

Encouraging. To encourage participation, the home visitor asks the teen what she has just seen her baby or felt her unborn baby do: "Let's see, now, Olga. What did we just see Miguel do?" If the teen hesitates, the home visitor shares her own observation. Encouraging is a mutual sharing, rather than a question-answer-question. The home visitor shares her observation as a hypothesis for the teen to consider—a kind of wondering out loud together, rather than a statement of fact: "Do you think that cloth feels soft to him?"

Discussing. To discuss, the home visitor combines whatever receptive posture skills are useful to help the teen recognize and understand what is happening between her and her baby, as well as the development of her unborn and then newborn baby: "Your baby stilled when you spoke to him quietly." In addition to inviting, elaborating, modeling, and encouraging, the home visitor uses alerting and inquiring to discuss with the young mother. To alert, the home visitor focuses the teen's attention: "Keep an eye open for what Megan does when you uncover her." To inquire, the home visitor asks if the teen has seen a particular behavior: "Have you seen your baby put her hand to her mouth?"

Guiding. To guide, the home visitor physically assists the teen in learning about her baby, conveying at the same time a sense of curiosity and adventure: "Let's see now, Teresa. If you hold your hand right about here, what happens?" (The home visitor helps to put the young mother's hands on her stomach as she attempts to soothe her active unborn baby.)

Guidelines for Using Receptive Posture Skills

Here are some practical guidelines for using your voice, eyes, body, touch, and mind in your work with young mothers. You may be more comfortable with some of these activities than others.

Using Your Voice

Use your voice to frame and mirror a mother's experience with her baby.

Framing

Framing an experience for someone works like this:

In this example, the home visitor puts a lovely golden frame around a big, beautiful experience of which the teen was only vaguely aware. Here, framing makes that experience stand out in a way that will make the second kick the mother feels very real to her. The home visitor adds to her experience of pregnancy and motherhood and helps provide a building block as she creates a home inside her for her baby.

The Teen:

"I don't know. I thought I felt the baby kick. It was probably indigestion. My friends say babies don't move . . . but I don't know . . . . I thought I felt the baby kick."

The Home Visitor:

"Let's think about this together, Ana. You say you thought you felt the baby move. When was it? How did it feel? Like a bouncing ball? Like a fish swishing its tail? You know, by 10–12 weeks inside you, the baby is really busy moving."

Mirroring

Another way to use your voice with a young mother is to mirror what she says. Mirroring makes her feel heard. It says to her, "I'm taking you seriously." Mirroring also says, "I am willing to hear anything you have to say. With me, you can speak your unspeakable thoughts." To mirror a teen's experience, use her own words. It works like this:

The Teen:

"I was sick this whole morning, like I was going to throw up. It's been like this for weeks. I feel so mad . . . just angry. I don't know . . . sometimes I think I'm mad at the baby."

The Home Visitor:

"I hear you, Cory; you've felt so sick, for so long. And you're mad at the baby for making you feel like this."

Mirroring works because it helps put scary or troublesome feelings on the table so that you and the teen mom can look at them together. There is strength in numbers. In this example, the home visitor is not encouraging the mother to be mad at her baby. Rather, she is encouraging the teen to let out feelings that might cause the teen trouble, feelings that might make her feel like a bad person. By mirroring, the home visitor gets this message across to the young mom:

> *"You're allowed many, many feelings during your pregnancy. At one time you may be excited, at another angry. Or you may feel these things all at once. You're allowed both sides of these feelings."*

Mirroring works when other approaches do not. Reassuring her, "You'll get over it," or presenting the experience as normal by saying, "All moms feel like that," or trying to teach her something such as, "Nausea is related to hormone changes," tends to make teens go silent.

At times mirroring is hard emotionally on the home visitor. It may be difficult to stay neutral. It's not easy to hear a teen mother say she is angry with her baby. It takes practice. Your fellow home visitors and your supervisor can be good sources of support.

Responsive Listening

Another way to use your voice is by not using it. Be still. Wait to respond. Listen for the meaning in what the young mother is saying. Take time for the two of you to be silent together.

Silence doesn't always create an empty space. Practice active listening with a colleague or supervisor through role-playing. Wait 10 seconds before responding. Those seconds of waiting can feel like an eternity to you, but for a young mother who is wrestling with her thoughts or just needs to be listened to, it can be a calming, enriching moment. Your engaged presence is all that really matters at those times. It works like this:

The Teen:	*The Home Visitor:*
"My boyfriend is acting differently towards me."	(all the while looking at the teen)
(pause)	"Um-mm."
"I think the baby is finally becoming real to him."	"Um-mm."
(pause)	"Um-mm."
"Maybe he's scared."	
(pause)	

Using Your Eyes

Maintaining gentle, frequent eye contact is an important way to build a relationship. It is a special way of saying, without words:

> *"I see you. You are held in my vision. In this noisy and sometimes chaotic environment, you are the most important person."*

Using Your Body

Your body language conveys the receptive posture. Your body becomes another tool to help you join with the young mother. Leaning gently closer to her can express that you want to hear her. A nod of encouragement or a gentle touch can reassure her and help connect the two of you. As she feels your presence, it will help you both become closer for the experiences to come. Chapter 6 discusses what it means to enter gently into the physical arrangements and boundaries created by teen parents.

Using Your Touch

Touch has power to soothe and regulate both babies and adults. Doulas—trained paraprofessionals who support the mother and child during pregnancy, delivery, and the weeks after birth—use touch both as a physical connector to pregnant and laboring mothers and as a physical source of comfort. The doula literature (Scott, Klaus, & Klaus, 1999) is a good resource on the power of touch.

Like the doula's touch, the home visitor's touch can be a model for the mother's own holding—both physical and emotional—of her child. For example, a home visitor can use her own touch to encourage a mother to put her hand on her abdomen when she feels the baby kicking actively. The home visitor then can put her own hand on top of the mother's: "What does the baby do, Gina, when you put your hand gently but firmly on your tummy?" (The baby may soothe and still.)

Home visitors must know a teen's comfort with being touched, even touched gently on the hand, and must respect their own comfort level in touching or not touching the young mother. Maintaining a mindful boundary—a respectful distance, both physically and emotionally from the teen—is an important way for the home visitor to maintain her credibility and effectiveness.

Using Your Mind

Jeree Pawl (1995), a gifted infant–parent therapist, stated, "Everyone deserves the experience of existing in someone's mind" (p. 5). Pawl continued:

> *Ten-month-olds . . . remember the objects behind them with which they have been playing and, without looking, reach for them with confidence and skill. This concrete image, as well as the cognitive/affective functioning it suggests, always brings to my mind a crucial internal sense that I see develop in infants who receive reasonable care. Babies feel that they exist in their caregivers' minds. The mother who is out of sight behind them is simultaneously holding and organizing them. When a child is held in mind, the child feels it, and knows it. There is a sense of safety, of containment, and, most important, existence in that other, which has always seemed to me vital. (p. 5)*

A home visitor helps a teen mom hold her baby in her mind by letting the young mother know that she is held in the home visitor's mind. Very likely, you do this instinctively and often. Here are some strategies for letting a teen know that you are thinking about her.

The Home Visitor:

(at all home visits)

"Last night I was thinking about what you said about . . . ."

"Do you remember when you told me about...? Let me tell you about something I saw that reminded me of that. . . . .

"Yesterday, I was wondering how things turned out with . . . ."

These strategies let a young mother know that in her absence you are thinking of her and remembering her—that she exists in your mind. She may grow to feel that she is "noted, noticed, spoken to over distance, rescued, protected, appreciated, and tethered across space and out of mutual sight" (Pawl, 1995, p. 5). What a gift! And what a gift for the mother to be able to pass on to her infant.

REFERENCES

Bromwich, R. (1978). *Working with parents and infants: An interactional approach.* Baltimore: University Park Press.

Pawl, J. (1995). The therapeutic relationship as human connectedness: Being held in another's mind. *Zero to Three, 15*(94), 2–5.

Scott, K. D., Klaus, P., & Klaus, M. (1999). The obstetrical and postpartum benefits of continuous support during childbirth. *Journal of Women's Health & Gender-Based Medicine,* 8, 1257–1264.

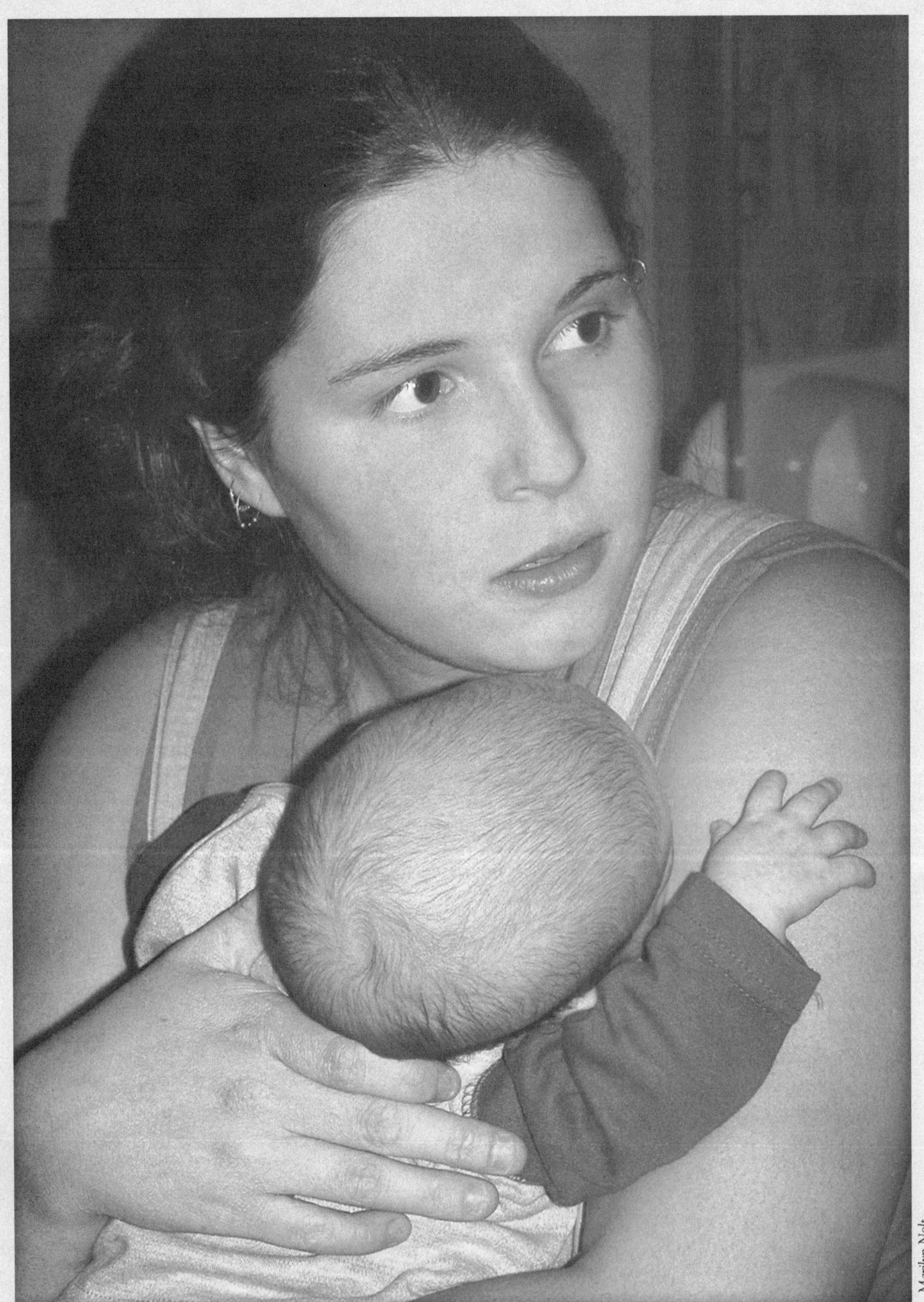

Marilyn Nolt

CHAPTER 3

KNOW THE TEEN

Just as you seek to know yourself, you must also seek to know the young pregnant woman whose home you visit regularly. Who is she? How do you come to know the answer to this question? That is what this chapter is all about.

A DUAL BIRTH

The time surrounding pregnancy, labor, delivery, and the first months postpartum bears witness to a dual birth. First, there are the many changes that occur in the mother's body and self-perception, expectations, dreams, fears, ambivalence, relationships, and knowledge. Then, there are the dramatic changes in the growth and development of the unborn baby and, later, infant. In the newborn infant, biological and behavioral changes in learning and in emotional and physical development occur with breathtaking frequency (Emde, Gaensbauer, & Harmon, 1976).

When the experience of new motherhood occurs within the context of adolescence—when the mother herself is undergoing similar and equally dramatic biological and behavioral shifts—the home visitor witnesses a coming together of two powerful events. You are witnessing a dual birth! Every time you visit a teen mother you are supporting her growth and "birth" as much as you are supporting her baby's growth and birth (J. Osofsky, personal communication, October, 2000).

ADULT AND TEEN MOTHERS

Flanagan, McGrath, Meyer, and Garcia Coll (1995) described adult women who are about to become mothers as having a reliably evolving sense of the following:

- Who they are—for example, friendly, smart, shy, short, or tall.
- Their short- and long-term future plans—being a homemaker, student, or perhaps teacher.
- How life has changed since their pregnancy or delivery—their enjoyment at feeling fetal movement or their inability to sleep as well.
- What becoming or being a mother means to them—their need for patience, listening for the baby crying, talking to the baby.

- Who their unborn baby/newborn is—"he's really active inside me," "she kicks a lot," "he calms down inside me when I sing," "she has big, smart-looking eyes."

But, teen mothers are teens first! And the normal state of development for many teens is that they are changing. Teens typically have many strengths: vigor, reactivity, a need for action, a desire (or not) for affiliation, a desire to be absolutely the same and absolutely different from peers. How can these special attributes be channeled into "good enough," or able, mothering?

Your task as a home visitor is to determine where a young mother is along the dimensions of self-knowledge, future plans, life changes, perception of motherhood, and knowledge of her baby. And—once you have come to understand all of that—how do you tailor your home-based care to make the best possible use of that knowledge? It is a complicated process because teens are so very different. Surprisingly, whether a teen is 13 or 19 doesn't seem to be as important as how she thinks about things.

Knowing how she thinks helps you help a teen feel like an "okay" mother, that is, a mother who feels good about her efforts and takes pleasure in the messages from her baby that say, "I like it here," a mother who doesn't feel as if she has to be a perfect A-plus mother. An okay mother instead can enjoy some serenity in her role and feel that doing okay is good enough. Mothers have staying power!

We know that there are specific interventions that help young mothers develop this sense of being an okay mother. One way to help mothers arrive at this point is to help them develop the story of their life with their infant even as they are living it. This is a way for them to keep things straight, make some order out of what they are going through, and, most important, feel like strong and able mothers. You will find other ways throughout this guide.

Finding Out How She Thinks and Feels About Things

There are at least three important aspects of a teen's life to keep in mind as you get to know her:

- The thinking processes she uses to think about her life
- Her usual mood state and her mood state today
- Her receptivity to intervention—her desire to learn from and be guided by you or to guard her autonomy. Either one is normal for the developing teen.

You can ask specific questions that will help you get to know a teen mother and know how to help her use her skills. Asking these questions and developing a sense of who she is and how she thinks, however, cannot occur in just one home visit. This assessment should occur naturally, within the context of your relationship with each other.

Your home-based interventions should be shaped to be within or just a little beyond the young mother's growth and development. For example, if a teen's developmental level makes her comfortable thinking concretely in the here and now, trying to engage her in thinking of the future can lead to frustration for both of you.

How She Thinks—The Questions

The five questions presented next, which are adapted from Flanagan and her colleagues (1995), help elicit information about how a young mother thinks along a continuum of concrete to abstract thinking, present to future orientation, and self-absorbed to other focused (see Figure 3.1). They are meant to alert you not only to how a teen views herself but also to how she thinks about how she views herself. So, listen for two things as you talk with her:

- The content of her answer and
- What her answer tells you about the kinds of thinking processes she uses.

Knowing these two things will help you individualize your interventions.

Figure 3.1

How She Thinks—The Questions

1. What can you tell me about yourself?
2. What do you see yourself doing in a few years?
3. How has your life changed since you became pregnant (had your baby)?
4. What do you think makes a good mother?
5. What have you learned about your baby so far?

As for the timing of the questions, asking them at different points in the teen's journey to motherhood helps you see where she is on the continuum of thinking about herself and her baby. With this approach, you will be able to notice whether her way of thinking is changing. The three key times are at the beginning of your relationship, as the teen nears her delivery date, and after the baby is born.

Let's look at each question and consider what a young mother's answers might mean.

1. What can you tell me about yourself?

This question helps you get a picture of the teen mother's thinking process in terms of the continuum from concrete to abstract. As you reflect on her answers, consider the extent to which they do the following:

- Focused on concrete, physical characteristics—"I'm tall. I have blue eyes."
- Focused on concrete traits and actions—"I'm tall, and I'm good at running."
- Action oriented only—"I'm a good cook. I've been to Great America. I walk my dog."
- Focused on action and abstract traits—"I'm a runner, and I'm friendly."
- Abstract only—"I'm thoughtful, patient, friendly."

2. What do you see yourself doing in a few years?

This question helps you get a picture of the teen mother's thinking process in terms of present to future orientation. As you reflect on her answers, consider the extent to which she exhibits the following:

- Does not answer or answers in a flip way
- Shares unrealistic goals with no plan for achievement
- Shares goals but with no plan of action
- Shares solid goals but with an unrealistic action plan
- Shares goals with a good action plan.

3. How has your life changed since you became pregnant (had your baby)?

This question helps you identify the teen mother's thinking process in terms of the range from self-absorbed to other focused. As you reflect on her answers, consider the extent to which she responds as follows:

- Is unaware of why this question matters
- Says that there are no changes
- Focuses on limitations and the things she can no longer can do, or begins to focus on a relationship with the baby
- Appreciates the larger responsibility of raising a child

4. What do you think makes a good mother?

This question also helps you identify the teen mother's thinking process along the continuum of self-absorbed to other focused. As you reflect on her answers, consider the extent to which she understands the following:

- The demands of caring for the baby—"I have to change her, feed her."
- That her life will change in relation to the baby—"Maybe a good mother has to get up when the baby cries."
- That self-denial helps the baby—"A good mother doesn't spend money on beer or makeup, she buys stuff for the baby."

- That she has to give of herself for the baby's sake—"A good mother is still and quiet when her baby is in her arms, even if she wants to be running around."
- That she must be emotionally available, patient, and loving with the baby

5. What have you learned about your baby so far?

This is another question that helps you assess the young mother's thinking process, ranging from concrete to abstract. As you reflect on her answers, consider the extent to which she does the following:

- Focuses on the baby's physical characteristics—short, fat, thin, tall, etc.
- Focuses on passive actions—"He sleeps a lot."
- Focuses on actions—"She laughs a lot, and she eats a lot."
- Describes personality traits without elaborating—"Oh, he's just a bad boy."
- Gives a rich description of personality traits—"She's so curious. She looks around all the time. She's really thinking about things, even if she can't talk."

How She Thinks—Using What You Learn

Shape your interactions with the young mother according to where her thinking falls along the dimensions of concrete–abstract, present focused–future focused, and self-absorbed–other focused. For example, if her thinking is mostly concrete, self-absorbed, and present oriented, a useful way to heighten her interest in the baby growing inside her is to relate to the baby through the teen. Greet her, saying, "Hello, Rosa," then, look directly at her growing midsection and say, "Hello, Rosa's baby."

If the baby inside her is very active, relate that to her own activity level. Does she prefer laid-back activities such as watching TV or reading a book? If she does, wonder aloud what it feels like to have such an active baby. If the teen is very active, think aloud with her about how she calms herself down. In effect, you are asking her how she soothes herself, which is a very good lead in to how she might soothe her unborn baby—talking softly to her baby or rubbing her hand gently across a part of the baby that she can identify.

Make use of how the teen thinks. There is no right or wrong way for a teen to be. The important thing is that you enter her sphere of development. If right now she is a concrete thinker, very present focused and self-absorbed, that's not only okay, but it's also pretty normal! As she gets a little older and becomes ever more attached to her baby, her thinking likely will become more reflective and abstract, more future oriented in relation to herself and her infant than it is now.

How She Feels—The Questions

Understanding the typical and current feeling state a teen is living with helps a home visitor understand where to focus, how to gently approach topics that may be troubling her, how to share in her happy states, and, most important, how to help her regulate herself. One of the teen's most important tasks after the birth of her baby will be to help her baby regulate himself. In your prenatal time with her, model this process.

There are three major feeling states to be aware of—anxiety, well-being, and sadness and/or depression. Frame the questions about the teen's feeling states in the context of her everyday life (see Figure 3.2). Asking her, "How do you feel?" may elicit a "fine," and you won't have learned very much.

Figure 3.2

How She Feels—The Questions

1. When you looked in the mirror this morning what did your face tell you about how you're feeling today? Were you feeling pretty good? Sad? Worried?
2. Is this usually what your face tells you when you look in the mirror? Or was it different today from most other days?
3. Let's see if you can help me understand where that feeling is coming from.

Let's look at each question and consider what a young mother's answers might mean.

1. When you looked in the mirror this morning what did your face tell you about how you're feeling today? Were you feeling pretty good? Sad? Worried?

This question helps you get a sense of the young mother's emotional state at the moment. As you reflect on her answers, consider the extent to which she accomplishes the following:

- Is able to describe how she looks but is not able to verbalize her feelings
- Is aware that her appearance may be an expression of a more inner self
- Understands that by discussing what she sees in the mirror she is describing how she feels
- Adds a narrative describing why she looks the way she does.

2. Is this usually what your face tells you when you look in the mirror? Or was it different today from most other days?

This question helps you explore whether the teen's emotional state at the moment is typical or whether something has happened to make her feel differently today.

As you reflect on her answers, consider the extent of the following:

- Her ability to discuss the ebbs and flows of her emotions and her inner changes that are expressed outwardly.

3. Let's see if you can help me understand where that feeling is coming from.

This request helps you explore whether the teen can associate her emotions with a cause and effect. As you reflect on her answers, consider the extent to which she accomplishes the following:

- Is or is not able to express a connection between events in her life and how they cause her to feel
- Describes narratively what she is feeling but has difficulty attaching herself to the emotions in her narrative
- Both experiences and describes her feelings in a way that helps her and you have a fuller understanding of why she feels the way she does.

Ask this question regardless of the feeling state the teen reports. It is especially helpful to know what makes her feel good.

Asking these questions repeatedly over time and in the context of your developing relationship with the teen mom helps you understand her typical mood state and fluctuations in mood state as she responds to events in her life. Although fluctuations in mood are normal in adolescence, all of us have a certain characteristic temperament and a certain outlook that need to be respected. This is especially important for teens.

How She Feels—Using What You Learn

Whatever the typical or current feeling state the teen presents, bear witness to it. Use a receptive, relaxed posture and absorb with full attention what she tells you. Maintain eye contact.

Let the teen know that you are willing and able to absorb what she has to say without being devastated by it and without passing judgment. To help her keep herself together, you remain regulated—which means you keep yourself together—in the face of her grief, joy, depression, or anxiety, no matter how overwhelming any of those emotions may be for her. For some teens, this is what distinguishes you from the other people in her life, who may be critical or overreactive, or who may bring their own agendas to her behavior and feelings. She knows that you have joined with her. She knows that you have entered the sphere of her experience as she attempts to cope with pregnancy, life events, and her own rapidly changing development.

Fully acknowledge her feeling states. Use the same skills discussed in chapter 2; frame the resources she has inside her to cope with her feelings (see Figure 3.3). It helps to have someone draw a strong frame around the helping resources that exist in her life right now—resources inside or outside her that help her cope with what she is living through.

Figure 3.3

Framing Resources

- "You've got a lot of heavy stuff on your mind right now, but you're so good at telling me about it—that's a really special strength."
- "I'm happy for you that you have [name of the baby's father, and/or friends or family members] in your life and that it makes you feel better to be around them."
- "Let's plan together how we can make this a little better."
  (This says, "Don't forget I'm an important resource in your life now.")

This is very hard to do! If the teen is highly anxious, your job is to help absorb some of that anxiety. But that doesn't mean that you should walk around with her anxiety. Practice leaving it at the door when you leave after a home visit. Talks with your supervisor and colleagues can help you rid yourself of your concerns for this teen. In fact, you and your supervisor should develop strategies for ridding yourself of work-related anxiety. Doing so does not mean that you are not an empathetic or compassionate person. It is the only way to keep yourself regulated, and ready and refreshed for your next visit.

Depression. Sometimes the teen's feeling state is depression. This is a complex issue that requires consultation with your supervisor. Depression has many faces. Depression can masquerade as anger. It also can manifest itself in eating or sleeping too much or too little, but always consider the context in which you see these behaviors, as teens can overeat or sleep too much simply because they are teens.

Young women who have experienced physical, sexual, or verbal abuse can appear depressed. They may also appear stunned or in shock and, in fact, they may be experiencing a form of posttraumatic stress syndrome. When the teen's daily life approaches being governed by these symptoms, it is time for a referral to a community mental health agency.

Sadness and grief. What may look like depression may actually be great sadness and grief. One of the first things to consider and ask the teen about is her relationship to the baby's father. Is he a part of her life still, or did visits and phone calls stop after he became aware of the pregnancy or birth? The relationship to the baby's father may have been the teen's first intimate experience. The pregnancy may even have resulted from an attempt to hold on to the relationship.

The shock and grief of losing such a relationship are overwhelming at any age, but they are monumental in adolescence, when there is often little perspective. It may feel to the teen that no one will ever love her again, and her self-esteem may feel shattered. She may express some of these feelings as anger and threats, but it is important to remember that beneath the bluster and bravado may be her first experience with grief and mourning.

After you've known the teen for a while, you can say, "I'm so sorry you have lost this important relationship. It must feel like the loss (or death) of a very important person." At this moment, think of what you do as grief counseling—acknowledge the loss, help her sustain the grief, hold her hand. In effect, mourn with her.

There are other events in the teen's life that can trigger grief reactions—the loss of a maternal or paternal relationship because of the pregnancy, having to leave school life, or not knowing how to relate to childhood friends on new terms.

The Need for Autonomy

Teens express the need to become their own unique person in a variety of ways for a variety of reasons. As a teen matures, she becomes increasingly aware that she has the ability to define herself. Defining herself as different and separate from her family of origin is an inborn drive as compelling as the drive to walk: as a toddler, she had to walk, because she could.

While a teen works hard at developing an identity that is uniquely her own, she is working equally hard at redefining how this newly emerging self will stay connected to her family of origin (Apter, 1990; Debold, Wilson, & Malave, 1993; Jordan, Kaplan, Miller, Stiver, & Surrey, 1991). This is a difficult developmental task—one full of anxiety, excitement, hope, and worry.

An Autonomy Checklist

There is a broad normal range by which teens exhibit their internal struggles with autonomy and connectedness. Observable behavior may go from openly rebellious and sullen to resentful to no changes in behavior at all. The checklist in Figure 3.4 is a guide to things to consider.

Figure 3.4

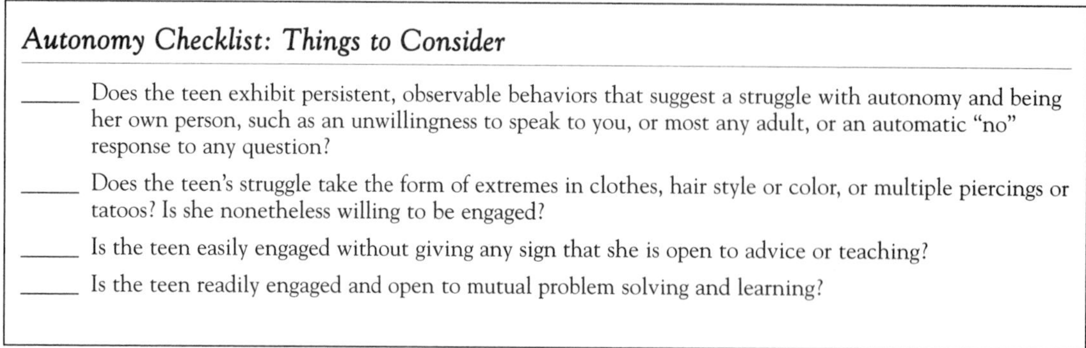

Autonomy Checklist: Things to Consider

_____ Does the teen exhibit persistent, observable behaviors that suggest a struggle with autonomy and being her own person, such as an unwillingness to speak to you, or most any adult, or an automatic "no" response to any question?

_____ Does the teen's struggle take the form of extremes in clothes, hair style or color, or multiple piercings or tatoos? Is she nonetheless willing to be engaged?

_____ Is the teen easily engaged without giving any sign that she is open to advice or teaching?

_____ Is the teen readily engaged and open to mutual problem solving and learning?

The Need for Autonomy—Using What You Learn

Wherever the teen is on this continuum, keep in mind that she is struggling with defining how she can be herself and still be connected to you, to the father of the baby, to her parents, and to her friends. As you respect her need for both uniqueness and relational connectedness, you are helping her define the real meaning of intimacy. It is this capacity to enter into intimate relationships that helps her become and stay attached to her baby. It is a lifelong process. Help her do this by shaping your interventions to where she is.

If a young mother is behaviorally rebellious and unengageable, respect that at the same time that you explain to her the nature of your job, "As your home visitor, it's my job to be here with you as you await the birth of your baby. I can see this doesn't make you happy, and it may not be what you want. But if I do my part by not asking a lot of questions that you don't want to answer, will you do your part by just letting me through the door?" Or, "Would you like to have the father of the baby or a friend with you when I come to visit? All I want to do is show you some pictures of what your baby might look like inside of you right now."

Reflect on her mood state. You can say almost anything you wish, so long as your own mood state remains even and regulated. What she does not need is to detect anger or disapproval.

Of course, never escalate into the mood state she is living in. That would destroy any hope of her trusting you. Imagine a ladder of mood states, with her rebelliousness and apparent anger being the uppermost rung. Remain always at the lowest rung. She will come to count on that.

If the teen is willing to be engaged but displays extremes in hair color or clothing style, her appearance should be acknowledged. This acknowledgment says that you have seen her; she is not invisible to you. You might say, "I see you had your nose pierced. Tell me what that means to you. Where did you have it done?"

These strategies can lead to a growing sense of mutuality. Regardless of how she behaves, she may come to feel that you are on her side.

Remember, adolescents, in general, do not think it is necessary or feel it is cool to have close, visible relationships with adults. At the same time, they may yearn for the safety, comfort, and acceptance of an elder or a mother-like person. These caring relationships do not necessarily come easily for many adolescents who bring their own histories of past relationships to this relationship.

In some instances, these past relationships have been fraught with experiences that lead teens to mistrust or discount the other. In many ways, when you meet a teenage program participant and begin to build your own new relationship with her, you are also meeting and working through all of her past caring relationships. Her history informs the present and guides the future.

References

Apter, T. (1990). *Altered loves: Mothers and daughters during adolescence*. New York: St. Martin's Press.

Debold, E., Wilson, M., & Malave, I. (1993). *Mother–daughter revolution: From betrayal to power*. Reading, MA: Addison-Wesley.

Emde, R., Gaensbauer, T., & Harmon, R. (1976). Emotional expression in infancy: A biobehavorial study. *Psychology Issues: A Monograph Series*, *10*(37).

Flanagan, P., McGrath, M., Meyer, E., & Garcia Coll, C. (1995). Adolescent development and transitions to motherhood. *Pediatrics*, 6, 273–277.

Jordan, J., Kaplan, A., Miller, J., Stiver, I., & Surrey, J. (1991). *Women's growth in connection: Writings from the Stone Center*. New York: Guilford.

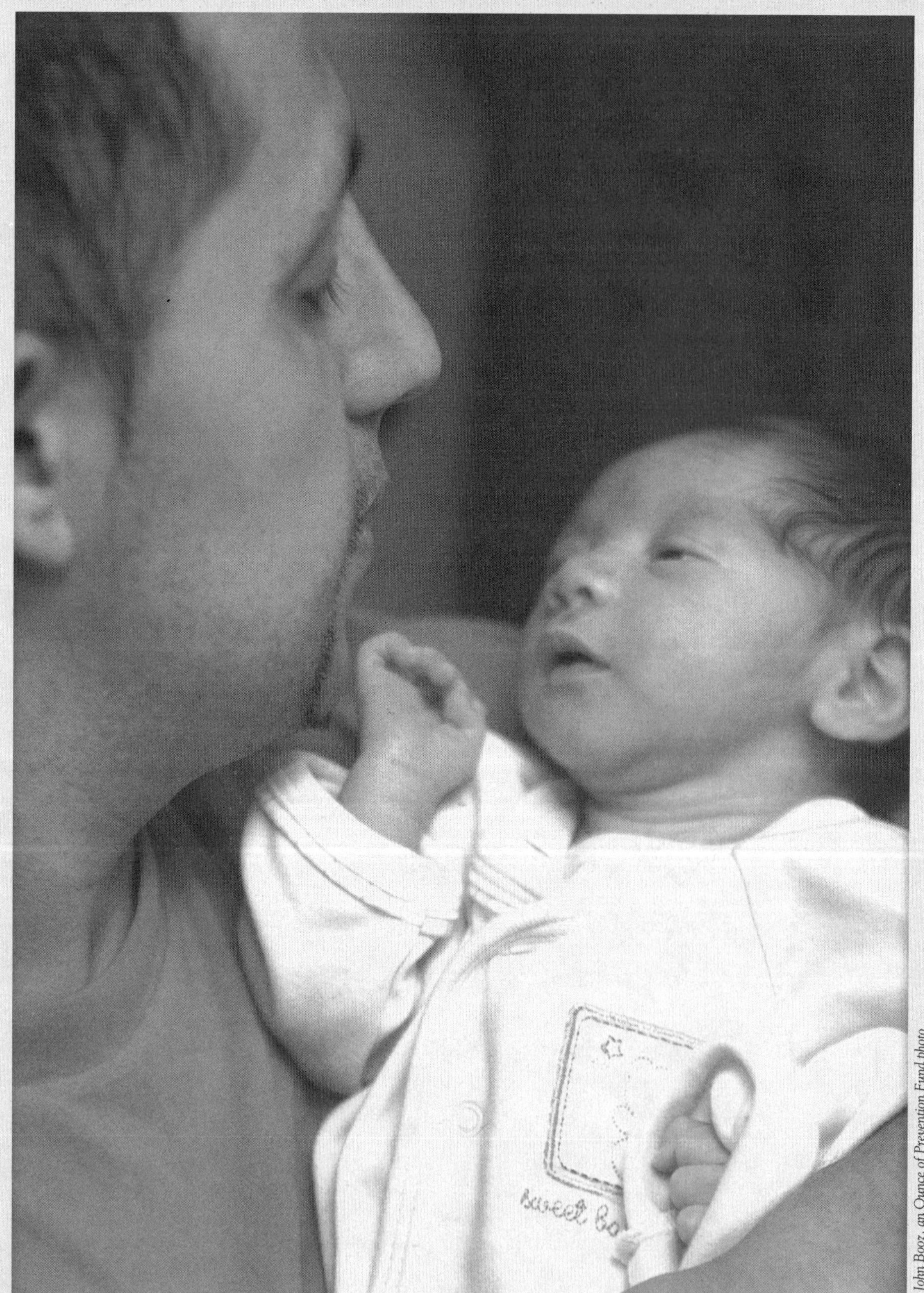

John Booz, an Ounce of Prevention Fund photo

CHAPTER 4

CONNECTING WITH FATHERS

Connecting with fathers is a wonderful outgrowth of facilitating the Community-Based Family Administered Neonatal Activities (FANA) with some young families. With others, the father is unavailable or the teen mother chooses that he not be involved. But, whether or not he is in a snapshot of the moment, the father is always a part of the family picture. As Kyle Pruett, a long-time researcher on fathers and their children, likes to say, "There is no such thing as a fatherless child" (Pruett, 1997, p. 3).

This chapter outlines guiding principles for engaging fathers through the Community-Based FANA and discusses some of the challenges and rewards for the home visitor.

DETERMINING FATHERS' INVOLVEMENT

Be sensitive to the mother's implicit and explicit cues as to her desire to have the father involved in home visits. This is best discussed when you first learn about the mother's living situation and her plans for caring for the baby.

The father's presence during the first visits usually indicates that he wants to be involved at some level. His physical proximity and degree of participation are a guide to whether he just wants to check out the situation or wants to really participate. Fathers who participate in Community-Based FANA home visits typically say that—more than anything else—having the home visitor ask them directly what they think or feel and encourage them to take a turn in an activity were the factors that influenced them to get involved.

When both parents seem invested in taking part, build a separate relationship with each. The same style and techniques of engaging and intervening are useful with both parents. Helping relationships based on acceptance, understanding, and a desire to support parents and infants are meaningful to both men and women.

Figure 4.1

Guiding Principles and Key Practices for Engaging Fathers in the Community-Based FANA

Guiding principle. Infants benefit from having a positive relationship with their mother and father, but building or maintaining the parents' relationship with each other is not the role of the home visitor.

Key practice. Work to build a meaningful relationship between mother and child and between father and child.

Guiding principle. Connecting with his baby is the ultimate prize for a father, as it is for the baby herself.

Key practice. Actively support a father's efforts to connect with and be responsible for his baby.

Engaging Fathers

Many young fathers share a common desire with mothers—that their children have a chance to grow safely, be healthy, and have more opportunities than they themselves experienced. In fact, both parents often have lofty dreams without much understanding of how they can make these dreams a reality. Home visitors can play an important role with each parent.

New parents—both father and mother—often experience great anxiety concerning their ability to provide for their baby. Accepting and coming to terms with the pregnancy and the future life can stir up strong feelings of both happiness and panic. Fathers often experience fears of the unknown, both of the unknown baby and the unknown changes that may occur in his relationship with the baby's mother and, certainly, the changes in his own life.

By the second trimester and the recognition of fetal movement, most young mothers have begun building a relationship with their unborn child. Pregnancy—the intimate and constant contact mothers have with the developing baby—becomes the laboratory for this developing relationship. Fathers do not have this opportunity. The months of pregnancy leave the father experiencing few of the reminders and happy experiences that draw the mother into a fond relationship with the new baby.

The Community-Based FANA serves as a conductor along the railroad of parenthood. Because the mother carries the baby within her, a father starts out at a greater distance than the mother and has fewer tracks leading to the child. This distance makes the home visitor's role as guide more difficult and, at times, more urgent with fathers. It is intrinsically easier for fathers to reverse direction and move away from the child than it is for mothers. Therefore, you may need to work harder to keep a father traveling forward on that parental railroad.

A father begins his relationship with his child through the reactions and responses of the baby's mother and, often, her family. Depending on his experience, the new baby can be the source of excited anticipation or of dread, burden, and anger. Although the imminent birth of a child can represent grand hopes for the future, it can also represent the ultimate loss of independence.

These feelings can challenge a father's fight-or-flight reaction to stress. It is not uncommon for fathers of babies born to teen mothers to flee. Teenage mothers are predominately single parents for at least some time during their child's early years. The situation is made more complex by the fact that the father is often not a teen himself. More than half of fathers of babies born to teen moms are in their 20s (Landry & Forrest, 1995).

When a father makes himself available and indicates an interest, and when the mother indicates that she wants his involvement, the Community-Based FANA creates opportunities for the dad to develop a close relationship with his baby. By the time the unborn baby reaches the last trimester, she is demonstrating many behaviors easily experienced from the outside. Her movements, her responsiveness, her periods of rest and activity are all available for the father to experience directly, although he may need a crash course in getting involved as the birth approaches. He has not had the same 6-month head start that the mother has had. As a home visitor, you are in an excellent position to be a guide on this urgent, incredible journey.

Fathers who are both welcomed and have the opportunity to be present during the birth and in the days after can begin to establish more deeply those ties essential to binding them together (Pruett, 1997). On first meeting their newborn, fathers report similar emotions as mothers. They touch and explore the newborn in the same pattern and manner, and they use the same high-pitched voice to catch the baby's attention. Studies indicate that an infant, just days old, can differentiate and anticipate his father's presence as well as his mother's. Kyle Pruett (1997) described one young father's experience:

> *A 17-year-old brand-new father was "blown-away" when his baby opened her eyes wide in response to his reaching down to pick her up. He asked his daughter, "I'm not your momma—and you still want me?" This tiny bit of encouragement from his baby touched him and kept him coming back for more.* (p. 5)

Fathers who are involved at birth or immediately after also tend to stay involved (Pruett, 2000). The postnatal Community-Based FANA can help a father root his feelings and observations in the behaviors of his child. These behaviors not only have the potential to excite him and make him proud but also can elicit a genuine and gratifying sense of profound connection. Fathers now get to feel for themselves a special and unique relationship.

Playing with his just-born baby, watching and feeling her incredible capacities, experiencing the sense of intimate care in being able to calm his newborn, and having the opportunity to express his parental feelings all contribute to building the father's growing sense of mastery. These experiences reassure dads that staying involved was worth the wait and that now they will have the opportunity to care for another.

For young men, becoming a father represents a dual birth as well. His child's first cries of life mark his own birth as a dad. Using the Community-Based FANA to promote strong feelings of empathy and attachment between father and child enables home visitors to help organize the father's emotions and behaviors in relation to his new role. In time, if the opportunities continue in a positive manner, that sense of internal organization can spread from the inside out, growing from emotional connection to social connection, responsiveness, and, ultimately, responsibility.

Preparing Fathers

Just as there are questions and activities that home visitors can use to prepare mothers and support their participation in the Community-Based FANA, there are a variety of ways that you can prepare and support fathers. If you are working with an expectant father in the first trimester, focus on acceptance. Support his efforts to accept the pregnancy and the developing baby; accept himself as a father and his responsibility to his baby; accept the baby's mother and be accepted by her; accept his feelings about what kind of father he will be; accept his loss of freedom and independence; and accept his excitement and hope at becoming a father at the same time that he accepts his doubts, confusion, and fear.

Figure 4.2 offers guidance that home visitors can share with fathers in the second and third trimesters. In the second semester, focus on living with the baby. In the third trimester, focus on getting ready to be with the baby.

Challenges

Recent studies indicate that more than half of teen pregnancies result from sexual relations with older men. Although a 2- or 3-year difference is most common, it also appears that the younger the mother, the greater the age gap with the father. Additional studies indicate that an alarmingly high rate of teen mothers report earlier experiences of sexual coercion or assault, and many young mothers are survivors of abandonment or abuse (Boyer & Fine, 1992).

Figure 4.2

Guidance for Fathers

Second Trimester

Hear your baby's heartbeat.

Wonder what kind of father you will be.

Create positive and exciting dreams about the future.

Find accepting, caring people to talk with about your feelings and the changes you're going through.

Find other fathers to talk with about this new experience.

If possible, talk with your own dad or father-figure about what it was like for him when he was waiting for you to be born.

Think about how you want to take care of and raise your baby.

Talk about the changes in your relationship with the mother of the baby.

Find books, movies, and magazines about babies and being a father.

Live with happiness, guilt, anticipation, ambivalence, and frustration.

Third Trimester

Begin to spend more time with your baby's mom talking about how you can share raising him.

Be patient and understanding of the mother's point of view.

Appreciate the huge emotional, physical, and hormonal changes that the mom is experiencing because of the pregnancy.

Talk, talk, talk with the baby's mother about the changes that the pregnancy is putting you through. Talk about what excites you, what scares you, and what makes you uncertain. Talk about her parents and your parents.

Find other dads to talk with about their experiences, and share your feelings with them.

Be flexible in your views; the baby changes everything!

Discuss with the mom if and how she would like your support during labor and birth. Discuss attending a prenatal or birthing class, either with her or on your own.

If your baby's mother is comfortable with your touch, now you can feel the baby move.

Imagine what the elbows, feet, and hands that you feel kicking will look and feel like once the baby is out.

Begin to play with the baby, even before he is born. If it's okay with his mother, gently push one side of her abdomen. The baby will move to respond. Then try the other side.

Count the baby's kicks and feel how active she is now. Wonder what she will be like once she is born.

Talk, read, and sing to your baby while he is still inside his mom. The more you talk now, the more he will recognize your voice once he is born.

Think about what you will want to read and sing to the baby after he is born. Remember the songs and stories that you're enjoying with him now.

Massage the baby gently through her mother's skin, if the mother feels like having you do that.

Think about how your schedule will work with the baby's schedule once he is born.

Try calming the baby with your voice during a time that she is really active inside her mom, if that's okay with the mom.

Think about how you will calm your baby after he is born, and remember how you were calmed. Decide how you want to calm, guide, and discipline your own baby.

(Source: Adapted from Brott & Ash, 1995)

In situations in which the baby's father was responsible for that coercion, abuse, or abandonment, home visitors are challenged to help the mother separate her feelings toward the baby's father from her feelings toward her unborn and then newborn baby. It is easy for her to transfer feelings and to attempt to hurt the father through the baby, or even to punish herself in reaction to the shame, guilt, or pain she may have experienced. Home visitors find themselves in a balancing act, taking every opportunity to foster connectedness between the father and baby, while at the same time creating a safe zone for the mother by also helping her maintain a sense of separateness in her mind, a reminder that the baby is not the father.

It is also easy for home visitors to transfer feelings. When you hear of or witness unhealthy relationships, your own feelings of disapproval or anger toward the father may churn up. As with other emotions, it is important to explore and plan how to handle these feelings with your supervisor. Remember, your work is about that mother and that baby, and that father and that baby, not about you and the baby.

Opportunities

This chapter is a reminder of how complex relationships are—men and women, men and children, and even your own relationships with the fathers you meet while doing your work. New relationships also bring opportunities for personal growth and relating to others in a new way. Involving fathers in the Community-Based FANA activities can be life changing. A father can be helped to build a relationship with his child that reaches toward his dream of being the best that he can be.

Your work promoting secure relationships between children and their parents benefits both the children and parents. A father once said, "Having this child in my life not only taught me about being a dad, but also taught me how to be a better man."

REFERENCES

Boyer, D., & Fine, D. (1992). Sexual abuse as a factor in adolescent pregnancy and child maltreatment. *Family Planning Perspectives*, *24*(1), 4–11, 19.

Brott, A. A. & Ash, J. (1995). *The expectant father*. New York: Abbeville Press.

Landry, D. J., & Forrest, J. D. (1995). How old are U.S. fathers? *Family Planning Perspectives*, *27*, 159–165.

Pruett, K. D. (1997). How men and children affect each other's development. *Zero to Three*, *18*(1), 3–11.

Pruett, K. D. (2000). *Fatherneed: Why father care is as essential as mother care for your child*. New York: The Free Press.

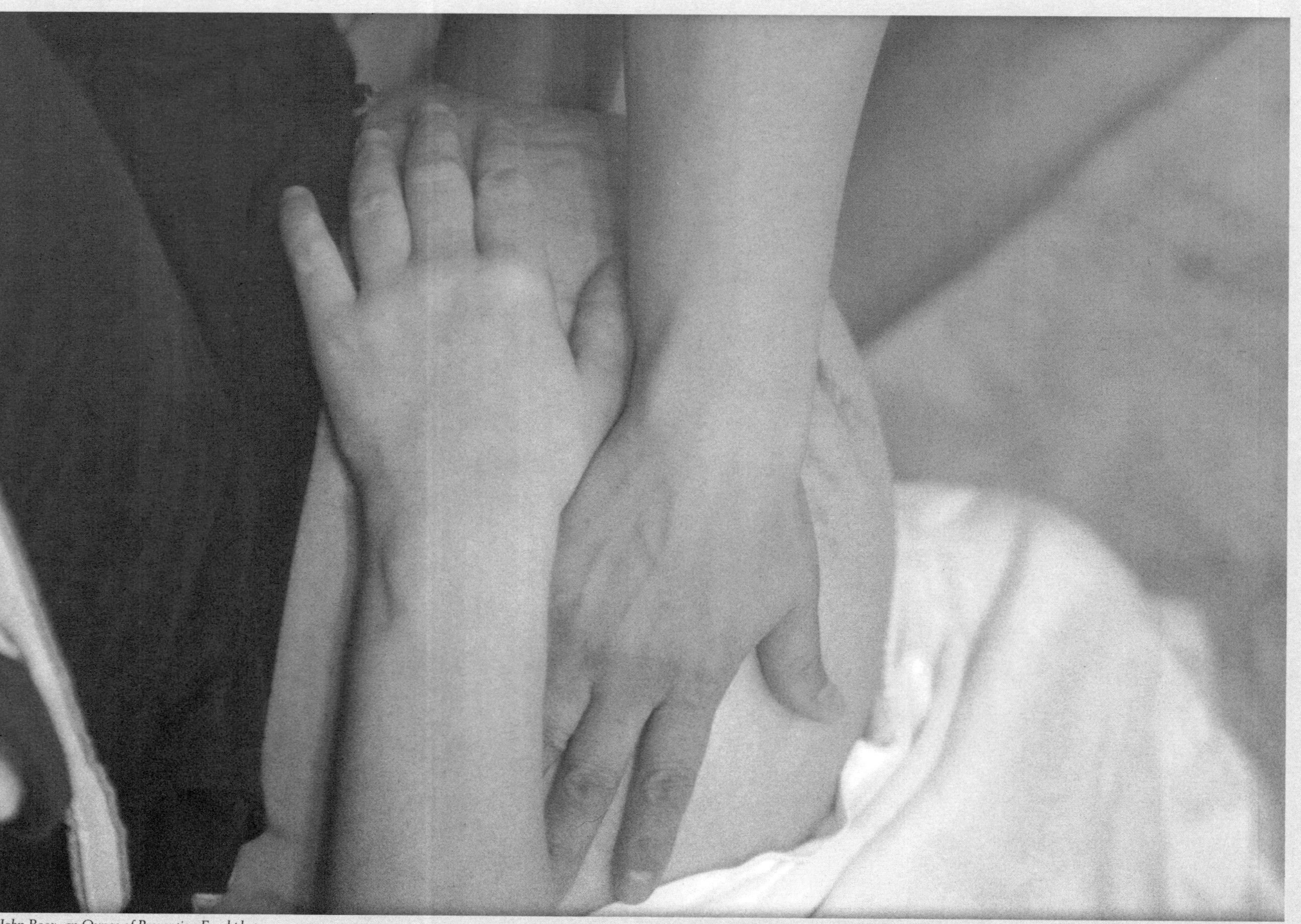

John Booz, an Ounce of Prevention Fund photo

MUTUAL GROWTH: THE TRIMESTERS OF PREGNANCY

As she moves through her adolescence, every teen's body changes dramatically, both inside and out. But the pregnant teen's body changes faster and in more observable ways as the baby inside her grows and makes his presence felt in many, many ways. All of this makes for a pressure cooker of change, with new developments unfolding at breakneck speed!

This chapter is meant to supplement your knowledge of the teen's developing pregnancy. It summarizes the physical changes in the teen mother and the growth of the fetus in each trimester, as well as the social and emotional issues a pregnant teen faces and the home visitor's role in relation to these issues. By design, this chapter is more didactic than the others so that you can have at your fingertips a resource on the trimesters of pregnancy.

Information in this chapter is organized within the following categories: physical changes in the teen mother, growth of the fetus, and social and emotional issues. Although the chapter offers you information for each trimester, the Community-Based Family Administered Neonatal Activities (FANA) covers only the third trimester—months 7, 8, and 9 of the pregnancy. Guidelines for sharing third trimester information with parents are included in chapter 6, "The Birth," and chapter 9, "Welcome Parents: The Prenatal Home Visits." A summary of prenatal development especially relevant to each prenatal home visit is included in the activities.

PHYSICAL CHANGES IN THE TEEN MOTHER

Consider this description: "There is a disruption of basic physiological processes such as sleep, digestion, and appetite, and hormonal surges regularly affect mood and cognition" (Cohen & Slade, 2000, p. 20). It sounds like a description of the teen years, doesn't it? But, as you've no doubt guessed, it is really a description of pregnancy.

Physical changes in adolescence are not individual, isolated events. They take place over a long period of time, from about age 10 to about age 20. Physical changes vary considerably from individual to individual, both in the amount of change and the length of time over which change takes place. One thing that is nearly universally true of teens is that they worry about their bodies. They show tremendous concern about whether their bodies are or will be right. There is great variability in the timing of physical changes in puberty—such as pubic hair growth, breast size, phallus size, and height and weight (Hermann-Giddens et al., 1977).

That gives teens plenty to worry about. When a teen sees herself as developing too fast or not fast enough, problem behavior can develop. In one study, late maturation resulted in an increase in girls' social problems, and very early maturation resulted in withdrawn behavior. For boys, early maturation led to a decrease in social problems and increased attention span (Laitinen-Krispijn, Vander Ende, Hazebroek-Hampschreur, & Verhulst, 1999).

The teen mother is growing before your eyes. She may well grow taller during this time, very likely within the months you are visiting her. Even apart from the pregnancy, there are enormous hormonal changes—the greatest changes and surges since infancy. The physical changes of pregnancy (see Figure 5.1) plus the normal physical and developmental changes of adolescence all add up to a lot of change. That is why your work helping pregnant teens maintain a sense of balance and perspective is so important.

As you prepare to understand and empathize with rapidly developing teens, Figure 5.2 offers some statements for you to think about and complete. Keep in mind your responses as you prepare yourself to understand the internal world of the young mother.

THE GROWTH OF THE FETUS

During the 9 months of pregnancy, the baby is incredibly busy. The baby is growing, moving, listening, and responding to the world around him. It has been said that the only truly new newborn behavior is the birth cry. All else has begun to emerge before birth: sucking, swallowing, breathing movements, kicking, sleeping, and even being awake.

The baby is an active participant in her development, even before birth when many of her needs are taken care of for her. The mother supplies oxygen and nutrients. There is plenty of stimulation from the sounds inside and outside the womb and from the mother's activity. Why is the human infant so active before

Figure 5.1

Physical Changes in the Pregnant Teen

First Trimester

- Fatigue and sleepiness
- Frequent urination
- Nausea, with and without vomiting
- Food aversions and cravings
- Slightly bigger breasts, sore breasts

Second Trimester

- Appetite increase as morning sickness goes away
- Return of energy
- Heartburn and constipation
- Continuing breast changes
- Significant midsection growth and need for maternity clothes
- Stomach skin beginning to stretch and itch
- Backaches and difficulty standing for long periods

Third Trimester

- Vaginal discharge
- Lower abdominal aches
- Shortness of breath
- Strong contractions as early as a month before delivery
- Leg cramps

birth? Activity or experience is fuel for the brain (see Figure 5.3). Fetal activity helps to build connections in the developing brain (H. Als, personal communication, May 23, 2000).

Human infants need three environments in order to develop: (a) the mother's womb before birth, (b) her breast and body after birth, and (c) the family's social group after birth (Hofer, 1997). We are an inherently social species. We need to seek out others in order to survive and grow. The baby's genetic code does not contain all the information that he needs to grow and develop. Interaction with others is required for development to proceed.

Humans are made so that we expect to have certain experiences—to see, to hear, to move, to be protected and nurtured. Even before birth, the baby depends on the mother's care—on what she eats, what she does, and even what she feels. The baby and the mother are in contact with each other and influence each other, right from the start.

Figure 5.2

Empathizing With the Rapidly Developing Teen

- When I was 15 years old, my physical appearance could best be described as . . .
- My greatest concern about my body was . . .
- My medical problems during adolescence were . . .
- One of my greatest misconceptions about the opposite sex was . . .

(Source: Adapted from Neinstein and Kaufman, 1996, p. 37)

What is your image of the womb? Most of us picture a peaceful place, certainly more calm, quiet, predictable, and stable than our hectic lives on the outside. The reality of this blissful state is quite different (Maurer & Maurer, 1988). The womb is positioned beside three relatively loud organs—the heart, the intestines, and the lungs. The womb can be booming, bumpy, and full of tastes and smells!

Most of the time, the baby finds the environment varied, changing from minute to minute as the mother walks, talks, eats, or gets worried or happy. This variability may help prepare the baby for the changing world on the outside, where sounds come unexpectedly and his mother cannot get there to feed him right away. Before birth, babies begin to experience—perhaps even adjust to—the ups and downs of everyday life.

The First Trimester—Months 1, 2, and 3

By the end of the first month of pregnancy, the earliest beginnings of the brain, heart, lungs, liver, stomach, and pancreas are present, as are arm and leg buds. Blood circulation is well established. All the fingers and toes are formed—even fingernails! The eyelids are fused closed and will stay that way until 25 weeks. By the end of the first trimester, the genitalia are present, and it is clear whether this littlest of persons is a girl or a boy. During this period, the baby floats in a state of

Figure 5.3

Understanding Fetal Development

- Newborn behavior is not new. Babies begin almost all the behaviors we see at birth while they are still in utero.
- Genes are not enough. The unborn baby actively stimulates development.
- It is varied inside the womb. The baby experiences continual change as the mother moves, talks, and goes about her daily life.
- The mother's behavior affects the baby. The baby's growth and development are affected by the mother's health habits.

relative weightlessness, like an astronaut. The pregnant teen does not experience the baby moving at any time during the first trimester.

In the first month, the baby is a tiny embryo, about the size of a grain of rice. Although the pregnant teen does not experience movement at any time during the first trimester, by the end of the third month the baby—now called a fetus—will be about 3 inches long, weigh about 0.5 ounce, and be developing many organs, as well as hands, feet, ears, and eyelids (Eisenberg, Murkoff, & Hathaway, 1991).

Brain development. During the first trimester, the neural tube forms and closes, and the brain cells begin to divide and multiply. By birth, 100 billion nerve cells will have formed—about as many stars as there are in the sky!

Whole body movements. The baby is moving by the end of the first trimester, even though the mother cannot yet feel it because the uterus has no sense of touch (Maurer & Maurer, 1988). When the baby is large enough that movements can be felt by the abdomen wall—during the second trimester, at about 16 weeks—the mother is able to feel the baby move.

When exactly does the baby start to move? It happens very early, about 7.5 weeks after conception (Hofer, 1981). The first movements are those that take place when the baby moves his head away from a stimulus (Hofer, 1981). Thus, the baby's first movements are protective, or away from a stimulus. About 2 weeks later, the baby will move toward the stimulus (Hofer, 1981). Toward the end of the first trimester—10 to 12 weeks—the baby is busy. Four patterns of behavior can be seen:

- Playing possum—periods of no movement, probably lasting no longer than 5 minutes because the baby is so active during this early period;
- Acrobatics—periods of rolling, flexion and extension, and head rotating that involve the whole body;
- Waving—periods of arm and leg movements; and
- Hiccups—strong, pulsed movements, such as hiccups.

(Van Dongen & Goudie, 1980)

Also by 12 weeks, head movements, stretching, and yawning are present. In the beginning of pregnancy, all these movements seem to be random. They do not occur in any particular order or at any particular time.

Hand movements. By 10.5 weeks, the baby's fingers are semiflexed and can move individually. Her hands can open. Her index finger has less of a tendency to bend—her pointer finger is already in action. By the end of the first trimester, hand-to-face contact begins.

Mouth movements—sucking and swallowing. The sucking reflex begins during the third month. By 12 weeks, the baby has begun to swallow amniotic fluid. What a lot of practice babies have sucking and swallowing before they are born! This early sucking probably helps to develop the lung buds and the digestive tract—another way that the baby plays a role in his own development (Moessinger, 1988).

Eye movements. Eye movements can be seen during the third month in utero. However, the baby's eyelids are fused and do not open until the third trimester, and the baby is not yet sensitive to light.

Touch. Touch is the first sense to develop. The mouth and face are the first areas to become sensitive to touch (Hofer, 1981). Sensation begins in the lips, then the inside of the mouth, nose, chin, and eyelids. Next to become sensitive are the palms of hands, genitalia, and soles of the feet, followed by the arms and legs and chest (Hofer, 1981). Bigger areas of the brain are devoted to the regions of the body that develop sensitivity to touch first, such as the face. Humans are very sensitive around and in the mouth. Consider how a paper cut would feel on your gum compared to one on your arm or leg. Think about the increased sensitivity of these vital body parts. And it all begins in the first months of life.

The Second Trimester—Months 4, 5, and 6

The most dramatic development of the second trimester is that the mother is able to feel the baby move. This is called quickening, and it can be experienced in many different ways, such as a slight fluttering like butterflies in the stomach, or a twitch. The baby is now 6 to 7 inches long and weighs about 5 ounces. His skin is pink and transparent. As this trimester progresses, the baby begins to move from side to side. At the end of the sixth month, the baby is covered with fine, soft hair, and his eyelids begin to part. Sleep and wake cycles are beginning to emerge; by the third trimester, they will be much more defined (Hofer, 1981). The baby may weigh as much as 1.5 pounds.

Size and appearance. During the second trimester, the position of the baby's head is likely to be down because it is heavier and also because she experiences a reduction in blood flow to her brain when her head is up, and she may therefore be more comfortable when her head is down. There is a lot of activity during the second trimester. Many position changes may occur, especially around 13 to 15 weeks. As the baby gets bigger and the space available to move gets correspondingly smaller, fewer position changes take place after 15 weeks.

Brain development—laying down of the cortex. During this period, billions of nerve cells move to their proper locations. Six layers of the cortex are formed, in exquisite order. Myelination of the nerve cells begins. Myelin is a fatty sheath that coats the nerve cells and speeds up messages between them.

Body movements. Most of the movements that the baby can do at birth are present by 14 weeks. During this trimester, movements become organized into longer stretches of activity. By about the middle of the second trimester—20 weeks—the periods of movement may be as long as several minutes, with definite periods of rest between. At this time there is also more of a daily pattern to fetal movements, with activity often peaking in the late evening.

Hand movements. During the second trimester, the baby's thumb and fingers begin to coordinate into a reflexive or automatic grasp. This is the same grasp that parents can feel right after the baby is born if they put a finger into her palm.

Sucking and swallowing. At 13 weeks, the baby can be seen sucking his thumb in an ultrasound image. Toward the end of the second trimester, the baby swallows up to an ounce of fluid an hour, or the equivalent of an 8-ounce baby bottle in an 8-hour day. Think how much practice an infant has sucking before birth! Fetal sucking regulates the amount of amniotic fluid, and the protein and nitrogen the baby take in also may have value.

Breathing. By 13 weeks, breathing movements begin. Here again, the baby practices basic movements and behaviors long before birth. Infants born prematurely during the second and early third trimesters cannot breathe on their own and will be helped to breathe in the Neonatal Intensive Care Unit (NICU).

Touch. By 14 weeks, the whole body is sensitive to touch. About this time, ultrasound shows the baby self-initiating touch by sucking her fingers and bringing her hands close to her face. Because very premature infants are sensitive to touch, care must be taken not to overstress them with too frequent, too rough, or unaware touch. Even in the earliest stages, though, a premature infant can be comforted by a gentle hand on her feet, or a familiar hand on her head. A preemie is especially attuned to her parents' touch and often relaxes and becomes more medically stable when a parent is with her.

Taste. By 16 to 20 weeks, taste buds start to develop. The baby will have 7,000 taste buds by birth and only 2,000 at age 60. What does amniotic fluid—water, salt, urine, sugars, fatty acids, and cholesterol—taste like when the baby swallows it? The baby likely experiences all four tastes: sweet, sour, bitter, and salt. As he varies how much he urinates and how much he drinks, the ratio of fluid to urine changes, and these changes create different tastes in utero, which may help stimulate his sense of taste. This is another example of the way that the fetus affects his environment and influences his own development.

Even in utero, it appears that the fetus has a sweet tooth. Doctors discovered this in the 1930s when they tried to develop a treatment for mothers who have too much amniotic fluid (DeSnoo, 1937). They tested how much amniotic fluid a baby would drink if it was injected with saccharine. The babies definitely drank more when the sweetener was added but only for a while. They became saturated with the sweet-tasting fluid and stopped gulping it down (Maurer & Maurer, 1988).

Hearing. Week 24 marks the beginning response to sound; premature babies born after 24 weeks can hear. Therefore, the hospital environment must be carefully monitored so that the sounds premature infants hear are not too loud or too sudden. The soft sounds of parental voices and regular caregivers become familiar sources of comfort to the premature infant, even during this very early period.

Vision. Eye movements continue, but response to light will come in the third trimester.

The Third Trimester—Months 7, 8, and 9

The information just covered on the first two trimesters is intended primarily for your own knowledge and preparation, but the following will help you directly with the Community-Based FANA.

Internally, the baby now actively kicks and stretches, responds to light and sound, and weighs about 3 pounds. By the end of this trimester, the baby will weigh between 6 and 9 pounds. It's all systems go for delivery!

Size and appearance. The baby is most likely positioned at the bottom of the amniotic sac, in constant contact with the uterine wall. In this way, the baby more fully experiences the changes in the mother's breathing rate and movements. Most premature infants are born during the third trimester.

Brain development. During this period, the brain cells form connections between cells. The brain goes from smoothness to characteristic hills and valleys. This is a tremendous period of brain growth.

Movements. Movement patterns change in the last trimester. There are fewer big movements for two reasons. First, space is at a premium. When the baby cannot move his whole body at once because he is too big, he begins to focus on smaller movements: fidgeting his arms and legs, playing with his fingers, or sucking his thumb. The baby is constantly touching the wall of the uterus and himself. He often bumps into the umbilical cord. The fetus shifts positions more when the mother is still. All the motor patterns seen in utero can still be seen after birth.

Premature infants born in the beginning of the third trimester—26 weeks—exhibit basic reflexes. These include pulling away from a heel stick and the hand grasp, toe grasp, rooting, and stepping reflexes. The Community-Based FANA guides you in looking at some of these reflexes with parents after their baby is born.

It seems to be a general principle of the nervous system that the "go," or activity, systems, develop before the "slow," or inhibitory, systems, and a second reason that there is less movement later in pregnancy is that as the baby matures the earlier high-activity level is replaced by more mature patterns of modulated, more controlled activity (James, 1997). A high, continuous level of fetal activity all through pregnancy may be a sign that the nervous system is not developing properly. As the pregnancy progresses in the last trimester, movements may be absent for larger periods of time—up to 45 minutes—a dramatic shift from earlier trimesters (Nijhuis & Tas, 1991).

Hand movements. By 27 weeks, a preterm infant's grasp is almost strong enough to support her weight. The hand grasp is one of the ways that the newly born infant—whether preterm or full term—has to hold on to her parent. You will be able to help parents discover the psychological power of this grasp using the Community-Based FANA. More babies suck their right hand than their left hand in utero, and, as newborns, they tend to turn their head when lying in the crib to the same side as the hand that they preferred to suck in utero.

Breathing. The baby breathes about one half to one third of the time now, working hard to develop the breathing muscles in his diaphragm. Fetal breathing seems to have a daily rhythm—more in the morning and less in the evening. Breathing often takes place in combination with mouth opening and swallowing. The amount of fetal breathing is affected by the fetal environment and fetal activity. The baby breathes less when the mother is smoking and drinking, for example, and less when oxygen deprivation, or hypoxia, occurs, such as when the cord is pulled tightly around the neck. The baby breathes more when active. Toward the end of the third trimester, the baby begins to breathe less, perhaps storing up energy for the journey ahead.

Sucking, swallowing, and rooting. At this point in the pregnancy, the baby sucks and swallows more than a quart of fluid a day. Between 26 and 32 weeks, coordination of sucking and swallowing increases. Babies born before 26 weeks cannot coordinate sucking and swallowing and must be tube fed until they can learn to suck from a nipple and swallow. By 32 weeks, swallowing improves, partly because muscle tone for swallowing is improving. Typically, all the oral reflexes are mature and ready to go by 37 weeks.

Smell. There is intense movement of fluid through the nose; the baby takes in twice as much fluid as she swallows. The mother's diet changes the smell of the fluid, which gives the baby varied experience with smell (Schaal, Orgeur, & Rognon, 1995). Shortly after birth, the infant prefers the smell of her mother's breast pad to that of another mother (Macfarlane, 1975). There is also some evidence that after birth the infant prefers the smell of another mother's breast milk to the infant's own formula (Porter, Makin, Davis, & Christensen, 1992). Speculation is that the infant may have some memory for in utero smells, which would be more similar to breast milk than to commercial formula.

Vision. At 24 to 25 weeks, eye activity in utero increases in response to light. By 29 weeks, the preterm infant's eyes open. By 32 weeks, the baby turns his head to light in utero. As the mother's skin stretches over her belly and becomes thinner, letting more light into the uterus, the baby perhaps gets a bit of experience seeing. Infants do not see like adults do until they are 4 to 6 months of age.

Hearing. In the third trimester, the baby begins to hear. Mothers are sure this is the case because they can feel the baby jump when there is a loud noise. What does the world sound like to babies before they are born? Do they hear like we hear? Sounds are not heard exactly as we hear them. Current thinking is that body tissues absorb all tones higher than a man's voice (Maurer & Maurer, 1988). The baby hears primarily the low tones. To the baby, the fetal world may sound like what we experience when living in an apartment building and hearing a stereo from a neighboring apartment. We hear the bass booming through the floor while the higher tones are inaudible. The baby's ability to hear low tones may give fathers an advantage in soothing a very active baby in utero.

Does this mean that the baby cannot hear his mother? Not at all. He certainly hears his mother. Her voice not only goes out but also vibrates down her throat and into her lungs. Even though the high tones may be absorbed, the rhythms and patterns of her speech become very familiar to her baby. In fact, fetal heart rate will slow during maternal speech, showing that the baby is taking in the stimulus. Shortly after birth, most newborns can turn to and find a source of sound. Now you know how they learn to accomplish this amazing feat!

Memory. DeCasper and Spence (1986) probably conducted the earliest literacy study. They asked 16 women to read a story aloud twice a day during the last 5 to 6 weeks of pregnancy. Then they tested the babies 3 days after birth to see if they recognized the story that the mothers read to them before they were born. Thirteen of the 16 babies did remember the story. They showed this by sucking more on a pacifier when they heard the familiar story. Do babies hear before they are born? Yes! Do they remember the patterns in some of what they hear? Yes!

Behavioral states. What is a behavioral state? A behavioral state indicates a level of arousal and associated motor, breathing, and heart rate patterns (see Figure 5.4). Sometimes, states are referred to as "sleep–wake cycling." After babies are born, they basically have three states—awake, asleep, or in between—although six newborn states have been identified in more detail: quiet sleep, active sleep, drowsy, quiet alert, active alert, and crying.

Researchers believe that before birth babies have four states (see Figure 5.4) that are similar to the following newborn states: quiet sleep, active sleep, quiet alert, and active alert (Nijhuis, 2003). Each of these states has a particular pattern of eye movements, body movements, and heart rate patterns.

Figure 5.4

Fetal Behavioral States

State 1: Similar to Quiet Sleep in the Newborn
- Stable heart rate; heart rate speeds up only with movements
- Eye movements absent
- Occasional, brief body movements; mostly startles

State 2: Similar to Active Sleep in the Newborn
- Continual eye movements
- Frequent body movements
- Heart rate more changeable

State 3: Similar to Quiet Alert in the Newborn
- Gross and small body movements absent
- Occasional eye movements
- Heart rate stable, but not as stable as State 1

State 4: Similar to Active Alert in the Newborn
- Most active state
- Vigorous and continual activity
- Many trunk rotations
- Continual eye movements
- Unstable heart rate

The closer the baby is to delivery, the more she is in States 1 and 4. If a baby is born before 37 weeks, she will not have as clearly developed states as a full-term infant. It will be harder to tell if she is awake or asleep. Her alert states may not be the bright, shiny-eyed alertness of a full-term infant. Rather, she may be hyperalert, with a frantic, wide-eyed look accompanied by stiff arms and legs (high tone) or hypoalert, with a glassy-eyed, dazed look and limp arms, legs, or facial muscles (low tone).

Habituation—getting accustomed to repeated stimuli. By 27–28 weeks, babies begin to be able to tune out repeated sounds, such as a vibrating electric toothbrush placed on the mother's abdomen by the baby's head (Leader, Baillie, Martin, & Vermeulen, 1982). Some babies are more able to tune out quickly—after just one to nine sounds—and others take as much as 50 sounds. Individual differences begin before birth. Fetal state influences ability to respond, but, if a sound is strong enough, the baby will respond regardless of state, whether awake or asleep (Leader, 1995).

Social and Emotional Issues for the Teen Mother

The social and emotional issues of pregnancy in general and adolescent pregnancy in particular are enormous. Many excellent books, chapters, and articles have been devoted to the topic. For a list of recommended readings, see the Resource List in Appendix A.

Four issues are of particular importance to home visitors learning to use the Community-Based FANA:

- The teen's perception of her changing body
- Her acceptance of her pregnancy
- The changes in relationships with her family, the father of the baby, and her friends
- The role of the home visitor in supporting the mother during this time

Following is a summary of these issues for each trimester of pregnancy.

The First Trimester

The teen's perception of her changing body. Be careful not to generalize about how teens see themselves, pregnant or not. All teens are different. Some relish exploring life's options as they see their bodies changing with advancing pregnancy. Others see their lives becoming limited as their clothes become tighter. Some teens simply refuse to acknowledge their growing midsection and wear clothes that are increasingly tight and uncomfortable. These teens need more time than others to accept all these changes.

Acceptance of the pregnancy. Going hand-in-hand with acknowledging her changing body is the teen's readiness to acknowledge the pregnancy. In the first trimester, she has only just learned that she is pregnant. Perhaps she has done multiple home pregnancy tests. As an adult, you already know how to read and trust your body, but a teen doesn't know what to expect. Is she pregnant or not? (N. Sinclair, personal communication, March, 2000).

It can be hard to tell if it was a teen's choice to become pregnant. She may not know herself. Musick (1993) noted that sometimes the first conception is for the teen's own mother. The teen's unconscious self may be seeking ways to become reconnected to her own mother, and she may be eager to rekindle the sense of being cared for by her mother.

Also, peer pressure can be both enormous and subtle. Sometimes teens get pregnant because all their friends are having babies. One young mother didn't show much interest in her pregnancy or in the baby when he was born. Fifteen of her friends were either pregnant or recently delivered when she became pregnant. Was the purpose of her pregnancy to remain a close member of her friendship group? She honestly did not know herself.

Changes in relationships. In this very important first trimester, huge changes in the teen's relationships begin to unfold. She meets new people in the medical profession as she begins prenatal care. Doctors and nurses who care for her during this time may be understanding, or they may show subtle or not-so-subtle signs of judging her because she is pregnant. The teen's parents come to know of the pregnancy, so does the baby's father, and so do her friends. Some teens withdraw emotionally in the face of such an overwhelming array of highly charged interactions. Other teens relish the attention.

This can also be a time of enormous emotional ups and downs. The teen begins to integrate the opinions of others with her own feelings. This is never an easy task, and it can be daunting in adolescence.

The home visitor's role. Be patient with the teen's ambivalence, apparent indifference, or lack of acknowledgment of her pregnancy. There are complex factors at work here that have a great deal to do with her choice—conscious or not so conscious—to become pregnant. Her feelings might be all over the map at this critical time. Your role is to help her understand and accept these feelings.

The Second Trimester

The teen's perception of her changing body. When the teen looks in the mirror now, she definitely sees a changing body. She needs clothes that accommodate her growing midsection, but she may not be ready yet to buy maternity clothes. Many teens are part of a peer group where pregnancy is acceptable and even expected. Such a teen may enjoy her changing body. Other teens may be devastated by what they feel is a very sudden turn in their physical appearance.

Acceptance of the pregnancy. Acceptance of the pregnancy depends on many things, including her acceptance of the physical changes and how much support she receives from the people in her world.

Changes in relationships. Now, at the midpoint of the teen's pregnancy, the reality of the pregnancy is likely very clear to the adults in her life—her mother, father, grandmother, and aunts, for example. What is happening to the teen's own mother through all this? What kinds of changes might the pregnancy trigger in this most central of relationships? Wakschlag and Hans (2000) spoke of "counter-transitions," that is, "a life in transition caused by someone else's life events" (p. 131). Is this pregnancy disrupting the prospective grandmother's life plans? How is she feeling about her daughter because of this disruption? What about the father of the baby? Has he remained in the picture? How is he facing the daunting reality of fatherhood, perhaps for the first time?

The home visitor's role. The end of the second trimester is a good time to suggest a tour of the labor and delivery area of the hospital where the teen will be having her baby. This is a good way of easing her into facing the reality of her pregnancy—if she is struggling with that—while at the same time presenting birth as very doable. Engage her chosen labor coach in this tour, as well as anyone else she wishes to have present.

This also is a time to ease generational relationships. The prospective grandmother may find this a good time to reminisce with her daughter about her own labor and delivery. Mother and daughter can look at any ultrasounds together and oooh and aaah over the coming baby.

There is so much going on right now. Remember, being fully present is powerful—whether the teen is sharing her concerns, becoming withdrawn, or being happy. No one can fix all the complexities in the teen's life. But you can help her blow off steam and regain her sense of control over herself. Reviewing "The Receptive Posture" in chapter 2 may help you prepare for home visits during this period.

Third Trimester

The teen's perception of her changing body. By now, the teen isn't comfortable unless she is wearing maternity clothes. Clinical experience teaches that this may be the time when a teen experiences sadness, even depression, if hers was not a planned pregnancy. The reality of the pregnancy is stronger now than any strategies she may have used to deny it. She is definitely less mobile and may feel physical discomfort. She also may be more dependent on those around her for help with everyday chores and activities.

Acceptance of the pregnancy. Even this late in the pregnancy, the teen still may not have accepted the pregnancy emotionally. This may be true even when the teen fully acknowledges the reality of the pregnancy and the upcoming birth. The push of the developmental tasks of adolescence doesn't stop because of pregnancy. The teen mother wants autonomy and connectedness at a time when all she is experiencing is dependence on the people around her (Wakschlag & Hans, 2000). Of course, there is enormous variation in all of this. Many 15-year-olds have made easy and healthy transitions into motherhood.

Changes in relationships. Relationships continue to change for the teen mother. The baby's father may or may not be actively involved with her. He has had most of the pregnancy to get used to this reality. How he is handling things now is key and affects the pregnant teen, for good or ill. He may be fascinated by the coming new life, or he may seem uninterested. This is a key time for changes in the teen's relationship with her mother as well.

If the teen is going to be bringing the baby to her parents' house, her family should by now be preparing their home for the baby's arrival. For some, this is a happy time, with plans for a baby shower underway or other signs of glad anticipation. For other teens, tensions and negative relationships in the home may become magnified around this time, as may positive relationships.

The home visitor's role. Unless you are working with a young woman who is already a parent, it is likely that you will begin your work with most expectant teens during this trimester. This is the time that you and she have to get to know each other and to establish your patterns and expectations of working together. There are many intriguing parallels to recognize about this time: the baby is practicing inside for life to come on the outside; the parent is creating patterns of attention, affection, and interaction with the developing baby; and you and the parent are creating your own ways of understanding, appreciating, and being together.

The work that you do with the young mother, the baby's father, and the maternal grandmother during this period takes on great importance, as it sets the stage for your ongoing relationships. Remember, first impressions really do make a difference. Your ability to listen and to understand others, your genuine interest and concern, and your consistent demonstration of being nonjudgmental can steady the mother and others while their lives are undergoing rapid and dramatic changes.

In building these new relationships, take time to consider how the young parent—and each of the other family members you meet—may be feeling, not only about the imminent birth but also about you. Be ready to be tested. You are not the first helper the teen has met during this pregnancy, and she will want to know from your actions, not only your words, how you will be with her. She will need to find out for herself if she can count on you to really understand her and her developing baby, as well as her evolving family situation. She will want to know that you are watching her back without being in her face. Remember that she is a teenager—expect exasperating as well as exhilarating times!

References

Cohen, L., & Slade, A. (2000). The psychology and psychopathology of pregnancy: Reorganization and transformation. In C. Zeanah (Ed.), *Handbook of infant mental health* (2nd ed., pp. 20–36). New York: Guilford.

DeCasper, A. J., & Spence, M. J. (1986). Prenatal maternal speech influences newborn's perception of speech sounds. *Infant Behavior and Development*, 9, 133–150.

DeSnoo, K. 1937. Das trinkende Kind im Uterus. *Monatschrift für Geburtshilfe und Gynäkologie* 105: 88–97. Cited in D. Maurer, & C. Maurer. (1988). *The world of the newborn*. New York: Basic Books.

Eisenberg, A., Murkoff, H., & Hathaway, S. (1991). *What to expect when you're expecting*. New York: Workman.

Hermann-Giddens, M. E., Slora, E. J., Wasserman, R. C., Bourdony, C. J., Bhapkar, M. V., Kock, G. C., et al. (1977). Secondary sexual characteristics and menses in young girls seen in office practice: A study from Pediatric Research in Office Settings Network. *Pediatrics*, 99, 505–512.

Hofer, M. (1981). *The roots of human behavior*. San Francisco: W. H. Freeman.

Hofer, M. A. (1997). Early social relationships: A psychobiologist's view. *Child Development*, 58, 633–648.

James, D. (1997). Fetal behavior. *Current Obstetrics & Gynaecology*, 7(1), 30–35.

Laitinen-Krispijn, S., Vander Ende, J., Hazebroek-Hampschreur, A., & Verhulst, F. (1999). Pubertal maturation and the development of behavioral and emotional problems in early adolescence. *Acta Psychiatrica Scandinavica*, 99, 16–25.

Leader, L. R. (1995). Studies in fetal behaviour. *BJOG: An International Journal of Obstetrics and Gynaecology*, *102*(8), 595–597.

Leader, L. R., Baillie, P., Martin, B., & Vermeulen, E. (1982).The assessment and significance of habituation to a repeated stimulus by the human fetus. *Early Human Development*, *7*(3), 211–219.

Macfarlane, A. (1975). Olfaction in the development of social preferences in the human neonate. *Ciba Foundation Symposium*, 33, 103–117.

Maurer, D., & Maurer, C. (1988). *The world of the newborn*. New York: Basic Books.

Moessinger, A. C. (1988). Morphological consequences of depressed or impaired fetal activity. In W. P. Smotherman & S. R. Robinson (Eds.), *Behavior of the fetus*. Caldwell, NJ: Telford Press.

Musick, J. (1993). *Young, poor and pregnant*. New Haven: Yale University Press.

Neinstein, L., & Kaufman, R. (1996). Normal physical growth and development. In L. Neinstein (Ed.), *Adolescent health care: A practical guide* (3rd ed., pp. 3–39). Baltimore: Williams and Wilkens.

Nijhuis, J. G. (2003). Fetal behavior. *Neurobiology of Aging*, *24*(Supplement 1), S41–S46.

Nijhuis, J. G., & Tas, B. A. (1991). Physiological and clinical aspects of the development of fetal behaviour. In M. A. Hanson (Ed.), *The fetal and neonatal brain stem: Developmental and clinical issues*
(pp. 268–280). New York: Cambridge University Press.

Porter, R. H., Makin, J. W., Davis, L. B., & Christensen, K. M. (1992). Breast-fed infants respond to olfactory cues from their own mother and unfamiliar lactating females. *Infant Behavior and Development*, *15*, 85–93.

Schaal, B., Orgeur, P., & Rognon, C. (1995). Odor sensing in the human fetus: Anatomical functional, and chemoecological bases. In J. P. Lecanuet, W. P. Fifer, N. A. Krasnegor, & W. P. Smotherman (Eds.), *Fetal development: A psychobiological perspective* (pp. 205–237). Hillsdale, NJ: Lawrence Erlbaum.

Van Dongen, L. G. R., & Goudie, E. G. (1980). Fetal movements in the first trimester of pregnancy. *British Journal of Obstetrics and Gynecology*, *87*, 191–193.

Wakschlag, L. S., & Hans, S. L. (2000). Early parenthood in context: Implications for development and intervention. In C. Zeanah (Ed.), *Handbook of infant mental health* (2nd ed., pp. 129–144). New York: Guilford Press.

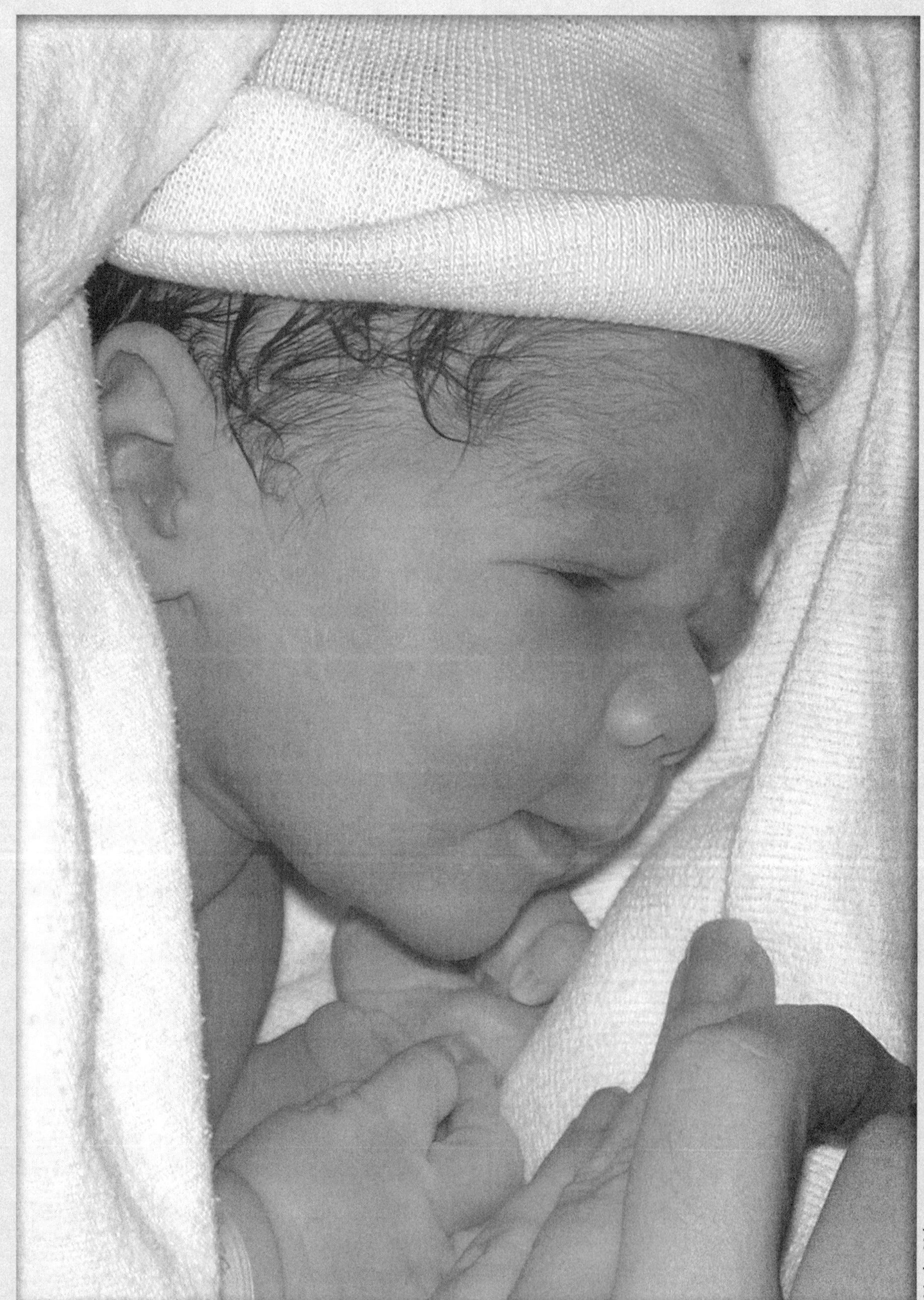

Marilyn Nolt

CHAPTER 6

THE BIRTH

It is never too soon to help young parents begin to prepare for the birth, but this topic—as all others—must be approached within the context of the parents' own development and beliefs. Birthing is an enormously sensitive and dynamic issue. There is no one right way to approach it. You can bring up labor and delivery in every home visit, but use your own good judgment about how and where to enter the discussion.

Some teens are very ready to talk about labor and delivery. It stills their anxieties to know more. Others never fully allow themselves to talk about it. Some want to see the hospital unit where they will deliver but refuse to discuss the physical mechanics. Others want to focus on their support person for labor but do not want to think about medications. As in every other aspect of her life, a young mom needs to be her own person with respect to birthing.

This chapter raises questions for home visitors about young parents' plans for labor and delivery and highlights important things for you to consider for each question. The Community-Based Family Administered Neonatal Activities (FANA) does not include activities or other interventions for the birth itself. But because your work with an expectant family brings you to important discussions and activities that support and help parents prepare for the birthing event, the chapter offers guidance in areas that you should explore with parents.

THE TEEN MOTHER'S PERCEPTIONS AND READINESS

The most important thing to discover is whether a young mother is ready to talk about labor and delivery. Many teens find it difficult to accept the reality of the baby growing inside them. For such a teen, labor will be the farthest thing from her mind.

Baby? What baby? Sometimes the motive or emotional drive for the pregnancy is not linked to the reality of a baby coming. A teen mother may desire a close, intimate relationship with the father of the baby, she may think that pregnancy will help her hold onto the relationship, or she may want to escape a tough home or school situation. She may be looking for a sense of fulfillment, affection, and conflict resolution. Labor? What labor? There are times when the pregnancy is a way of defining a teen mother's role in the world; being a parent can profoundly define that role, as it does with an adult mother.

Labor and Delivery Checklist

Go slowly. For each young mother, consider what you know about her thinking style and how best to approach her. Find out also about the ethnic and cultural norms about birth with which she has grown up.

To help the teen mother prepare for her birthing experience, consider the questions in the checklist in Figure 6.1. You do not need to address all of the questions with her directly, but you should make sure that she has addressed them with her doctor, midwife, doula, you, or another support person by the end of 36 weeks gestation.

Figure 6.1

Labor and Delivery Checklist

- What is the young mother's understanding of labor and delivery?
- Who is her support person who will be present at labor?
- What is the physical arrangement of the birthing unit?
- How will she recognize the onset of labor?
- How will she get to the hospital?
- What are her plans for pain medication?
- How aware is she of the changes her body will undergo during labor?
- What does she expect to happen and what does she expect to see when her baby is born?
- How does she plan to feed her baby—breast or bottle?
- Has she chosen a pediatric care provider?
- Where and to whom will she and the baby come home after being discharged?

Understanding of Labor and Delivery

The only thing that some teens may know of delivery is what they have seen on television, where labor is sometimes shown as enormously painful and other times shown with no pain at all. Sometimes a cast of 10 or 12 others is present; sometimes no one but a doctor is there. Rarely is the full reality of birth conveyed.

The best place to begin is by asking the teen, "What are your thoughts about labor and delivery?" Other helpful questions include the following:

- Have you ever been present at a birth, or heard all about one?
- What have your friends told you?
- Have you ever seen a birth on television?

Follow her lead. She may be afraid of the birth. She may be well-informed or full of misconceptions. That is why it is important that home visitors have a basic, accurate knowledge of labor and delivery. The resource list in Appendix A includes several reference materials that can tell you what you need to know. Encourage the teen to elaborate by asking her to tell you more about where she learned something. Corrections should come gently, as in, "That's so interesting, but really very different from what I've heard. Can I tell you what I learned? (or what I learned from my own experience?)."

The Mother's Support

As early as possible in the pregnancy, help the teen identify the person or people who will support her during labor. Hospitals used to allow only one support person in the delivery room—not so anymore. However, many hospitals still allow only two people to be present, and if a teen is being supported by a doula, encourage such hospitals not to count the doula as one of those two people.

The pregnant teen may choose the father of the baby, her own mother or grandmother, an aunt or cousin, or any combination of people important to her. Help her decide who her supporters will be, and invite that person or people into the experience early on.

Some teens choose a person with whom they do not have a steady relationship—or even a person who objects to being there. Those teens may need help resolving difficulties before the birth, or they may need help choosing someone else. Sometimes a young mother chooses someone who has herself had a traumatic labor and delivery or perinatal loss. In that situation, the support person serves the mother best when she is able to work through her own experience first, or the teen may want to choose another support person.

If at all possible, meet with the teen mom and her labor coaches together a few times before birth. During these meetings, communicate the mother's desire that her chosen supporters be with her during labor, and highlight for the coaches how very important they will be to the teen in labor. If they are eager to be there but anxious and uncertain about their role, provide training and reassurance. Training can be as simple as suggesting that a coach hold the teen's hand and wipe her brow throughout labor.

The Birthing Unit

Strongly encourage the young mother to visit the hospital birthing unit she will be using, even if she does not want to address any other aspect of the birth. The hospital visit is a concrete, visual practice session that allows the teen to see the halls she will walk, the doors she will go through, and the friendly faces of labor and delivery nurses and other personnel.

It is best if she, one of her supporters, and you as the home visitor make this visit together. Very often, the hospital visit dispels misconceptions from the made-for-TV deliveries she may have seen. More often than not, delivery is not an emergency. She will see from the pace of the unit that things generally happen systematically and fairly routinely in labor and delivery. Point out all this to her. As you tour the unit, ask her what she hears and what she sees.

Recognizing When Labor Starts

Encourage the teen mother to bring up the very important topic of the onset of labor with her doctor, midwife, nurse practitioner, or doula. Guide her in getting the following specific information:

- Physical changes she can expect, such as what happens if her water breaks, the length and spacing of contractions, and what contractions actually may feel like;
- Emotional changes that occur normally during the labor, such as comfort, excitement, irritability, anger, a sense of not being able to go on, and exaltation; and
- Social changes during the course of labor, such as needing to be alone for a while, needing constant companionship during hard labor, becoming angry at her coach, and becoming tearfully grateful to her coach. (Adapted from Humenick, 1998.)

The Trip to the Hospital

Once a teen recognizes that she is in labor, what then? Help her and her coach make a plan. Some of the questions to plan for include the following:

- Who will call the doctor and the doula or other support person?
- Is a phone readily available at home or at a neighbor's? Can this neighbor be counted on in the middle of the night?
- Who will take her to the hospital?

Putting these plans in writing can reassure and relieve the teen mother and even organize the people in her household.

Plans for Pain Medication

Young mothers may not know that they have a choice in pain medication for labor. Help the teen get the information she needs by encouraging her to talk to her doctor, midwife, nurse practitioner, or doula. Guide her in making a list of questions for these health care professionals such as the following:

- What are my choices for pain medication?
- Are there different types of medication that are used at different stages of labor?
- What are the advantages and disadvantages of some of the most commonly used medications and methods, such as Demerol or an epidural?

Learning about this aspect of labor can give the teen some sense of control over an experience that is not easily predictable.

Changes in Her Body During Labor

Labor is not a unitary experience. Knowing the different experiences in different stages of labor can help minimize the teen's element of surprise and anxiety. The best source of information is her doctor, midwife, nurse practitioner, or doula.

Expectations for the Moment of Birth and Immediately After

What are the practices of the hospital in which the teen will give birth? Will she be encouraged to hold and feed her baby immediately after he is born? Will the baby be separated from her for several hours to be bathed, have footprints made, and temperature and other vital signs assessed?

What will the teen mother expect to see? Has she ever seen a newborn? Does she know that the baby will be covered with the fluids of delivery? In the last few years, pregnant teens have been able to watch real births on television and see all that there is to see. Find out what each teen knows and what she expects.

Breast- or Bottle-Feeding

Young mothers need to think carefully before they deliver about whether they will breast- or bottle-feed. Family practices, the influence of her friends, and her life circumstances will shape what she chooses to do. For example, will she work full time or be a full-time student after the baby is born?

Explore this with her, and, once again, encourage her to explore this crucial question with her doctor, midwife, nurse practitioner, doula, or pediatrician. Although this is an issue you might feel strongly about, make it clear to the mother that you will support whatever decision she makes.

Choosing a Pediatrician

One of the first questions maternity floor nurses will ask the young mother after birth is where the baby will get his first well-baby checkup. With mothers and babies going home from the hospital so quickly after birth, sometimes within 24 hours or less, having a pediatrician to count on immediately after discharge is very important. She will need to know who and when to call with her questions about infant care and well-being.

Ideally, a teen mother can choose her pediatrician and meet him or her before the birth. Experiencing that connection will minimize obstacles for her as she seeks the best possible care for her baby. However, choosing a pediatrician is a luxury not available for many young mothers who receive care through public health clinics or hospitals. You can guide the teen mother on this essential matter by helping her find out what her choices are. You may also need to explain the difference between an obstetrician, who takes care of the mother and baby before birth, and the pediatrician, who cares for the baby after birth.

Going Home

Planning the details of going home after birth before she even checks in to the hospital leaves the young mother free to experience more of the magical, wondrous aspects of bringing new life into the world. The following list highlights some things to plan for:

- What is the mom's and baby's discharge environment going to be like?
- To whom will they be going home?
- Who will drive them home?
- Who will help her out once she and the baby are at home?

Complex Emotions

How a mother perceives birth is an individual phenomenon and must be respected as such. Some mothers—by every objective measure—experience long, difficult labors, but nonetheless describe their labor as "easy." Others have very short labor and effective pain medication, yet say it was a horrifying experience. Prior experiences with injury or physical abuse, pain thresholds, and social supports all contribute to mothers' perception of the childbirth event.

There are times, however, when things happen that by any measure carry with them a weight of sorrow, conflict, anger, or an array of other complex feelings. The home visitor must be prepared to support the parents during this time (see chapter 7).

Reference

Humenick, S. (1998). Flow, flow, flow a birth: Pathway to an optimal experience. *Journal of Perinatal Education*, *7*(1), v–vii.

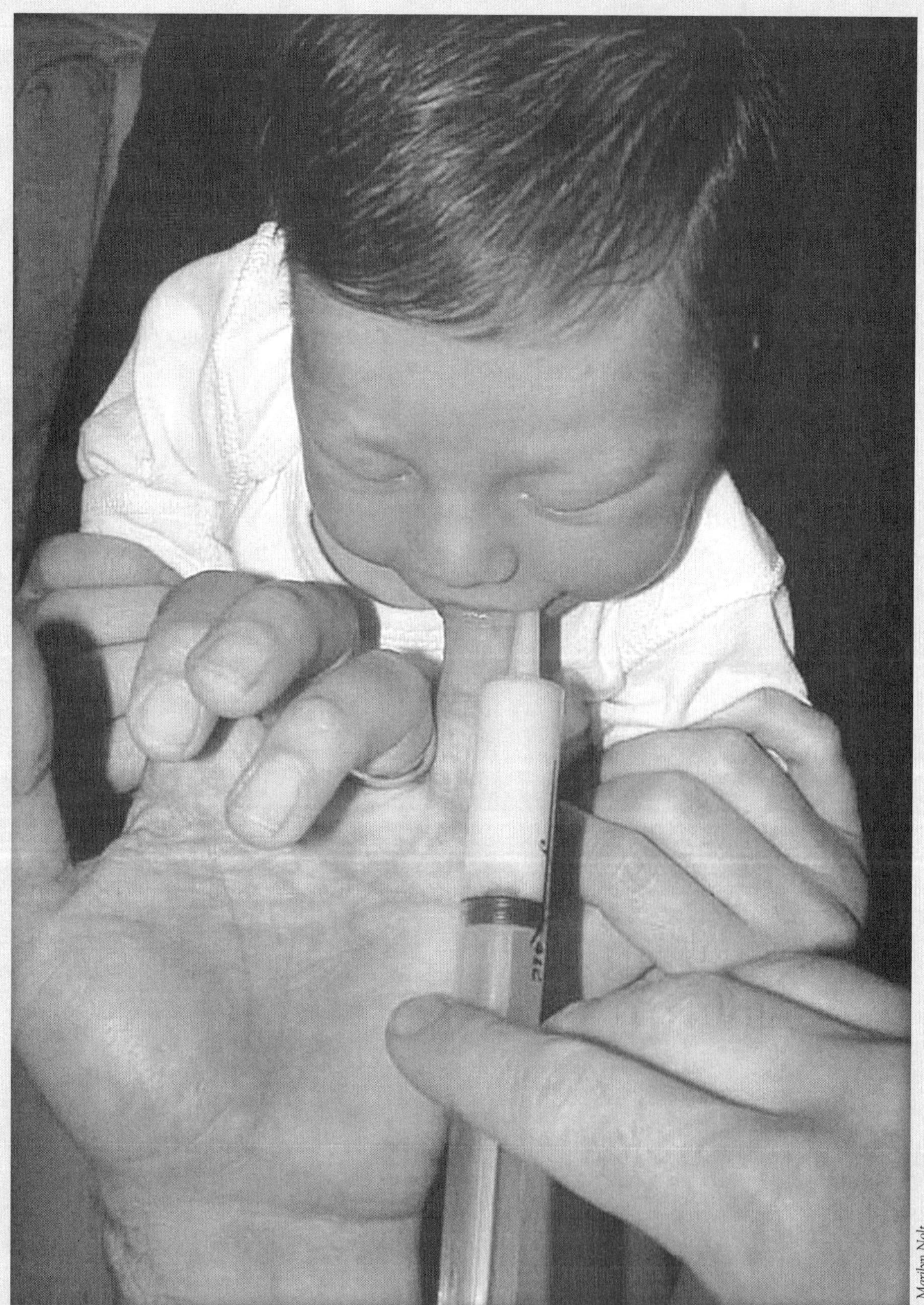

Marilyn Nolt

CHAPTER 7

When Things Don't Go as Planned

Sometimes the unexpected happens, and the outcome of a pregnancy is not the birth of a healthy baby. Two of the most difficult outcomes to understand and cope with are the death of a baby and the birth of a baby with serious problems. This chapter guides the home visitor in how to support parents in these circumstances.

Relying on the Receptive Posture

Home visitors who enter into the intimate experiences and life changes that accompany pregnancy and childbirth are touched by the emotions that families experience throughout this period. Being aware of your own feelings and reactions is essential during these times. The receptive posture that characterizes all your work with the Community-Based Family Administered Neonatal Activities (FANA) becomes even more important in such times of internal upheaval. It provides you with a center for your approach with families—to hear and observe, to understand to your fullest capacity, and to be available to hold others' feelings with them so that they will be more able to hold these feelings when you're not there to support them.

When a Baby Is Born With Serious Problems

Sometimes the outcome of pregnancy—even the pregnancy of a healthy teen mother—is a baby born with serious health or developmental problems. David Cromer and David Ingall described the challenge one such developmental disability presents to parents and health care providers:

> *The unexpected delivery of an infant with Down syndrome is an event that challenges families and staff to call upon reserves of strength and coping abilities rarely faced in day-to-day experience. Simultaneously, there is the reality and wonder of a new life, a son or daughter who has just entered the world, and the fact that this is not the expected child. It is this clash of reality and expectation that creates an intense and oftentimes confusing array of feelings in all of us. (Cited in Cardone, Kraft, LaPata, Lawrence, & Salafsky, 1991, p. iii)*

Although they are writing about Down syndrome, a genetic disability that results in mental retardation, the same clash of expectation and reality occurs with any serious problem evident at birth.

Although most common in older mothers, babies with Down syndrome are born to teen moms, too. Very likely your first enormous task is to explain what Down syndrome is. You don't need to be an expert to do this. A very simple statement of fact is that babies with Down syndrome learn, but not as quickly as other children their age. They likely will need special attention from teachers and therapists in infancy and throughout school. But babies with Down syndrome are as engaging and fun and loving and challenging as any other children!

Supporting the Parent–Child Connection With Preterm Infants

Prematurity is not an unusual outcome of teen pregnancy. Babies who are born prematurely are likely to spend their first days in a Neonatal Intensive Care Unit (NICU). Although it may not be possible to conduct an entire postnatal Community-Based FANA with the parents and infant in the NICU, there are many activities that you can facilitate even in that environment, especially Parent Time activities (see chapter 10). NICU staff also are valuable resources to these new parents' early experiences with their newborn.

Telling their birth story and sharing their perceptions of their newborn can help parents come to accept the baby that they have, rather than the baby they planned for. The receptive posture that you are learning helps you explore and understand the parents' story and hold their emotions with them. These moments of coregulation—helping the parents keep themselves together—are important to parents who are coming to terms with what has happened to their young family.

Babies born early are not as developed as full-term babies, so some of their systems may not be ready yet for all of the postnatal Community-Based FANA activities, even once they are home. However, some of the activities can be done with premature infants. The hand and toe reflexes, especially the toe and finger grasps, often can be completed and can bring great comfort to the parent.

Many NICUs encourage parents to hold their baby in skin-to-skin "kangaroo care." This is an ideal time for parents to get to know their infant through touching, caressing, and soothing. There are studies that indicate that sensory stimulation, touch, sound, and gentle movement in particular are safe and benefit premature infants' development (Hernandez-Reif & Field, 2000).

Other studies illustrate that parents of premature babies benefit from support in understanding and responding to their infant's cues (Hernandez-Reif & Field, 2000). You can use the postnatal Community-Based FANA to help parents better appreciate their infant's unique ways of letting them know what level of activity, interaction, and stimulation she can tolerate and when she needs a break. Because premature infants may more easily become overstimulated, it is even more important to help parents read, understand, and respond to their baby's cues without personalizing them. Your gentle support and guided information can help parents make sense of experiences that might otherwise frustrate them and interfere with growing closer to their baby.

As a premature baby's systems mature, he is able to tolerate more interaction (Hernandez-Reif & Field, 2000). Such experiences can help parents more fully appreciate how much their infant has changed and developed during his time being cared for in the NICU. Because Community-Based FANA activities are designed to highlight what infants and parents can do, new families who start out with concerns about what their baby cannot do often benefit tremendously from participating in these activities.

When a Baby Dies

The harsh reality is that sometimes babies die, even babies of young mothers. Babies may die early in the pregnancy; before 20 weeks gestational age this is usually called a miscarriage. They may die in utero prior to birth; after 20 weeks this is called an intra uterine fetal demise, or IUFD. They may die at the time of birth; this is called a stillbirth. Or they may die within a few hours or days after birth; this is called infant death.

There are as many responses to these perinatal losses as there are teen mothers and fathers. For teens who have developed dreams and shaped their futures around the coming baby, infant death carries with it unspeakable sorrow. For those who were deeply conflicted about the pregnancy—including young mothers who carried the baby under duress from family or the baby's father—feelings can be very complicated and may include guilt, relief, anger, and sorrow.

There is no easy way to enter into the life of a mother and father who are experiencing the death of a baby. Every time feels like the first time. Schedule meetings with your supervisor after each home visit with parents who have suffered perinatal loss. Discuss, in an unhurried way, the content of your talks with the parents, and explore your own response to what you have seen and heard. You may find yourself walking a very fine line—on the one hand being flooded by sorrow of your own and a sense of failure, and on the other hand maintaining the helpful protective distance that allows you to be fully there for the parents and to bear witness to their grief.

The kinds of things you do with and for young parents at this time depend, in part, on when they experience the loss. If it is very early in the pregnancy, a teen mother may wish to talk about the actual experience of miscarriage, which can be frightening at any age. A miscarriage, even very early in the pregnancy, can be experienced as a profound loss. Well-meaning family members or friends may try to help a teen mother recover from her loss by ignoring it. Remember that simply holding her hand and saying, "I'm sorry," can go a long way toward affirming the depth of her feelings.

When young mothers go into labor and deliver between 17–24 weeks, remember that they have already felt the baby move. Often mothers report this time as the first real indicator of the baby's humanness.

Mothers, fathers, and families may need guidance in how to approach this event. As soon as possible after the birth, while the teen is still in the hospital, help her find out about prenatal loss services that may be available through the social work or pastoral care department of the hospital. Trained grief counselors are invaluable in these circumstances. If there are no services, guide the parents in thinking through the kinds of things they may or may not wish to do now. Knowing what their options are now minimizes regrets later. What parents choose to do is up to them; the important thing is that they know they have choices.

Figure 7.1 lists things that may be helpful to explore with parents when they experience perinatal loss. Two booklets that mothers, fathers, and extended family members may find helpful are "When Hello Means Goodbye" and "Miscarriage." They are available from The Centering Corporation (see the Resource List in Appendix A).

Figure 7.1

Perinatal Loss: Questions to Explore With Parents

Miscarriage

- Was she alone when it happened?
- Did she have some idea of what was happening to her?
- How does she feel about the pregnancy ending?
- How are the important people in her world responding to the miscarriage?
- Are they treating it in a way that is consonant with how she feels about it?

After 17 Weeks

- Do the parents wish to see and hold their baby? (After 17 weeks, and sometimes 16 weeks, a dead baby can be swaddled and held.)
- Do they wish to have nursing staff take a picture of them with their baby?
- Have they named the baby?
- Do they want to keep mementos of birth, such as the receiving blanket or wrist and ankle ID bands?
- What do they wish for the body? Hospital disposal? (They will not be able to retrieve ashes.) Funeral home cremation? (They will be able to retrieve ashes.) Burial? A memorial service?

REFERENCES

Cardone, I., Kraft, S., LaPata, R., Lawrence, P., & Salafsky, I. (Eds.). (1991). *A hospital-based, multi-disciplinary approach to the unexpected delivery of an infant with Down syndrome*. Evanston, IL: Evanston Hospital.

Hernandez-Reif, M., & Field, T. (2000). Preterm infants benefit from early interventions. In J. Osofsky & H. Fitzgerald (Eds.), *WAIMH handbook of infant mental health* (Vol. 4, pp. 296–325). New York: Wiley.

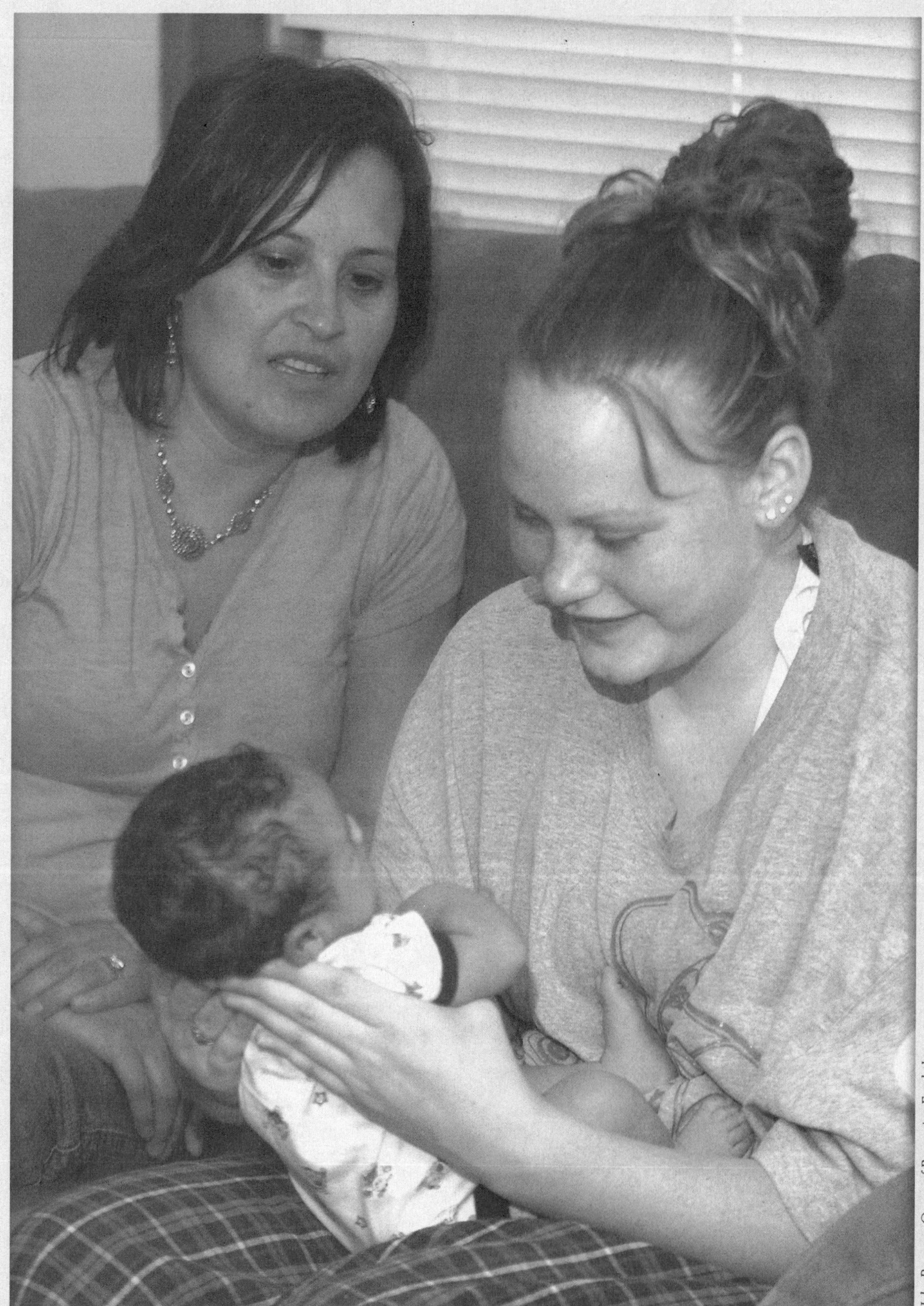

John Booz, an Ounce of Prevention Fund photo

COMING THROUGH THE DOOR: THE STRUCTURE OF THE COMMUNITY-BASED FANA

The Community-Based Family Administered Neonatal Activities (FANA) offers home visitors an organized way to actively engage expectant and new parents in an exploration of their baby's development and of their expectations for parenthood. Each of the prenatal and postnatal FANA home visit sessions has the same basic structure: Preparation, Parent Time, Parent and Baby Time, Family Time, and Reflection and Writing to the Baby (see Figure 8.1).

This chapter outlines and explains that structure and offers five guiding principles and key practices for using the Community-Based FANA. It also explores a variety of special circumstances—such as when the baby is born with problems or when the mother is considering adoption—and offers suggestions for adapting the home visits and the Community-Based FANA structure and activities to support young parents in these challenging circumstances.

More information on principles and practices for using the Community-Based FANA prenatally and during the 4 weeks after birth are presented in chapter 9, "Welcome Parents," and chapter 10, "Welcome Baby."

THE FANA HOME VISIT

The Community-Based FANA is designed for use during home visits that take place twice a month, beginning prenatally at about 26 weeks and continuing through the 4 weeks after the baby is born. It can be easily adapted for use in other settings, such as a center-based program, or on another schedule, such as weekly visits.

Preparation

Preparation occurs before each visit and generally takes 15–20 minutes. Preparation is a "state transition" time for the home visitor. It is a time to set aside other tasks and concerns and shift attention to this family—this mother, this father, this baby—and to prepare physically and psychologically for the visit. Most important, it is a time to reflect on what you already know about the mom, dad, and the people who are significant to them. Anticipate and plan for who might be present for the visit.

Figure 8.1

Community-Based FANA Home Visit Structure

Prenatal Visits

Preparation

- Review what you know about mother, father, and family
- Select prenatal activities and gather materials
- Ready yourself physically and psychologically

Parent Time

- Greet and reconnect with mother, father, and family
- Explore baby's name
- Elicit and validate parents' observations of baby

Parent and Baby Time

- Explore baby's present behavior
- Position
- State
- Facilitate prenatal activities
- Fetal movement and newborn behavior
- Hearing
- Behavioral states
- Touch
- Smell and taste
- Vision

Family Time

Reflection and Writing to the Baby

Postnatal Visits

Preparation

- Review what you know about mother, father, and family
- Select postnatal activities and gather materials
- Ready yourself physically and psychologically

Parent Time

- Greet and reconnect with mother, father, and family
- Review labor and delivery experience
- Discuss baby's name and its significance
- Elicit and validate parents' observations of baby

Parent and Baby Time

- Explore baby's present behavior
- Position
- State
- Facilitate newborn activities
- Staying asleep (habituation to sound and light)
- Muscle tone
- Foot reflexes
- Rooting
- Soothing
- Looking at and following
- Hearing and turning to sounds

Family Time

Reflection and Writing to the Baby

As you prepare for the home visit, consider how the young mother learns, her psychological and physical stage of pregnancy, and her perceptions of her baby and of herself as a mother. Review the appropriate sections of the prenatal or postnatal Community-Based FANA and select activities to use with the parents during the upcoming home visit. Then gather any necessary materials for those activities. Think creatively about what will appeal to this mom and dad. Anticipate their responses, and modify the activities to suit the parents' needs and your own style.

Review your assessment of the teen mother's learning style. Where along these dimensions does she fall?

- Concrete → Abstract
- Present orientation → Future orientation
- Self-absorbed → Other focused

Knowing these things about the mother's learning style helps you frame the home visits. For example, a young mother who is a concrete thinker and very present orientated may not respond much to a question such as "How do you feel?" Answering that question fully takes a certain reflective process, an ability to gauge and compare past and present feeling states. The teen who is a present thinker and not yet reflective may simply say, "Fine," without further elaboration. That leaves you not really knowing much about the teen. With a concrete/present-thinking teen, a better question might be, "Now let's see. Let me take a good look at you. I need to look at your eyes for a second. Is there a tired person in there?"

Think about what you know about the father and others whom you have met who are significant in the mother's life. If you are working with the father, knowing about his learning style is equally helpful. Finally, think about your own needs and readiness for a moment:

- Are you hungry?
- Is there a nagging call you have to make?
- Do you need to get directions to the teen's home?
- What is your mood?
- How emotionally available are you for this home visit?
- What is the quality of your attention right now?
- What do you need to do to get ready to focus on this mom and dad and their baby?

Take some time to prepare yourself mentally, emotionally, and physically for the visit.

Parent Time

Each home visit begins with time to greet and reconnect with the mother, father, and others important to the parents. The Community-Based FANA (see chapters 9 and 10) provides specific questions and their rationales for use during every aspect of the home visit. During Parent Time, for example, ask about the parents' well-being and listen attentively. Explore changes that have occurred since the last visit. During the home visits after the baby's birth, give the mother and father plenty of time to tell the story of labor and delivery.

As a bridge to Parent and Baby Time, ask the parents what they have noticed about their baby—whether in utero or after birth—and validate the parents' observations of her. In both prenatal visits and the first visit after the baby is born, ask parents about the baby's name and what the name means to them (see chapters 9 and 10).

Parent and Baby Time

Parent and Baby Time helps the parents become fascinated with their baby and intrigued by his developing competencies. Begin by observing and talking about what the baby is doing at the present moment, whether that is in utero or after birth. Then initiate an active, joint inquiry about the baby's behavior and emerging developmental capacities.

Now, during Parent and Baby Time, is when home visitors introduce Community-Based FANA activities. While the teen is still pregnant, Parent and Baby Time focuses on activities of the unborn baby—and there are many! After the baby is born, Parent and Baby Time uses the postnatal activities to engage the parents with their newborn. Many of these postnatal activities allow parents to see in action what they have already learned about their baby during pregnancy.

The prenatal Community-Based FANA highlights one area of fetal development during each home visit as an opening to broader consideration of the parents and baby together. It also enables you to preview with parents newborn behavior and parenting challenges in the same developmental domain.

The postnatal FANA shows you how to guide parents in a hands-on exploration of their newborn's reflexes and motor abilities, capacity for social engagement, and preferences for soothing and consoling.

Remember that your goal is not to get through a certain number of activities in a home visit. Your goal is to join with the parents, meet them where they are, advance their experiences and understanding a bit, and then wait for them to incorporate the new ideas into their own way of holding their baby in their minds—their own way of thinking and feeling about their baby. That means that in any given home visit, you may not even use some of the ideas and activities that you prepared ahead of time.

Be sure not to overwhelm the parents. One or two activities will probably be enough during any one visit. If the parents have more compelling things to talk about, it's okay not to use any activities at all during that home visit. Matching your intervention to what's happening with the parents at the moment is the art of home visiting.

Family Time

Family Time is a pause in the home visit that creates a special time for parents and baby to be together. Pleasant, familiar routines and rituals are comforting to the baby and enjoyable for the parents. Parents can begin to create these positive times for themselves and their baby during pregnancy.

In prenatal home visits, encourage parents to choose a special way of being with their baby. That special way could be reading a story, singing a song, playing music, massaging the baby, or just talking to her. Encourage parents to repeat the same routine for each visit so that they have practice providing a predictable, consistent experience for the baby and themselves. The rituals begun during the prenatal FANA home visits can become a family's way of life after the baby is born.

Reflection and Writing to the Baby

The Community-Based FANA concludes with time for reflection on the home visit and for the parents to write to their baby. Reflection and Writing to the Baby, like the other Community-Based FANA home visit components, promotes the teen's recognition of her developing unborn baby and her attachment to and interest in her newborn.

Reflection. Invite the parents to pause and think about what you have just done together. Step back to consider their feelings, thoughts, and actions. When you do this, you offer young parents a model for reflecting on their parenting. Use consistent questions to guide parents in reflecting and writing. Ask the following questions:

- What did you see or experience that surprised you?
- What did you see or experience that you expected?
- How did you feel about what we just did together?
- What do you think the next few weeks will be like?

Writing to the Baby. Writing to the Baby helps a young mother learn about herself and her baby. It is a time-honored and effective way for the teen to bring order into her life, to begin to establish some mastery over the breathtaking rapidity with which her life events are occurring. It is a time for her to pause, observe, acknowledge, and begin to create a coherent narrative for the child of his early beginnings.

Reflection and Writing to the Baby in the Community-Based FANA builds on an exciting research finding: Mothers who have put some of their own childhood experiences in order—both the good and bad experiences—are less likely to repeat the bad ones with their own children (Main & Goldwyn, 1984).

What does it mean to put life experiences in order? It means not letting our experiences just wash over us. It means paying attention to important events and relationships and making links between our actions and what happens because of our actions. And it means remembering, day-to-day, month-to-month, year-to-year, the lessons we learn from our lives.

Judith Musick (1993), a pioneer in the use of journal writing for teens at risk, noted:

> *No matter who the adolescent is or how she lives, personal writing can provide an authentic means of self-expression, a new and different route to self-awareness. For an adolescent at risk, it can also provide a certain distance between feeling and doing, a way to help her think before she acts. (p. 21)*

A father, too, can enjoy writing to his baby as a way to connect with her.

Be sensitive to parents' comfort with writing down their thoughts and feelings. Some parents would rather talk and have you write down what they say. The written document should stay with the parents in a safe place.

Special Circumstances

Many things that happen before and during pregnancy affect how a young mother will experience the Community-Based FANA activities. If you become aware of special circumstances—such as the teen having experienced interpersonal violence or problems being found with the baby in utero—be prepared to adapt your home visits and Community-Based FANA activities to accommodate these circumstances. As always, take your cues from the young family.

When a Problem Has Been Diagnosed Before Birth

Be guided by what the parents know and feel. Their comfort level with the news that their doctor has given them is your guide to how many and what kinds of prenatal activities to facilitate.

It is important not to overwhelm parents with too much exploration of their unborn baby. At the same time, however, do give them the opportunity to experience what their baby is able to do and to explore also what they are already experiencing with the baby. A strong kick, the awareness of sleep–wake cycles, or a response to a parent's touch or voice can be a potent, inspiring reminder that, even with difficulties, there is a child who has a growing capacity about to be born. Activities designed to preview the newborn present an even more sensitive challenge, as the parents likely will be filled with concern about the unknown and experiencing feelings of loss and grief as they begin to prepare themselves.

Let the parents' willingness and readiness guide your steps after the baby is born, too. Start with one of the prenatal activities from an early visit—movement, hearing, or state. Be sensitive to how the parents experience the activity. Leave time and space for their emotions to evolve and be shared.

As you think about your own role in these situations, consider your level of knowledge about the baby you will be meeting. Parents can share with you what their doctor tells them, but it is your responsibility to learn about developmental problems or specific conditions away from the family. Know as much as you can—not to make medical predictions or recommendations, but to better understand. Medical consultants, journals and books, and access to community advocacy and support associations for various conditions are all resources available to the home visitor in these circumstances.

Much of your prenatal work will involve making yourself wholly available to hear the parents' feelings and help them live with the emotional impact. Rather than initiating these discussions, it may be best to let the parents bring them up. They likely are already involved in many difficult and emotional discussions with medical providers and their own family and friends. Your receptive posture provides them a place in which they don't need to decide anything or care for others. You are there for them. This is a treasure.

Your own feelings are also moved by the journey you take with this family as they learn about and prepare for the future. These experiences can easily remind you of your own experiences, fears you may have had in the past, or worries about your own family's future. It is your responsibility to be aware of the effects that this work has on you and to use your own support system, especially your supervisor, to care for yourself. The better you do this, the more available you are to the family.

When the Pregnant Teen Is Considering Adoption

When a teen is planning for adoption, the home visitor may be confused about the direction to take. Because the Community-Based FANA is designed to promote attachment, the prospect of a separation by adoption brings with it questions about if and how home visits can be conducted in such a circumstance. Should you facilitate the Community-Based FANA with these young mothers? Is it appropriate to invite a pregnant teenager and the baby's father into experiences that are intended to bring the infant in utero closer to the parents' awareness and emotional involvement?

The first and most important factor to consider is what you know about the teen parent and how and why adoption has become an option. Being young, and perhaps single, the expectant mother is weighing all kinds of life decisions. As you get to know her, her support system, and how she copes with and organizes life events, you begin to have a better idea of how she will put the pieces of this puzzle together. Because the planned adoption may stir your own feelings, the Community-Based FANA's receptive posture offers guidance on how to avoid becoming part of the puzzle.

During the last months of pregnancy, while the mother may be still in the process of deciding about adoption, the developing baby is asserting his presence. The pregnant teen is experiencing a day-to-day relationship with the baby, even if the future relationship is still to be determined. No matter what the final resolution, having an opportunity to explore and express her relationship now can help with either the separation or the attachment that will come later.

Follow the pregnant teen's own comfort level with exploring the baby's prenatal development. Offer opportunities for the young parent to connect with the baby she has now. In such instances, you have a heightened responsibility. You must judge continually how much the teen wants to know and help her explore without bringing her to an emotional crisis in the midst of her decision-making process.

The previewing the newborn activities and discussions may be best saved for those times when the mother initiates interest. By following her lead and being responsive to her interest, the home visitor can use the prenatal Community-Based FANA to help the teen make informed decisions and be better prepared to live with the decisions she makes.

When the Teen Has Experienced Interpersonal Violence

As the relationship that you build with a teenager becomes closer, you sometimes are confronted by the harsh realities of her life. The very sense of empathy and openness that so effectively moves you closer to the pregnant teen can at times bring you face to face to bear witness to the pain present in her life. This is especially true when pregnant teens have experienced interpersonal violence.

The prevalence of acquaintance or date rape among teenagers is between 20% and 68% (Rickert & Weinmann, 1998), and as many as 13% of births to adolescents are a result of rape, incest, or some other coercive sexual relationship (Leiderman & Almo, 2001). Young women who remain in violent relationships may experience continued or increased harm during the months of pregnancy and during the postpartum period. One study found that among mothers between 13–17 years old, 26% experienced intimate partner violence in the first three postpartum months (Leiderman & Almo, 2001).

Because interpersonal violence is so prevalent, home visitors must be prepared to face this reality in the lives of the young parents with whom they are facilitating the Community-Based FANA. However, the emotional needs of these young women may well be beyond the scope of your program's home visits. There are many programs to support young women who are or have been victims of violence and to prevent future exposure. Learn about such local programs and develop contacts with advocacy, support, and mental health services designed for women who have had these experiences.

As with all special circumstances, being fully aware of how you are affected yourself is the first step in guiding your reactions and responses. This may not be easy for you. One third of all women have experienced sexual, physical, or emotional violence, and many more have loved ones who have experienced such violence. The circumstances that you encounter in your work as a home visitor can sometimes resonate with experiences you have had in your own life. Just as you keep your own excitement and joy about the new life you are meeting secondary to the parents' joy, so must you keep your own pain or anger separate from the mother's pain. When you are able to be attuned, available, and receptive to the teen's story, she will more easily trust your concern and become open to your efforts on her behalf.

The inner life of the pregnant teenager is never certain, and it is rarely fully clear what the relationship a young mother has with the father of her baby represents to her. This is even more confounding when emotional and physical violence are involved. Adolescents often experience adults in their lives as either not understanding how they feel or as telling them how they ought to feel. By holding back your own judgments, you strengthen your relationship with a young mother in these circumstances. The Community-Based FANA can create a safe and sensitive environment in which parents can feel as they really do about their baby, and this may change minute by minute.

As you work with a teen who has experienced interpersonal violence, explore and learn what meaning the baby has for her. Does the baby represent a painful experience, or does he represent positive hope for the future? Is it both? This can change during the course of the pregnancy and even after the baby is born. Stay open to the emotional ties you learn about, and be available for celebration and to provide comfort. You may be one of the only people who is aware of the intimacies of the young woman's life and yet is able to listen without judgment while she works on making sense of her changing life. Having someone who really cares and really listens makes a difference!

Remember that you cannot always do this work alone. As with other special circumstances, you, too, need a sensitive and safe place to process your own emotions. Supervision and discussion with peers can help when your works leads you to navigate others'—or your own—pain. Although this work can bring you face to face with personal histories and injuries, remember that your role is limited.

Guiding Principles and Key Practices for Using the Community-Based FANA

The Community-Based FANA is a tool for affirming or helping to develop parents' sense of connection to and responsibility for their infant. Through your home visits and the FANA activities, you promote parents' attachment to their newborn child by helping them begin to feel like "mother" and "father." The following principles should guide your use of the Community-Based FANA.

Guiding principle. Successful Community-Based FANA home visits depend on parents being comfortable having the home visitor in their home.

Key practice. Enter gently into the boundaries of the home and into the physical arrangements between parents and baby.

Enter the hospital room and home gently. Leave the setting as it is. Remember, you are a guest. During the prenatal period, let the parents show you where to sit during a home visit. After delivery, if the mother is holding the baby in a rocking chair, put your own chair as near hers as you can without disrupting her arrangement. If the father is holding the baby, greet him warmly and encourage him to stay just as he is. If the baby is in another room, talk to the parents alone first. If the baby is awake and lying in a bassinet with the parents sitting some feet away, respect this.

The environment people create and how they position themselves in physical relation to others, including their baby, can be an expression of either self-care or infant care. For reasons that neither you nor the parents may fully understand at this point, the grouping they have chosen is important.

Guiding principle. Young parents need to feel that they are in charge when it comes to their baby.

Key practice. Seek opportunities to empower parents by acknowledging and supporting their authority and their responsibility for their baby.

Always invite parents to try activities with you, rather than telling them what to do. Encourage parents to determine with you what will be most helpful to them during any visit. Ask their permission before adjusting the home environment or asking them to reposition themselves. For example, to make a prenatal video together, you may need space to set up the equipment. Asking, "Would it be okay with you if I put my equipment over here?" communicates respect for the parents and their environment and sets the stage for acknowledging their authority in relation to the baby.

After the baby is born, always ask permission to touch or hold the baby. This further encourages the development of the parents' sense of authority and responsibility for the baby. This may stand in sharp contrast to the parents' experience with their mothers, grandparents, aunts, or older siblings who may attempt to assume authority over the infant. Speak consistently of the baby as belonging to the mother and father. Ask permission each time before you interact with the baby: "May I pick up your baby?" "Would it be all right with you if I swaddle her? I just want her to be still and quiet for a moment while we talk to her."

Guiding principle. Parents' perceptions are the key to helping them integrate, or bring together, the dreamed of—or feared—baby with the baby who is right there before their eyes.

Key practice. Elaborate or reflect on every observation the parents initially make about themselves or their baby to help them explore their feelings.

Some observations may be off-base and difficult to hear. For example, a young mother might say during the last weeks of pregnancy, "This baby is killing me. I got a bad one. I can tell." As much as you might want to change those feelings, your job is not to do that. Instead, foster her relationship with you so that she feels safe enough to explore her feelings. Acknowledging the depth of her feelings is the place start. Your calm, careful listening conveys that she can say what she is feeling—bad or good—and that she can hold these feelings and you can hear them.

You can also ask the teen to share more: What is hard for her now? What worries or concerns does she have about herself? About her baby? Reassure her that you two can talk about this again if she likes and that you will be there to support her as she gets to know her baby after he is born.

After delivery, the real baby is present, and Community-Based FANA activities give the infant a chance to speak for herself. For example, if a father says to you, "My baby can't see or hear yet," you can acknowledge his statement and engage him in an upcoming activity: "Oh, so you're saying that your baby really can't hear or see yet. When we play with her a little later, let's see what she tells us about her ability to see and hear." Remember that nothing a teen mother and father say about their baby is wrong to them; those are their perceptions of their infant. It is the baby who either affirms these perceptions or says, "Hey, Mom! Hey, Dad! This is the real me!" through the Community-Based FANA activities.

Guiding principle. The baby's responses are the most powerful force in developing parents' identity as "mother" and "father."

Key practice. Use every opportunity to connect the parents and baby.

For example, if the teen is holding her infant in a face-to-face position and he begins to scan her face, you can say: "Look at this! He's saying, 'Mom, I love looking at your face!'" Or, if the baby soothes to the mother's attempts to console him, try speaking for the baby: "Thanks, Mom, that felt so good." Even in the absence of a particular infant response, you can use the words "Mom" and "Dad" a lot. This also works during the prenatal period. For example, if a teen shows you a special toy she bought for her baby, you can say: "What a thoughtful mother you are!" or, when a dad talks about how much fun it is to feel the baby kick, you can say: "How wonderful that you are already spending time with your baby! This is what your baby will want most—you!"

Guiding principle. Babies change the delicate balance in relationships, including the relationship between the parents and home visitor.

Key practice. Respect the changing reality and shape your interactions with the parents to reflect those changes.

Whether you have come to know the parents over the months before delivery or only in the last few days of pregnancy, the birth of the baby will change the relationship and shift how you relate to each other. There are many different forms this may take. The young mother may be suddenly shy or quite the opposite. She may be eager to show off her breast-feeding skills or worry that she will do something wrong. If you have children of your own, and the teen knows this, she may become dependent on you for information, or she may rebel against you as an authority.

It helps to anticipate these changes and respect them. Observing these changes also helps you understand how the teen mother may be affecting the people important to her in her home environment. Now is a good time to revisit what you learned about her—and yourself—through the "Know Yourself" and "Know the Teen" activities in chapters 2 and 3. Now, with the baby born, who have you become to the teen mom or dad, and how does that feel to you? Who has the teen become?

Using the Guiding Principles

These principles and practices are not always easy for home visitors to follow. If, for example, you see a young mother sitting several feet away from her baby, your first impulse is probably to move the bassinet closer to her. Or, if the baby is alert, you might be strongly tempted to immediately show the teen this state, or to pick up the baby and engage him. Most difficult is when a parent says something negative about the baby: "She's so mean and greedy. She wants to eat all the time." Your job is to use your observation skills to watch this scenario without attempting to change it.

References

Leiderman, S., & Almo, C. (2001, October). *Interpersonal violence and adolescent pregnancy: Prevalence and implications for practice and policy*. Bala Cynwyd, PA: Center for Assessment and Policy Development.

Main, M., & Goldwyn, R. (1984). Predicting rejection of her infant from mother's representation of her own experience: Implications for the abused–abusing intergenerational cycle. *Child Abuse and Neglect, 8*, 203–217.

Musick, J. (1993). *Young, poor and pregnant*. New Haven: Yale University Press.

Rickert, V. I., & Weimann, C. M. (1998). Date rape among adolescents and young adults. *Journal of Pediatric and Adolescent Gynecology, 11*(4), 167–175.

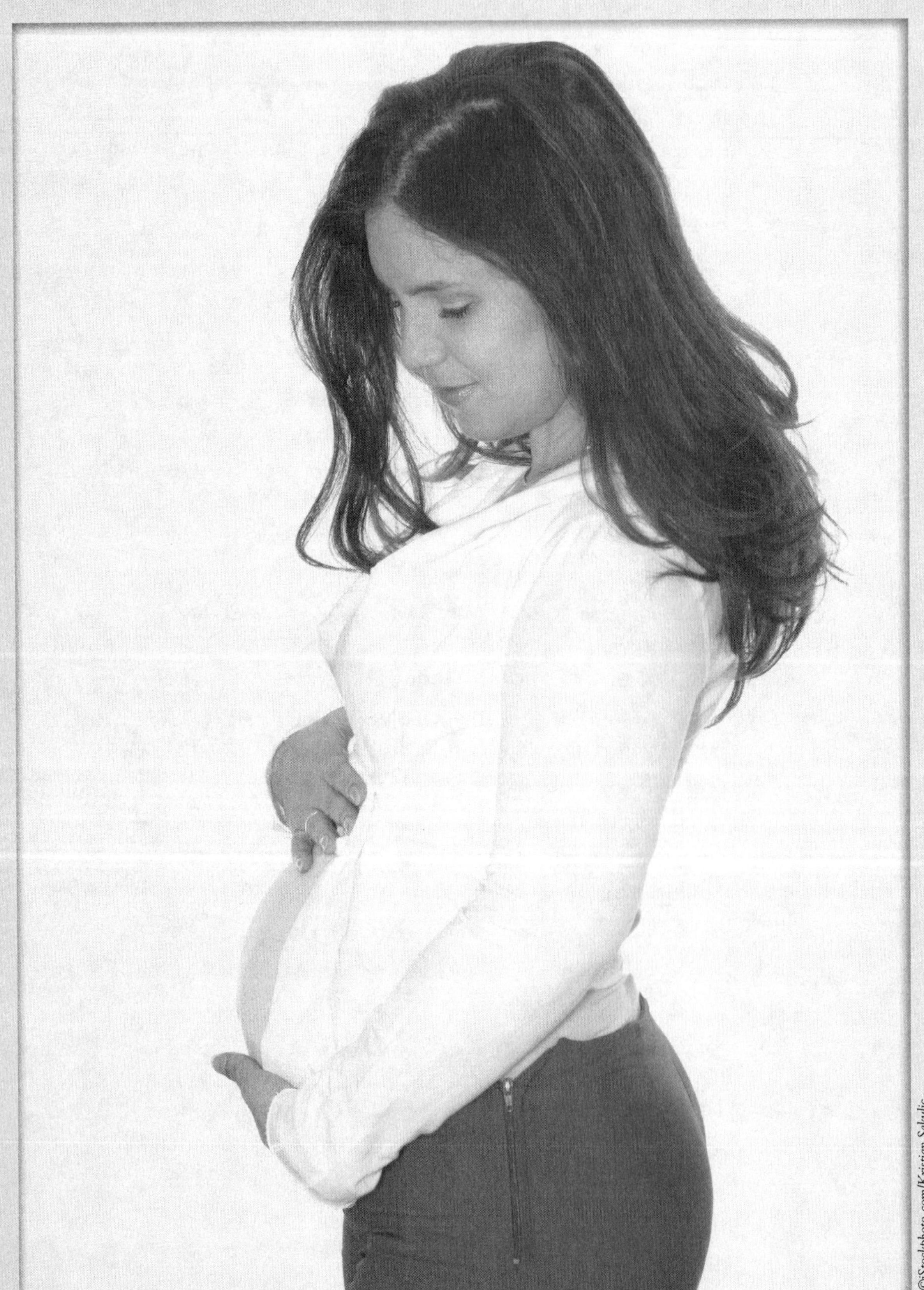

CHAPTER 9

Welcome Parents: The Prenatal Home Visits

There are so many things home visitors can do to help young parents attach to their baby during pregnancy! Now that you know the structure of Community-Based Family Administered Neonatal Activities (FANA) home visits and the guiding principles and key practices for making them happen, you are ready to use it with young families.

This chapter provides Community-Based FANA activities and instructions for six prenatal home visits, beginning in the 7th month of pregnancy, at weeks 26–27 gestation, and ending in the last month of pregnancy, at 36–37 weeks. By this time in the pregnancy, the baby is very real to everyone, and the activities help parents get to know their developing baby.

The home visit guides are designed for two prenatal visits per month, with activities tailored to where the mother and the baby are prenatally during those periods. Once you are familiar with the prenatal Community-Based FANA and how to use it as it was designed to be used, you can adapt it for other uses that fit your program's model and services.

The First Time

When you are ready to use the Community-Based FANA for the first time, start by reviewing the basic components of all Community-Based FANA home visits (see chapter 8).

Once you are confident that you know what each visit has in common, you are ready to take on the specifics of the Community-Based FANA home visits tailored to the prenatal period. Each home visit activity guide includes several possible activities for you to do with young parents. You have many choices and options for interactive discussions and activities for any specific week of pregnancy, beginning with the 26th week.

This is when everything you have learned about the expectant parents comes into play. Use what you know to think about which activities are best suited to them. Make sure that you leave plenty of room for parents to make their own choices from among possible things to do. That means that you must be prepared to use any of the FANA activities that seems best once you are with the parents. Remember to be flexible and come prepared!

Being flexible also means being willing to extend one component of the home visit and shorten another when that seems best. Remember, though, to keep the flow of the visit—the sequence of the components—consistent across the weeks before birth.

Before you jump into the home visit activity guides and make your first Community-Based FANA home visit, think through how to prepare for and facilitate a prenatal home visit.

The Prenatal Home Visit

Each prenatal home visit guide includes a focus on what the baby is doing now in one aspect of development and a parallel focus on what the newborn will be like in that same developmental area (see Figure 9.1). This helps the parents think about what the baby is like and able to do right now, and anticipate what the baby will be like as a newborn in terms of a particular sense, reflex, or capacity. For example, when the prenatal focus is on the baby's ability to suck in the womb, the corresponding newborn preview focus is on feeding.

Prenatal Preparation

To prepare for the prenatal home visit, review what you know about the young family, select the prenatal activities that you plan to use, gather the necessary materials for those activities, and ready yourself physically and psychologically.

Figure 9.1

The Developmental Focus of the Prenatal Home Visits

Week 26–27
Focus on the Unborn Baby: Movement
Previewing the Newborn: Newborn Behavior

Week 28–29
Focus on the Unborn Baby: Hearing
Previewing the Newborn: Maternal Speech

Week 30–31
Focus on the Unborn Baby: Fetal State
Previewing the Newborn: Newborn State

Week 32–33
Focus on the Unborn Baby: Fetal Touch
Previewing the Newborn: Holding and Soothing

Week 34–35
Focus on the Unborn Baby: Fetal Sucking
Previewing the Newborn: Feeding

Week 36–37
Focus on the Unborn Baby: Vision
Previewing the Newborn: Seeing Each Other

Reviewing What You Know

Physical and psychological stage of pregnancy. Remind yourself of the baby's gestational age and where the teen is in her pregnancy. Look over the relevant sections of chapter 5, "Mutual Growth: The Trimesters of Pregnancy," if you need the review. If this is not your first visit with the young mother, review your notes and think about how she was feeling emotionally and physically on your last visit. Picture her in your mind—where she was sitting, how she looked, and the mood she was in. Remember what engaged her the most. Think about her expectations and plans for the birth. How prepared is she for the coming event?

Mother's view of the baby. Review what the teen mom has said about her baby such as, "he's very active," "she has strong legs," "he doesn't quiet down very easily," or "she jumps when I sneeze." How have her thoughts of her baby changed over time? How do the father and other significant people in her life talk about the baby? All of these prenatal ideas are very important during the postnatal visits as you and the parents engage with the baby in a number of activities that will either confirm or challenge their prenatal views.

Be wholly available to receive the parents' points of view, and work toward understanding them. Avoid the temptation to try to teach parents what to think or feel or to try to undo what they already feel. Rather, continue to help them have meaningful experiences with their baby in utero and help them keep expressing themselves as they evolve into the kind of parents they want to be.

Choosing Activities and Materials

Review the suggestions for prenatal activities in the home visit activity guide for the appropriate gestational age. One or two of the newborn preview activities are probably enough for any one visit. Your goal is not to razzle-dazzle the parents or to question them relentlessly.

Be sure to choose activities from the appropriate weeks of the Community-Based FANA. Remember that the activities are designed to match what is happening developmentally in utero.

Gather the materials necessary for the activities you've chosen, as well as any other materials you plan to use during the home visit. Remember that the purpose of any material is to engage the parents and help them connect with their baby. Be careful not to overwhelm them with stuff. A variety of visual aids can help teens explore the world of their unborn baby, including the following:

- Pictures of pregnant teens
- Plastic models of the unborn baby at various gestational ages

- A teen mother's own ultrasound
- Pictures of a newborn baby
- Books that teen parents can read to their unborn baby and music that they can play for her

Prenatal Parent Time

Prenatal Parent Time is an opportunity to greet and reconnect with the young family, explore the baby's name and what it means to the parents, and elicit and validate their observations of their baby.

Connecting

Greet and connect—or reconnect—with the teen mother by focusing on her first. Figure 9.2 offers discussion points and questions you can ask to help make this connection.

Figure 9.2

Focusing on the Teen Mother

Concrete Areas to Discuss

- Her clothes
- Her hair
- Any major changes in her appearance

The Immediate Past

- What has your day been like so far?
- Have you had a doctor visit since I last saw you? What happened?
- How have your spirits been since I last saw you? Pretty cheery? Not so hot?

Primary Activities

- How was your time at school?
- Who did you eat lunch with yesterday?
- Has work been okay, or has it been pretty rough for you? What's your time there like?
- What has home been like? How is it going with your brothers, sisters, mom, dad, cousins? Do you have any special jobs at home?

Asking the teen mother about her well-being with respect to her pregnancy helps you connect with her. But it also bridges time spent focusing on her alone and time spent with her focusing on her and the baby together. Try the following questions:

- With everything you've just told me is going on with you, it must be hard to balance taking care of yourself and your baby. How have you been feeling?
- Have you felt any physical changes?

Exploring the Baby's Name

If the parents have already chosen a name for their baby, finding out what that name means to them may be another way of finding out what the baby means to them. Is the baby to be named after a beloved aunt, a brother, or perhaps a grandparent? Is the baby's name to be the same as the mother's or the father's? The answer can be another window into the parents' perception of this coming infant. If, for example, a young mother says that the baby's name is a family name or a combination of family names, that indicates connectedness. If a teen says that she hasn't chosen a name for the baby or that she let her mother choose, that may indicate distance. Try asking the following questions:

- Have you been thinking about names for your baby?
- Great! Tell me about the baby's name and what it means to you.
- Is there any special name that you use for your baby now? (If there is not, you may want to encourage the mother to call the baby by a name, such as "Sweetie," or any other name she chooses. Some mothers may not be ready for this yet. As with every aspect of your home visits, join with the mother where she is.)

Validating Parents' Observations

Ask the parents what they've noticed about their baby, and acknowledge everything that they have observed about their baby so far.

- What has your baby told you about herself this week?
- Has your baby changed in any way that you can tell?
- Were there times when you felt particularly close to your baby?
- Were there times when you were worried or concerned about him?

Prenatal Parent and Baby Time

Parent and Baby Time in prenatal home visits allows you to help parents do two exciting things—explore what their unborn baby is doing at that stage in her development and look ahead to what their newborn will be like. This is at the heart of the prenatal Community-Based FANA.

Some teen mothers will be comfortable learning—and some will be eager to learn—about the baby growing inside them. Others may be inhibited, uncomfortable, or frightened, and those reactions may appear to be indifference or hostility. Take it slowly. Proceed with respect for the care and development of each individual teen mom. The experiences she is having with the baby, and with you, all contribute to the creation of her parenthood. This is indeed a dual birth!

Exploring the Baby's Present Behavior

This is the time for the parents to connect with the baby. The first part of the visit focuses on the parent. Now it is time to complete the transition by focusing on the developing baby.

State. Begin by asking about the baby's state: "You have noticed so much about your baby already. Let's see what the baby is doing right now." Draw the mother's awareness to her baby's present fetal state by asking: "What do you think the baby is doing right now? Is he awake or asleep? Is he moving? What are those movements like?"

Ask the mother to touch her growing midsection—to hold and spend a quiet moment with her baby. Touching helps a parent connect with the baby in the moment by carrying her mind from wherever it might be right to the baby.

This is critically important as you and the parent play with and talk about the developing baby and what is to come. Touching is essential to infants' growth and development. Babies can't live without it. This moment in the prenatal home visit is the perfect time to establish patterns of gentle touch.

Ask the mom if her baby is awake or asleep, and ask her to tell you about the baby's behavior. Listen to her, and interpret the emotional tone of her response to help you decide how to proceed. Connecting with the baby has the potential to bring up a full spectrum of feelings—from excitement, anticipation, and joy to sadness, fear, and anger. Keep your work with each parent on track and in synch by matching your statements and behaviors with hers. It is so easy for you as a home visitor to express your own feelings—usually excitement—but this is a time for you to hear and hold the parent's feelings and emotional state.

For example, a young mother may appear uninterested in her baby's activity, whereas you are very excited about the baby's movements. Stay where the teen is, perhaps by asking, "What does that kick feel like to you?" As she makes the emotional and mental transition from experiencing self to experiencing baby, remain quiet, supportive, and available. This is what being fully present means, and this is a time to demonstrate that as you and she continue to work together, you will accept and respond to how she feels.

Position. To explore the baby's position, ask: "I wonder what position the baby is in?" Encourage the mother to touch her belly and trace the baby's position inside her. "Can you tell where the baby's legs are? How about her head?" The goal of these questions is not for the parents to be able to identify body parts or fetal position. It is to invite and support parents to make a space in their own emotions for their baby, as well as to be more aware of and attuned to the baby's state. These are abilities that parents will use to understand and help their babies after they are born.

Previewing the Newborn

Keep in mind that in the prenatal period you are setting the stage for what the mom and dad will see, feel, and hear after their baby is born. Your goal is to heighten their engagement with the baby growing inside the mom as a way to prepare them for engaging with their newborn.

By this time in the home visit, you and the parents have probably established a fun and lively rapport. After having spent time connecting with the mom and with the developing baby, you are in a good position to help move the parents' thoughts in yet another direction. This transition moves them from the baby as he is now to the baby they will see when he has finally arrived.

The prenatal visits—before sleepless nights and before the nervousness and uncertainty of being a new parent—also offer an ideal time to wonder aloud together about how the parents plan to care for their baby. The preview activities are a springboard to discussions that can help clarify their attitudes, beliefs, and expectations about parenting and inform their decisions. These activities allow some of the critical circumstances all new parents face to be discussed before the baby arrives, such as the breast-feeding or bottle-feeding decision, why infants cry, how to soothe and calm a crying baby, and the effect on the baby of hearing harsh and mean words around her as opposed to loving words.

As always, home visitors must be in harmony and balance with where each family is. Match your previewing the newborn activities to what each parent is ready to experience and explore.

Prenatal Family Time

Prenatal Family Time is an opportunity to help new parents establish patterns of parental behavior that are fun and meaningful. In time, these behaviors can become part of what parents and children learn to expect from each other based on the repeated experiences they have together.

Facilitating a Family Ritual

Children love to do special things over and over with their parents. Family Time during prenatal home visits is an opportunity to help parents build a family ritual that can continue throughout the baby's early years. Singing to the baby, listening to a favorite song, or reading a book all are great activities. Encourage the parents to do one or more ritual every day, and invite them to use this time in each visit to share the ritual.

If the parents do not have an idea for a family ritual, suggest reading together: "Reading together is one way to feel close to and help your baby learn. You can start to build this ritual between you and your child even before the baby is born." Invite the parents to choose a book—bring several with you to the home visit, including picture books without words—and then to read or tell their baby the story. Let the parents know that if they do this often with the same book during pregnancy, there is a chance that their baby will remember the way this story sounds and respond to it in a special way after birth. Give the parents quiet time during Family Time to read to their baby.

Prenatal Reflection and Writing to the Baby

Encourage the parents to start a family book for their child, even before the baby is born by offering: "We have talked so much—and you have thought so much—about your baby! Would you like to write some of these thoughts down and keep them in a family book for you and your baby? Either or both of you can write something now or later. If you like, you can tell me what you want to say, and I'll write it down." It may help some parents to have a template to get started.

The Prenatal Home Visit Activity Guides

The Activity Guides for the prenatal home visits provide Parent and Baby Time activities for six home visits, spanning the period from 26–27 weeks gestation to 36–37 weeks gestation. Required and optional materials are listed for all activities. Each activity guide also lists the home visit components and some relevant prenatal developmental milestones as a reminder for you when you are just getting started.

The Prenatal Home Visit Activity Guides are provided in the Appendix B Tool Kit on pages 125–154.

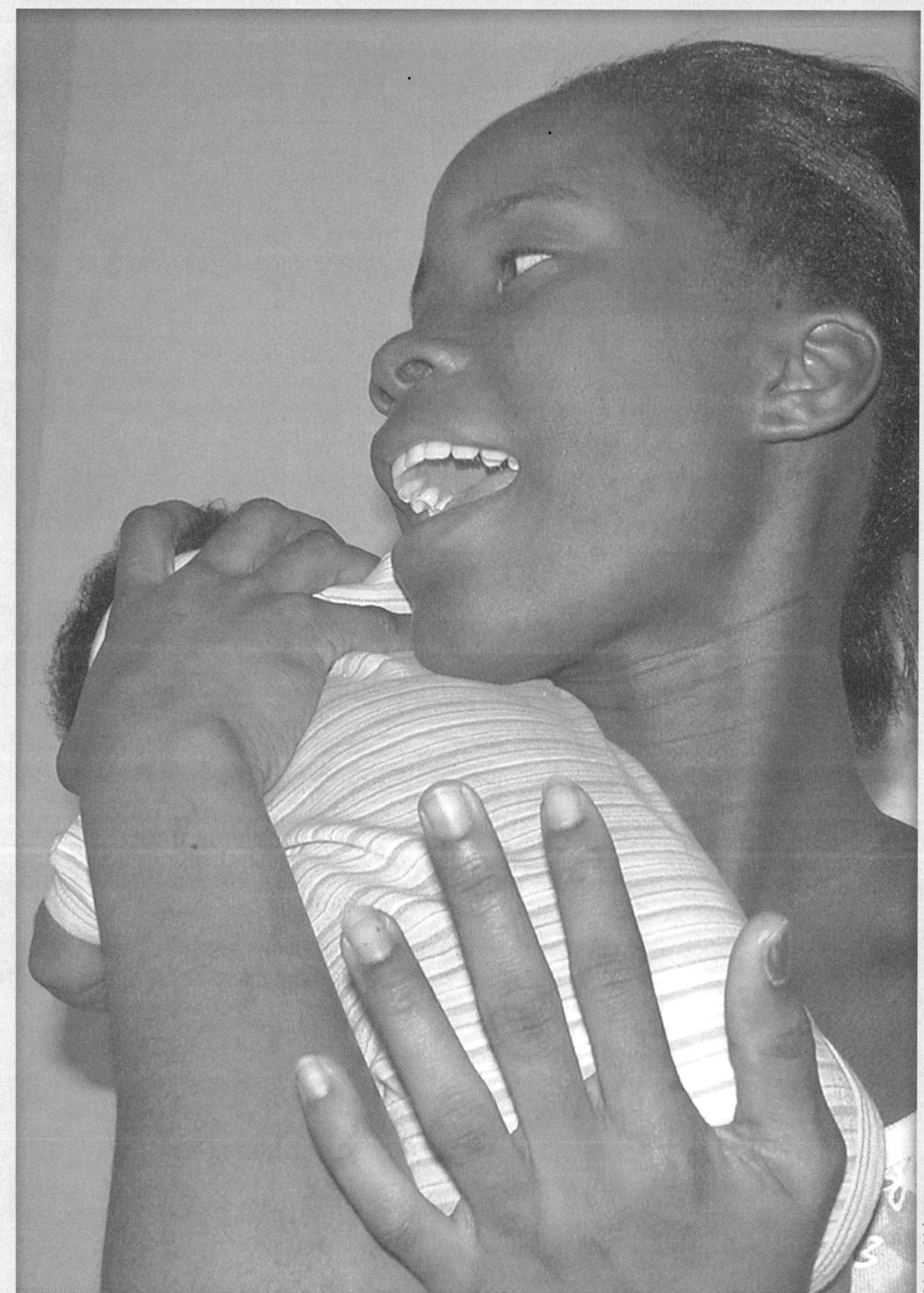

Marilyn Nolt

CHAPTER 10

WELCOME BABY: THE POSTNATAL HOME VISITS

Now is the mystical, magical moment when you meet the newborn baby! There are so many aspects of this experience that should be attended to—so where to begin?

This chapter answers that question with Community-Based Family Administered Neonatal Activities (FANA) and discussions for postnatal home visits, beginning with a first postpartum visit and spanning the first month of life outside the womb.

In many ways, the postnatal FANA home visits mirror the prenatal visits. For example, now you can speak of labor and delivery as it really happened. The focus on the newly born infant will parallel the many fascinating behaviors that you and the parents focused on when the baby was in utero. With the newborn right before their very eyes, the young family will learn all that he has to teach them about who he is!

The postnatal home—or hospital—visit activity guide offers in-depth discussions for you to facilitate with the new parents. Through a series of guided explorations with the parents of their newborn's capacities, postnatal activities focus on what the baby can do.

As with the prenatal home visits, the key to success is facilitating the postnatal visits following the same basic Community-Based FANA structure: Preparation, Parent Time, Parent and Baby Time, Family Time, and Reflection and Writing to the Baby.

POSTNATAL PREPARATION

Prepare for the postnatal visits in the same way that you prepare for prenatal visits. Review what you know about the young family, select the postnatal activities and discussions, gather the necessary materials, and ready yourself physically and psychologically for the visit.

Reviewing What You Know

Labor and delivery. Birth is a major developmental event. Providing the teen mother with an opportunity to talk about it—including all that was good, disappointing, or frightening—helps her reestablish a sense of equilibrium and mastery.

If this is your first postnatal visit with a family, review the mother's expectations and preparations for the birth.

- What was she expecting to feel at the first signs of labor?
- Who was she planning to call when labor started?
- How was she planning to get to the hospital?
- What did she expect the labor room, the doctors, and the nurses to be like?
- Did she share her thoughts about the kind of birth that she wished for or feared?
- Who were her coaches going to be?

Having these things fresh in your mind before the first postpartum visit will help you to contrast the real event with the wished-for event. If this is not your first postnatal visit with the family, then review the young mother's experience of the birth.

Mother's view of the baby. Now is the time when all the ideas that parents had about their baby in the prenatal period are either confirmed or challenged. As with the prenatal visits, be wholly available to receive the parents' points of view. Work toward understanding them. Do not try to teach parents what to think or feel, or try to undo what they already feel. Continue to help them express themselves as they evolve into the kind of parents they want to be.

Choosing Activities and Materials

Review the suggestions for activities and discussions in the postnatal home visit activity guide and choose the ones that seem right for this family at this time. Gather the materials for the activities you've chosen. As always, remember that the purpose of the materials is to engage the parents and help them connect with their baby. Necessary postnatal materials include the following:

- Receiving blanket the right size to comfortably and snugly swaddle the baby;
- Red rattle;
- Red ball; and
- Flashlight.

Although you choose activities ahead of time for each visit, be prepared to do whatever the baby is available to do once you arrive. Follow the baby's lead. Figure 10.1 links babies' states to the kinds of Community-Based FANA activities that lend themselves to those states.

Figure 10.1

What You Can Do When

Asleep	Awake	Crying
State	State	Soothing
Habituation	Reflexes	
Reflexes	Muscle tone	
Muscle tone	Orientation	

Postnatal Parent Time

Parent Time after the baby is born has the same goals as prenatal Parent Time. It is a time to greet and reconnect with the young family, explore the baby's name and what it means to them, and elicit and validate the parents' observations of their baby.

Connecting—The Postpartum Interview

Greet and reconnect with the teen by focusing on her first. A postpartum interview of the young mother says to her, "We have a fascinating baby right here before us, but you are equally important!" There are four interview topics, with questions to help you explore each one with the parents:

- Understanding the mother's physical and personal well-being
- Describing the labor and delivery experience
- Exploring the baby's name
- Eliciting and validating the parents' observations of the baby

Each topic relates to the next one in a deliberate manner and order developed from clinical experience. The goal is to guide the parents in an ever-widening circle of engagement with their own experience, their relationship with their baby, and their relationship with you, the home visitor. Although the interview questions are meant to be asked within the context of a quiet conversation, you nonetheless actively engage with the parents. Controlled but strong energy is a good way to think of your position.

Understanding the mother's physical and personal well-being. Begin the interview with a focus on the mother's well-being. Listen carefully. Explore changes that have occurred since the last time you talked with her about herself.

- What have these last few days been like for you?
- Let me look at you—are you really tired?
- Are you sore?
- Have you been drinking plenty of water? Eating enough? Napping as much as you can?
- How are your spirits?

Describing the birth experience. Why tell the story of the birth event? Telling any story helps us gain control over the events we are describing. By controlling the birth story, parents are able to get some control over what they have just experienced, including any negative aspects. Give the mother and father plenty of time to tell their story of labor and delivery. The new mother may wish to share a little or a lot. If it seems right, encourage the parents to begin the story now and elaborate later, if they choose.

In a simple, gentle way, try going back and forth in time, encouraging the new mother to compare what happened during birthing with what she expected: "That was pretty much what you expected, wasn't it?" or "You must have been very surprised, given what you expected."

- Let's start at the beginning. What time did you realize you were first experiencing labor pains?
- What form and where did the pains start—strong back pains, mild pelvic pain, indigestion? Was it like what you expected?
- Who did you call when you realized labor was starting? Was that person available? Was it the person you had planned to call? What was that like for you—were you...(glad, sad, angry, grateful, etc.)?
- What happened when you got to the hospital? Did the labor and delivery room look the way you expected it to look?
- What did you experience from . . . (nurses, doctors, the doula, etc.)? Did they help? How did it compare to what you thought it would be?
- What about pain medicine? What kind did you have? Did it help?
- Tell me about pushing the baby out—how long did it last? Who helped? Did you feel it? Were you exhausted by then?
- How long was it from the onset of labor to delivery?
- What did you see the first time you looked at your baby?

Exploring the baby's name. Just as in the prenatal home visits, finding out what the baby's name means to the parents may be another way of finding out what the baby means to them.

- How did your baby get her name?
- Was this a name you decided on yourself or did someone help you?
- Do you know any other people named (baby's name)?

Eliciting and validating the parents' observations. Ask the parents what they've noticed about their baby. Three things to keep in mind as you validate the parents' observations are (a) the parents' prenatal perceptions and expectations for the baby, (b) their current perceptions and expectations, and (c) what the new baby is telling the parents about himself.

Depending on the teen, you may have to be very concrete. No matter what the parents say, acknowledge everything they have observed about their baby so far: "You've noticed so much about your baby already!" or "You've probably noticed a lot more about your baby than you can even tell me about right now!"

- What has your baby told you about himself so far?
- What have you seen your baby do in these last few days?
- Have you seen your baby open his eyes?
- Have you seen your baby move his legs and arms?

Postnatal Parent and Baby Time

Parent and Baby Time in postnatal visits parallels prenatal Parent and Baby Time in that the focus is on helping parents explore their baby. After the baby is born, the emphasis is on the baby's state and what she can do. Parent and Baby Time flows naturally from the interview questions eliciting the parents' view of the baby, which creates a bridge from focusing on the parents alone to focusing on the baby together with them.

Exploring the Baby's State Through a Guided Exploration of Newborn Capacities

This is the time for the parents to connect with the baby. Gather the parents in an intimate circle around the baby and transition from the interview: "Let's see what else your baby will tell us about herself today. Let's start by looking at her together. What do you see her doing right now?"

Sleep/awake states. At some time during the postnatal visits, it may be possible to observe all five newborn sleep–awake states: deep sleep, light sleep (dream sleep), alert, fussy, and crying. Highlighting these states with the parents is an excellent way to help them begin to understand the subtleties of their baby's behaviors.

Begin by asking about the baby's state: "What do you see him doing right now? Yes, he looks very soundly asleep (alert, fussy, drowsy, crying) to me, too."

Engage the parents in discussing other states that they have seen. This is a good time to relieve parents' worries about very deep sleep, which can frighten some parents into thinking that their baby is not breathing: "Have you ever seen him when he's so sound asleep you don't even see his body moving with his breaths? That's a beautiful, deep, baby sleep-state. Maybe other times you've seen him when he looks asleep but you see his eye lids fluttering? Or maybe he's grimacing, or his hands are shaking?"

Many parents will respond, "Oh! Yes. I think he's having a nightmare." Explain that he's not really having a nightmare, because he's not really dreaming yet, but that what they see their baby doing lets them know that he will dream someday.

Ask parents: "Have you seen him with his eyes wide open, quietly looking around, maybe even looking right at you? Yes, that's a wonderful quiet-alert time for your baby. It's the time when he will most want to play, and as he gets older those quiet-alert times will get longer and longer throughout the day."

"What does he do when he's fussy? Have you heard him come up into a nice loud cry? Well, he's either blowing off steam, or he's hungry or wet. In a few weeks you will get to know those signals pretty well. Whatever the reason for his crying, he will always love being quickly held by you."

If the parents respond that they are afraid of spoiling the baby, reassure them: "From everything we know, you just can't spoil a baby by hugging him quickly and a lot when he cries. It lets him know that his cries are important and that he is important. What do you like best from the people around you when you cry or are sad?" Relate this back to prenatal discussions about the baby soothing himself. Also think back with the parents to strategies for self-care, expectations from others, and what feels good and what does not. Ask the mother to remember her prenatal experiences with the baby. For example, when the baby kicked in utero, did he stop kicking if the mother put her hand firmly on her abdomen?

"All babies are different. Some go from sleeping to crying to sleeping again. Others go from sleeping to a quiet-alert time, to fussy, and then back down to sleep. During Parent and Baby Time, we'll be able to watch together as your baby goes through these states."

Postnatal Family Time

Remember Family Time from the prenatal visits and recall how the mother and father were feeling and what that experience was like. Explore with them the possibility of continuing this ritual with their baby now that she is here. Invite them to do so now, if they like. Encourage the mother to find unhurried moments when she can just be with her baby, as she was before the baby was born. Mention that you will ask about this again in your next visit.

Postnatal Reflection and Writing to the Baby

Reflection. During the postnatal visit Reflection, help the parents look at their first perceptions of their baby and then link those perceptions with the baby they really saw during the Community-Based FANA activities. This is a time for you to help the new parents develop expectations and to provide guidance about any issues that have emerged. Take special care to be sensitive to the mom's emotions. Model for her the hoped-for parent–infant interaction by doing for her what you hope she will do for her baby.

Begin by summarizing briefly what the parents observed during the Parent and Baby Time activities: "Let's think about what we just did together. We saw…" Next, engage the parents in a series of open-ended questions designed to elicit feedback and give them an opportunity to check out what they saw the baby do.

- How do you feel about what you just saw?
- Did you see anything that surprised you?
- Did you expect to see most of what you saw?

Guide the parents in thinking about what they just saw and how that might be different from what they had originally thought. Relate their observations back to their original perceptions: "Remember in the beginning you thought your baby looked flimsy? What do you think now that he has told you a bit more about himself?" Then begin developing expectations for care: "Let's talk about what it will be like to care for your baby over the next few weeks."

During Reflection at the final home visit, congratulate the parents for completing the Community-Based FANA and express your pleasure at being with them during this very important time of life. You may wish to take several pictures of the mother and baby together and the father and baby together.

Writing to the Baby. At the end of the visit, ask the parents if they'd like to bring out the family book that they started before the baby was born. Invite the mom and dad to look at past letters they each have written and to write again to their baby, now that she is here!

The Postnatal Home Visit Guide

The postnatal home visit activity guide provides Parent and Baby Time activities and in-depth discussions for at least two home or hospital visits after the baby is born. The activities you do with parents and their newborns are drawn from the Brazelton Neonatal Behavioral Assessment Scale (1995). The guide can be used as often—and in as many postnatal visits—as desired. As with the prenatal activity guides, required and optional materials are listed for all activities, and each home visit component is listed as a reminder for you when you are just getting started.

Remember to be flexible. Rearrange the setting as little as possible. The postnatal interview can be done when the baby is either awake or asleep.

Although the postnatal activities can be done in any order depending on the baby's state, follow the basic structure of the Community-Based FANA home visit: Preparation, Parent Time, Parent and Baby Time, Family Time, and Reflection and Writing to the Baby. It typically takes about 40 minutes to facilitate the postnatal activities.

Because of natural events after the birth of a baby—the baby gets hungry, you run out of time, the mom gets very tired, company comes over—it may not be possible to complete the Community-Based FANA activities at the time of the first postpartum visit. It's easy at the next visit to pick up where you left off. Briefly summarize what was already completed and recall key aspects of the last visit. It is a good idea to take notes so that you know where to focus on the next visit if the current one is not completed.

The Postnatal Home Visit Guide is provided in the Tool Kit on pages 155–161.

Reference

Brazelton, T. B., & Nugent, K. (1995). *Neonatal Behavioral Assessment Scale* (3rd ed.). London: MacKeith Press.

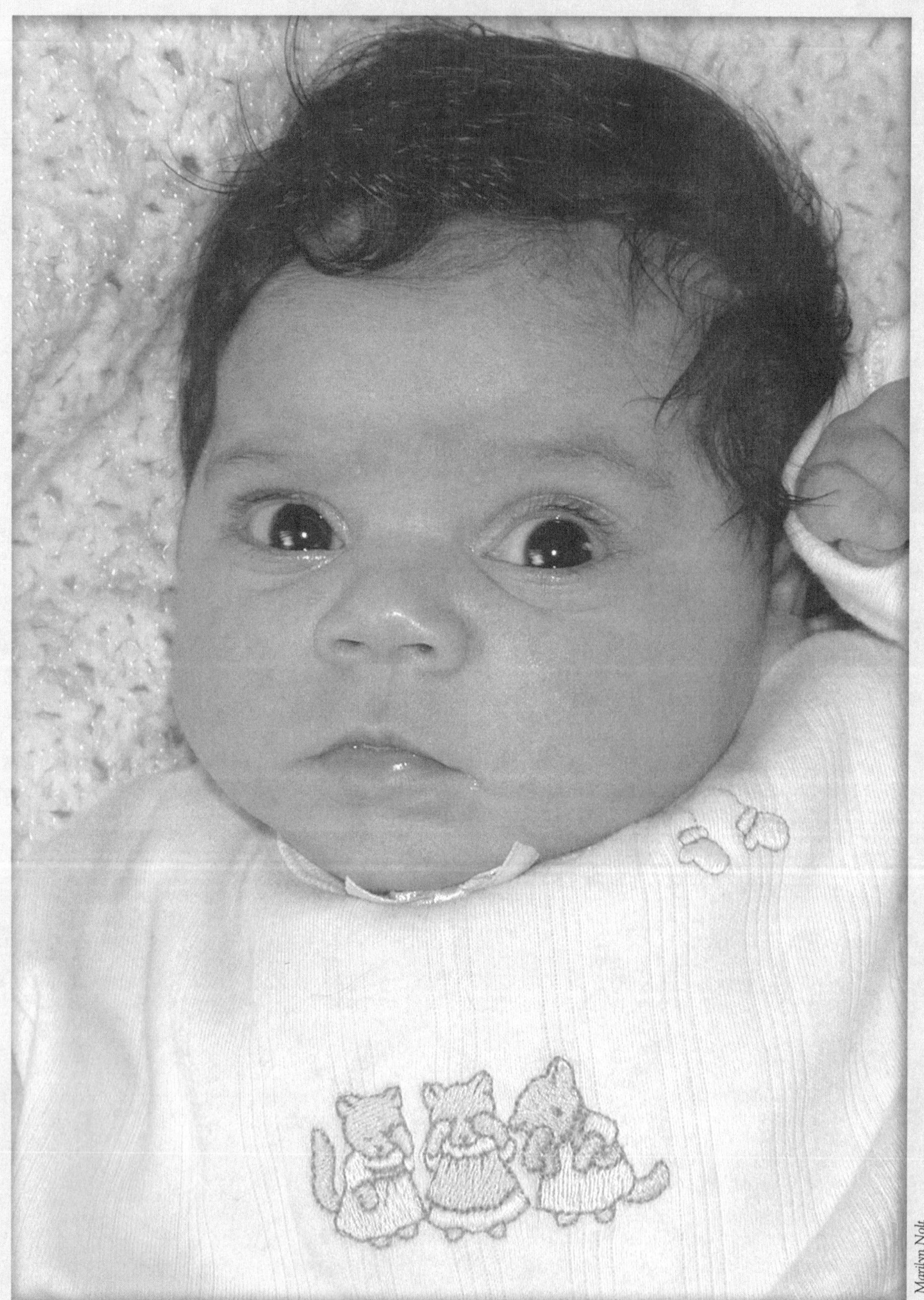

Marilyn Nolt

CHAPTER 11

Getting Started

Teenagers and Their Babies: A Perinatal Home Visitor's Guide ends almost where it began—with knowing yourself. Knowing yourself is the starting point for introducing the Community-Based FANA into your work with families. Knowing how you like to learn reminds you that parents also have ways that they learn best.

Now that you have completed this guide, you have much to think about and many activities to consider doing with families during the perinatal period. The Tool Kit in Appendix B includes the Home Visit Activity Guides, as well as all of the checklists, questionnaires, and other tools from througout *Teenagers and Their Babies* that will make your work easier.

You now face several challenges. The first is how to absorb and take in the information you've been exposed to while reading about, discussing, and practicing the Community-Based FANA. The second challenge is using the Community-Based FANA until it becomes a comfortable, natural part of your work with families. Third is practicing the receptive posture until you find ways to use what you know to guide new parents in their own discoveries about their child and their emerging relationship with him. Finally, experimenting with the various activities creates more and more vivid experiences for both parents and child, experiences that help build close connections.

A Balancing Act

Think for a moment about all of the conflicting feelings that expectant and new parents go through. This particular time of life is filled with first-time experiences. Many of these experiences come with their own push and pull of emotions, driven by what the parents already know and what they are uncertain about. Developing a healthy balance between knowledge and uncertainty and between confidence and lack of confidence marks a young parent's growth into parenthood. This balance brings an inner sense of parental self, a resilience that protects parents through rocky times as they learn about and live with their child throughout all the lifelong firsts.

You, too, are challenged by a similar tug of war. You may have many first-time experiences with this new intervention. You may feel confident and competent at times, shaken and inadequate at other times. You, too, benefit from being able to balance your own feelings. Learning from what you do and what you are experiencing with families builds a professional resilience. Much like the new parent, your own acceptance of where you are in the process of learning allows you to face new challenges with an appreciation for the moment and hope for the future.

As you build your Community-Based FANA skills, you may become aware of conflicting forces within you—the inherent tension between learning and doing. For this period, balance is a most important feature of your work. In time facilitating the Community-Based FANA will be as natural as falling in love with a newborn!

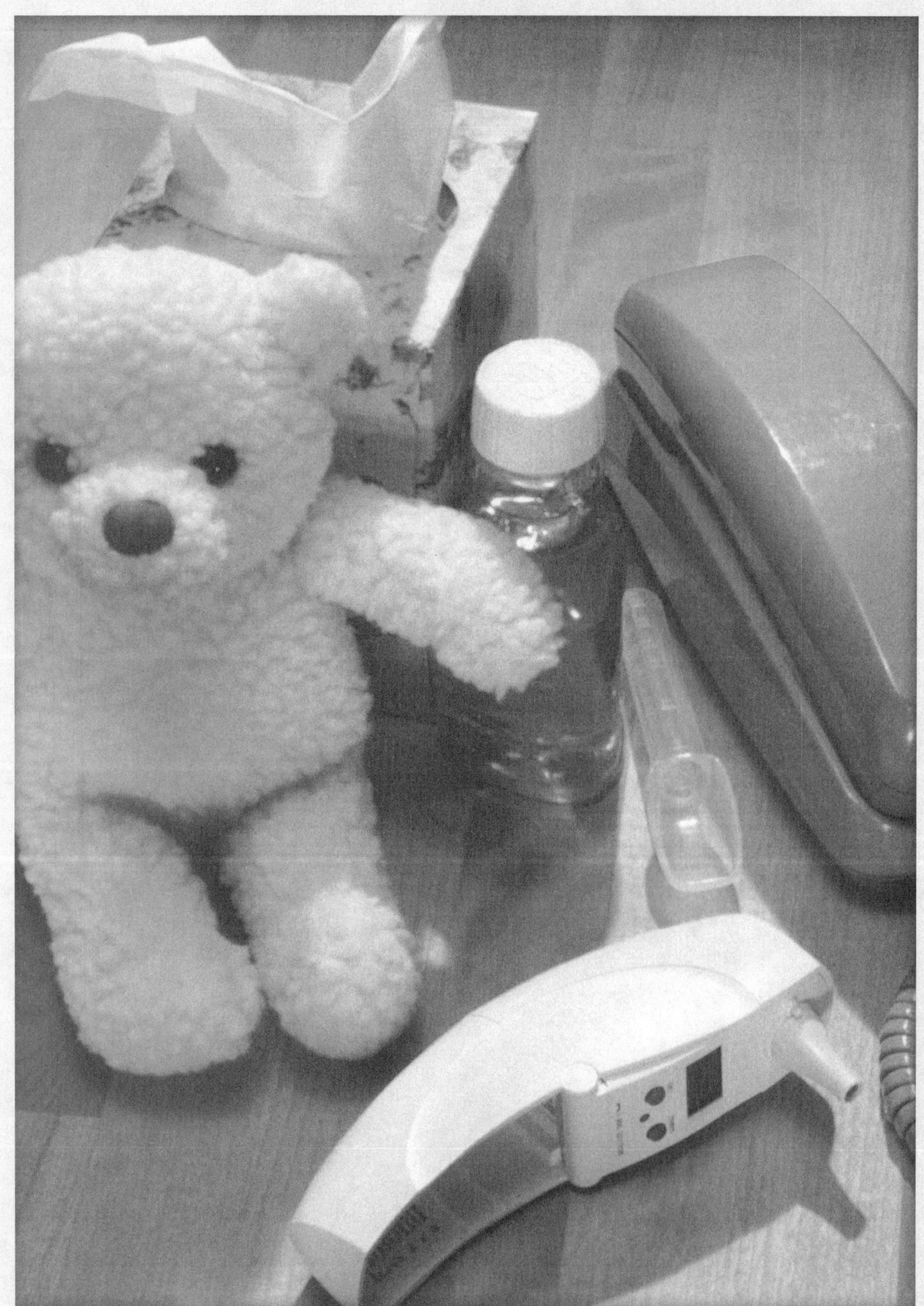

Comstock

Appendix A

Resources

There are many wonderful resources available for enriching the work you do with families using the Community-Based FANA. Here are some favorites.

Baby Basics: Your Month by Month Guide to a Healthy Pregnancy

Baby Basics is a publication of The What to Expect Foundation, which describes the guide as written to both a third- and sixth-grade reading level. It is a prenatal guide and literacy education tool with a special focus on low-income expecting families. For more information, including a look inside the guide, or to order *Baby Basics*, see www.whattoexpect.org.

The Centering Corporation

The Centering Corporation is a nonprofit organization whose mission is to provide education and resources for people who are bereaved. They have a wide selection of materials related to loss and grief. Especially useful may be "When Hello Means Goodbye" and "Miscarriage." For more information, see www.centeringcorp.com.

Childbirth Graphics

Childbirth Graphics is a company specializing in childbirth education. Their product list includes a variety of useful resources, from print materials to videos to teaching models. Some materials are available in Spanish. Among the most useful for this work are the following:

Timeline of Pregnancy (chart and tear pad)
Fetus Model Set
Your Pregnancy Week by Week
Fetal Development (chart and tear pad)
With Child (book and display version)
Life Unto Life (booklet)
Growing a Baby (chart and tear pad)
Newborn Baby Models

The Corner Health Center

The Corner Health Center in Ypisilanti, Michigan, is a comprehensive teen health center that offers medical care, health education, and support services to low-income young people ages 12–21 and their children. The Center produces several booklets for adolescent parents. The "You and Your Baby" booklets are especially helpful. For more information about the "You and Your Baby" booklet series or to order online, see www.cornerhealth.org/prevention.html#booklets.

DONA International

DONA International has a range of information and materials related to doula services, and the DONA Web site has a catalog of childbirth-related books. For more information, see www.dona.org.

FemmEd, Inc.

This company has a catalog specializing primarily in pregnancy, childbirth, and parenting, with a section devoted to materials for working with teens. Some materials are available in Spanish. For more information, see www.ChildbirthClasstoGo.com.

InJoy Videos

This company has a large selection of videos relevant to birth and parenting, including videos created specifically for teenagers. Some materials are available in Spanish. For more information or to order, see www.injoyvideos.com.

International Childbirth Education Association (ICEA)

ICEA has a list of training for childbirth educators and a catalog of valuable resources, including *Baby and Me: A Pregnancy Workbook for Young Women*. To find out more, including how to order a catalog, see www.icea.org.

Johnson & Johnson Pediatric Institute

The Johnson & Johnson Pediatric Institute has a variety of information and resources available, including booklets and monographs. Especially useful are the following:

Touch in Labor and Infancy: Clinical Implications
Nurturing Your Baby's Development (booklet)
The Importance of Touch: A Guide for Parents and Caregivers (booklet)
Your Baby's Development: A Parents Journal (booklet)

For more information about the institute or to order resources, see the Johnson & Johnson Pediatric Institute Web site at www.jjpi.com.

Nine Months and a Day: A Pregnancy and Birth Companion

This book was written by childbirth educator Adrienne B. Lieberman and physician Linda Hughey Holt and published by The Harvard Common Press. It is a pregnancy, labor, and delivery companion providing essential information from pregnancy to newborn care. *Nine Months and a Day* is widely available online and in bookstores.

Noodle Soup

This company has a large catalog devoted to helping to build strong families, with a wide range of materials from print to video. Some materials are available in Spanish. Especially useful is How Big Is My Baby Now? (actual size chart). For more information or to order, see www.noodlesoup.com.

Your Amazing Newborn

This book was written by physician Marshall H. Klaus and social worker Phyllis H. Klaus and published by Perseus Books. Focusing on the abilities of newborns, the book has over 100 beautiful photographs of babies in their first 2 weeks of life and includes some of the latest findings from research. *Your Amazing Newborn* is widely available online and in bookstores.

The book is also available as a 30-minute video, "Amazing Talents of the Newborn," available online from the Johnson and Johnson Pediatric Institute. For more information, see www.jjpi.com.

Appendix B

Tool Kit

This final section of *Teenagers and Their Babies: A Perinatal Home Visitor's Guide* includes all of the checklists, forms, interview questions, activities, and other tools that you will use in your daily work with families and the Community-Based Family Administered Neonatal Activities (FANA). They are gathered here in one place for your ease of use.

TOOLS FOR KNOWING YOURSELF

Guiding Principles and Key Practices for Knowing Yourself

Guiding principle. We are all—and always—in a process of growth.

Key practice. Seek to understand the special magic of your age, no matter what age that is, and connect to the teen with this understanding in mind.

Guiding principle. We change through our work with teens, and they change as they work with us. We are both in a process of becoming.

Key practice. Create a space to coexist with the new you that you're becoming and the new person that the teen is becoming. Build your relationship and structure your interactions with a young parent to foster the strengths of each of you as you co-develop and co-emerge.

TOOLS FOR KNOWING THE TEEN

How She Thinks—The Questions

1. What can you tell me about yourself?
2. What do you see yourself doing in a few years?
3. How has your life changed since you became pregnant (had your baby)?
4. What do you think makes a good mother?
5. What have you learned about your baby so far?

How She Feels—The Questions

1. When you looked in the mirror this morning what did your face tell you about how you're feeling today? Were you feeling pretty good? Sad? Worried?
2. Is this usually what your face tells you when you look in the mirror? Or was it different today from most other days?
3. Let's see if you can help me understand where that feeling is coming from.

Autonomy Checklist: Things to Consider

_____ Does the teen exhibit persistent, observable behaviors that suggest a struggle with autonomy and being her own person, such as an unwillingness to speak to you, or most any adult, or an automatic "no" response to any question.

_____ Does the teen's struggle take the form of extremes in clothes, hair style or color, or multiple piercings or tatoos? Is she nonetheless willing to be engaged?

_____ Is the teen easily engaged without giving any sign that she is open to advice or teaching?

_____ Is the teen readily engaged and open to mutual problem solving and learning?

TOOLS FOR CONNECTING WITH FATHERS

Guiding Principles and Key Practices for Engaging Fathers in the Community-Based FANA

Guiding principle. Infants benefit from having a positive relationship with their mother and father, but building or maintaining the parents' relationship with each other is not the role of the home visitor.

Key practice. Work to build a meaningful relationship between mother and child and between father and child.

Guiding principle. Connecting with his baby is the ultimate prize for a father, as it is for the baby herself.

Key practice. Actively support a father's efforts to connect with and be responsible for his baby.

Guidance for Fathers

Second Trimester

Hear your baby's heartbeat.

Wonder what kind of father you will be.

Create positive and exciting dreams about the future.

Find accepting, caring people to talk with about your feelings and the changes you're going through.

Find other fathers to talk with about this new experience.

If possible, talk with your own dad or father-figure about what it was it like for him when he was waiting for you to be born.

Think about how you want to take care of and raise your baby.

Talk about the changes in your relationship with the mother of the baby.

Find books, movies, and magazines about babies and being a father.

Live with happiness, guilt, anticipation, ambivalence, and frustration.

Third Trimester

Begin to spend more time with your baby's mom talking about how you can share raising him.

Be patient and understanding of the mother's point of view.

Appreciate the huge emotional, physical, and hormonal changes that the mom is experiencing because of the pregnancy.

Talk, talk, talk with the baby's mother about the changes that the pregnancy is putting you through. Talk about what excites you, what scares you, and what makes you uncertain. Talk about her parents and your parents.

Find other dads to talk with about their experiences, and share your feelings with them.

Be flexible in your views; the baby changes everything!

Discuss with the mom if and how she would like your support during labor and birth. Discuss attending a prenatal or birthing class, either with her or on your own.

If your baby's mother is comfortable with your touch, now you can feel the baby move.

Imagine what the elbows, feet, and hands that you feel kicking will look and feel like once the baby is out.

Begin to play with the baby, even before he is born. If it's okay with his mother, gently push one side of her abdomen. The baby will move to respond. Then try the other side.

Count the baby's kicks and feel how active she is now. Wonder what she will be like once she is born.

Talk, read, and sing to your baby while he is still inside his mom. The more you talk now, the more he will recognize your voice once he is born.

Think about what you will want to read and sing to the baby after he is born. Remember the songs and stories that you're enjoying with him now.

Massage the baby gently through her mother's skin, if the mother feels like having you do that.

Think about how your schedule will work with the baby's schedule once he is born.

Try calming the baby with your voice during a time that she is really active inside her mom, if that's okay with the mom.

Think about how you will calm your baby after he is born, and remember how you were calmed. Decide how you want to calm, guide, and discipline your own baby.

(Source: Adapted from Brott & Ash, 1995)

TOOLS FOR THE BIRTH

Labor and Delivery Checklist

- What is the young mother's understanding of labor and delivery?
- Who is her support person who will be present at labor?
- What is the physical arrangement of the birthing unit?
- How will she recognize the onset of labor?
- How will she get to the hospital?
- What are her plans for pain medication?
- How aware is she of the changes her body will undergo during labor?
- What does she expect to happen and what does she expect to see when her baby is born?
- How does she plan to feed her baby—breast or bottle?
- Has she chosen a pediatric care provider?
- Where and to whom will she and the baby come home after being discharged?

TOOLS FOR WHEN THINGS DON'T GO AS PLANNED

Perinatal Loss: Questions to Explore With Parents

Miscarriage

- Was she alone when it happened?
- Did she have some idea of what was happening to her?
- How does she feel about the pregnancy ending?
- How are the important people in her world responding to the miscarriage?
- Are they treating it in a way that is consonant with how she feels about it?

After 17 Weeks

- Do the parents wish to see and hold their baby? (After 17 weeks, and sometimes 16 weeks, a dead baby can be swaddled and held.)
- Do they wish to have nursing staff take a picture of them with their baby?
- Have they named the baby?
- Do they want to keep mementos of birth, such as the receiving blanket or wrist and ankle ID bands?
- What do they wish for the body? Hospital disposal (they will not be able to retrieve ashes)? Funeral home cremation (they will be able to retrieve ashes)? Burial? A memorial service?

TOOLS FOR COMING THROUGH THE DOOR

Community-Based FANA Home Visit Structure

Prenatal Visits

Preparation

- Review what you know about mother, father, and family
- Select prenatal activities and gather materials
- Ready yourself physically and psychologically

Parent Time

- Greet and reconnect with mother, father, and family
- Explore baby's name
- Elicit and validate parents' observations of baby

Parent and Baby Time

- Explore baby's present behavior
- Position
- State
- Facilitate prenatal activities
- Fetal movement and newborn behavior
- Hearing
- Behavioral states
- Touch
- Smell and taste
- Vision

Family Time

Reflection and Writing to the Baby

Postnatal Visits

Preparation

- Review what you know about mother,
  father, and family
- Select postnatal activities and gather materials
- Ready yourself physically and psychologically

Parent Time

- Greet and reconnect with mother, father, and family
- Review labor and delivery experience
- Discuss baby's name and its significance
- Elicit and validate parents' observations of baby

Parent and Baby Time

- Explore baby's present behavior
- Position
- State
- Facilitate newborn activities
- Staying asleep (habituation to sound and light)
- Muscle tone
- Foot reflexes
- Rooting
- Soothing
- Looking at and following
- Hearing and turning to sounds

Family Time

Reflection and Writing to the Baby

PREPARING FOR THE HOME VISIT

- Consider how the young mother learns, her psychological and physical stage of pregnancy, and her perceptions of her baby and of herself as a mother.
- Review the appropriate sections of the prenatal or postnatal Community-Based FANA and select activities to use with the parents during the upcoming home visit.

- Gather any necessary materials for those activities. Think creatively about what will appeal to this mom and dad. Anticipate their responses, and modify the activities to suit the parents' needs and your own style.
- Review your assessment of the teen mother's learning style. Where along these dimensions does she fall?
  - Concrete ➔ Abstract
  - Present orientation ➔ Future orientation
  - Self-absorbed ➔ Other focused
- Think about what you know about the father and others whom you have met who are significant in the mother's life.
- Finally, think about your own needs and readiness for a moment:
  - Are you hungry?
  - Is there a nagging call you have to make?
  - Do you need to get directions to the teen's home?
  - What is your mood?
  - How emotionally available are you for this home visit?
  - What is the quality of your attention right now?
  - What do you need to do to get ready to focus on this mom and dad and their baby?
- Take some time to prepare yourself mentally, emotionally, and physically for the visit.

Reflection

Use consistent questions to guide parents in reflecting and writing. Ask the following questions:

- What did you see or experience that surprised you?
- What did you see or experience that you expected?
- How did you feel about what we just did together?
- What do you think the next few weeks will be like?

TOOLS FOR PRENATAL HOME VISITS

The Developmental Focus of the Prenatal Home Visits

Week 26–27

Focus on the Unborn Baby: Movement

Previewing the Newborn: Newborn Behavior

Week 28–29
Focus on the Unborn Baby: Hearing
Previewing the Newborn: Maternal Speech

Week 30–31
Focus on the Unborn Baby: Fetal State
Previewing the Newborn: Newborn State

Week 32–33
Focus on the unborn baby: Fetal touch
Previewing the newborn: Holding and soothing

Week 34–35
Focus on the Unborn Baby: Fetal Sucking
Previewing the Newborn: Feeding

Week 36–37
Focus on the Unborn Baby: Vision
Previewing the Newborn: Seeing Each Other

Focusing on the Teen Mother

Concrete Areas to Discuss

- Her clothes
- Her hair
- Any major changes in her appearance

The Immediate Past

- What has your day been like so far?
- Have you had a doctor visit since I last saw you? What happened?
- How have your spirits been since I last saw you? Pretty cheery? Not so hot?

Primary Activities

- How was your time at school?
- Who did you eat lunch with yesterday?
- Has work been okay, or has it been pretty rough for you? What's your time there like?
- What has home been like? How is it going with your brothers, sisters, mom, dad, and cousins? Do you have any special jobs at home?

Asking the teen mother about her well-being with respect to her pregnancy helps you connect with her. But it also bridges time spent focusing on her alone and time spent with her focusing on her and the baby together. Try the following questions:

- With everything you've just told me is going on with you, it must be hard to balance taking care of yourself and your baby. How have you been feeling?
- Have you felt any physical changes?

Validating Parents' Observations

Ask the parents what they've noticed about their baby, and acknowledge everything that they have observed about their baby so far.

- What has your baby told you about herself this week?
- Has your baby changed in any way that you can tell?
- Were there times when you felt particularly close to your baby?
- Were there times when you were worried or concerned about him?

TOOLS FOR POSTNATAL HOME VISITS

Postnatal Home Visit: Reviewing What You Know About Labor and Delivery

On your first postnatal visit with a family, review the mother's expectations and preparations for the birth.

- What was she expecting to feel at the first signs of labor?
- Who was she planning to call when labor started?
- How was she planning to get to the hospital?
- What did she expect the labor room, the doctors, and the nurses to be like?
- Did she share her thoughts about the kind of birth that she wished for or feared?
- Who were her coaches going to be?

Postnatal Home Visit: What You Can Do When

Asleep	Awake	Crying
State	State	Soothing
Habituation	Reflexes	
Reflexes	Muscle tone	
Muscle tone	Orientation	

The Postpartum Interview

Understanding the Mother's Physical and Personal Well-Being

- What have these last few days been like for you?
- Let me look at you—are you really tired?
- Are you sore?
- Have you been drinking plenty of water? Eating enough? Napping as much as you can?
- How are your spirits?

Describing the Birth Experience

- Let's start at the beginning. What time did you realize you were first experiencing labor pains?
- What form and where did the pains start—strong back pains, mild pelvic pain, indigestion? Was it like what you expected?
- Who did you call when you realized labor was starting? Was that person available? Was it the person you had planned to call? What was that like for you—were you...(glad, sad, angry, grateful, etc.)?
- What happened when you got to the hospital? Did the labor and delivery room look the way you expected it to look?
- What did you experience from . . . (nurses, doctors, the doula, etc.)? Did they help? How did it compare to what you thought it would be?
- What about pain medicine? What kind did you have? Did it help?
- Tell me about pushing the baby out—how long did it last? Who helped? Did you feel it? Were you exhausted by then?
- How long was it from the onset of labor to delivery?
- What did you see the first time you looked at your baby?

Exploring the Baby's Name

- How did your baby get her name?
- Was this a name you decided on yourself or did someone help you?
- Do you know any other people named (baby's name)?

Eliciting and Validating the Parents' Observations

- What has your baby told you about himself so far?
- What have you seen your baby do in these last few days?
- Have you seen your baby open his eyes?
- Have you seen your baby move his legs and arms?

Prenatal Home Visit 1
Fetal Movement—Newborn Behavior
(26–27 Weeks Gestation)

Remember:

About Your Work

- Preparation
- Parent Time
- Parent and Baby Time
- Family Time
- Reflection and Writing to the Baby

About the Baby

- The baby starts to move very early, about 7.5 weeks after conception.
- About 9 weeks after conception, the baby can move her head, trunk, arms, and legs.
- During the second trimester, the mother is able to feel the baby move, and the baby begins to move from side to side.
- Most of the movements present at the end of pregnancy and after birth are present by 14 weeks.
- In the third trimester, space is at a premium. When the baby cannot move her whole body at once because she is too big, she begins to focus on smaller movements:
    - Fidgeting her arms and legs;
    - Playing with her fingers; or
    - Sucking his thumb.
- The baby shifts positions more when the mother is still.

Parent and Baby Time Activities—Exploring the Baby's Present Behavior

Activity: Your Baby Here and Now

Materials: *With Child*, Childbirth Graphics' large stand-up book; 10-, 15-, 20-, and 30-week fetal models (optional)

Before the home visit, review the movement sections of "The Trimesters of Pregnancy" in chapter 5. Invite the teen to look with you at the pictures of the mother and baby in the book. Start with the first trimester and move through the pictures in order. Talk about what the baby is able to do right now at the stage of development in each picture. Encourage wonderment about her baby! Let the mom hold the fetus models, if she seems interested. (Note that some teens do not like the feel of the models.)

Activity: Kick Count

Guide the mother in thinking about her experience with the baby's movements so far. Has she felt some hard kicks, or has she not yet identified kicks? Maybe she has been so busy with school, friends, and family that she hasn't been still long enough to feel kicks! This is a good time to introduce her to the idea of developing a quiet time with her baby. Frame the next few minutes for her: "You can start right now. Let's be very still for a minute or two and see what your baby does while you are still." Keep her responses as the central focus: "What did you feel? How did that feel to you?" If the baby is moving and kicking, introduce the idea of counting the kicks: "Wow, he is really moving! Let's see if we can count his kicks. Tell me when you feel a kick, and we'll keep track." If the baby is not very active, don't choose kick counting.

Ask the mother if she has names for the baby's different kind of movements. Share some things other mothers say such as "squirming," "rocking and rolling," and "kicking the heck out of me!"

Activity: Sharing Your Baby With Others

Ask the parents if the people important to them—their own parents, brothers and sisters, best friends—have felt the baby move. Let the mother know that if she likes she can encourage them to get involved. Share ideas on how to do that. One way is for the mom to lie still on the couch or bed after dinner. She can hold the baby and see if the baby begins to move. If so, she can invite others to feel the baby move. This can become a favorite evening ritual for the parents and the baby.

Activity: Playing With Your Baby

It is never too early to introduce parents to the idea that their baby is ready to interact with them right from the start—even while the baby is still growing inside the mother! Mothers can try several things related to movement 26 weeks into the pregnancy. She can help still a very active baby by gently stroking her own stomach and speaking softly. At a time the baby is moving, the mother or father can initiate interaction by gently pressing a hand on one side of the mother's abdomen two or three times and then moving it away. The baby likely will move to that side. They can try this on the other side, too. Encourage parents to talk to their baby as they play. If the baby does not respond, work with the parents to frame this response: "I guess the baby is not in the mood right now." Or: "We'll play later when you are awake, baby." Or: "I wonder what you're doing right now, baby? Are you asleep?"

Activity: Here's Looking at You

Materials: Ultrasound pictures; fetal models (optional)

Looking at an ultrasound picture together provides you with the opportunity to engage young parents in two very important activities.

- Engage the parents in a moment of shared attention and modeling—a wonderful introduction to what you hope the parents will do with their baby after the baby is born.
- Model a sense of wonder at the miracle of life—a fascination that you hope will carry over to parents' feelings about their baby after the baby is born. This might be a good time to use the plastic models of the baby at various stages of pregnancy, if the teen seems interested.

If the young mother has had an ultrasound, ask if she would be willing to show it to you. She may not be comfortable doing this, because the ultrasound itself may have been stressful. Enter this experience gently with her. Begin by asking what having the ultrasound was like for her. Was someone with her? What were some of her thoughts as she saw the picture of her baby come up on the screen? Was it easy for her to understand what she was seeing? If she was confused, you can make her experience seem more normal by sharing your own confusion with her: "I really didn't understand what I was seeing the first time I looked at an ultrasound."

If the teen is comfortable looking at the ultrasound with you, ask her to take you on a guided tour of what you are seeing—the baby's nose, chin, arms, hands, legs, and penis (if there is one). Ask her what she saw the baby doing. Did she see any physical movement? Did the baby put her hand in her mouth? Did the mom see the baby swallowing? Sucking her finger? If the mom saw the baby sucking her finger, you can begin to explore how she feels about this and can introduce the idea of self-soothing—that even the baby has ways to help herself be calm.

Wonder together about what the baby is experiencing, about how much she is growing and changing—just as the teen mother herself is growing and changing—and about what the baby's experience of the mom might be.

Activity: My First Picture

Materials: Ultrasound picture

Encourage the parents to put the baby's ultrasound picture in a frame or to carry it in their wallets.

Activity: Imagining You

Materials: 10- and 20-week fetal models or pictures of a developing fetus

Introduce parents to the idea that their baby has been moving since he or she was only 8 weeks old! Invite the parents to hold the 10-week model of a fetus. Say: "Your baby began to move when he was just this size—only 10 weeks old! By the time he was this size (show the 20-week model) he had already developed all the movements he will have when he is born. He can kick his legs, suck his fingers, and hold on to his umbilical cord. When he gets bigger—as he will in these next weeks—and has less room to move, you may feel him move less. He only has room to practice smaller movements, such as moving his fingers, opening and closing his hands, making small movements of his legs and arms, grasping his umbilical cord, and even sucking on his fingers.

"Your baby's movements are also becoming more coordinated as his brain and nervous system matures. His movements are less random and more on purpose. He can put his fist in his mouth, cross his legs together, and tuck up against one side of the uterine wall. His movements also are less frequent during the last few weeks because there is less room for him to move.

"During these last months of pregnancy, your baby's muscle tone is building. His reflexes are developing. These are the same reflexes that you will see when your baby is born—his grasp, his ability to 'root,' which means to turn his head when he is stroked on his cheek.

"All the movements that your baby does on the inside, he will also do on the outside. When the baby is born, you will be able to see what he has been doing for all these months!"

Parent and Baby Time Activities—Previewing the Newborn

Activity: Newborn Baby Movement

Materials: Newborn baby doll

Now that you and the parents have an appreciation of fetal development fresh in your minds, show the parents a newborn baby doll. Talk together about what the newborn can do—kick her legs, turn her head, open her eyes and look at her parents, suck on her fingers, root, suck, and swallow. Remind the parents that you will be there with them after their baby is born and that you will look together at their very own amazing newborn and all that she can do!

Prenatal Home Visit 2
Hearing
(28–29 Weeks Gestation)

Remember:

About Your Work

- Preparation
- Parent Time
- Parent and Baby Time
- Family Time
- Reflection and Writing to the Baby

About the Baby

- In the third trimester, the baby begins to hear.
- Week 24 marks the beginning of response to sound.
- The baby does not hear sounds as we hear them. He hears primarily sounds in the low tones.
- The baby hears his mother, though, because her voice not only goes out but also vibrates down her throat and into her lungs, and the rhythms and patterns of her speech become very familiar to him. Fetal heart rate slows during maternal speech, showing that the baby is taking in the stimulus.

Parent and Baby Time Activities—Exploring the Baby's Present Behavior

Activity: First Sounds

Parents often say that hearing their baby's heartbeat for the very first time is one of the most important moments in their lives. It certainly is a sound that forever marks a change in their lives. Young parents also say that this is a single moment that motivates changing their own behaviors in order to better care for another—their baby!

Explore with the mother and father their experience and feelings on first hearing their baby's heartbeat. Consider the following questions:

- What do you remember about the first time that you heard your baby's heartbeat?
- Who was with you at the time?
- What feelings do you remember having when you listened to her heartbeat?
- What did it make you think about?
- Was there anyone else who you wanted to be able to hear your baby's heartbeat? Was that person able to hear it?

Activity: Hey, World—I Hear You!

The teen mother may already sense that her baby is able to hear in utero. Explore this with her. Following are some questions to ask:

- Have you ever noticed your baby reacting to sounds?
- What kind of sounds? Loud, sudden sounds? Music?
- How can you tell if your baby has a favorite song or prefers a special kind of music?

Activity: Hearing What Baby Hears

The parents can experiment with how their baby might hear different sounds by putting their fingers in their ears and being aware of sounds as they walk around. Parents can try listening to their own footsteps as they walk, jump, or dance. This approximates how their baby probably hears sounds in utero.

Activity: Dad, I Know You Are There

Encourage the father to talk to the baby in utero at a time during the home visit when the mother recognizes that the baby is very active. Ask her to describe how the baby reacts. Be careful, though, to explain that the baby's reactions do not mean that the baby prefers someone else's voice to her own. In fact, the baby pays most attention to the rhythms and patterns of the mother's speech. You can help the mom see this after the baby is born.

Although the baby knows the mother's voice best, the dad's voice probably can be heard in utero, too, because of the baby's ability to hear low tones. Maybe this is a way that nature prepares babies to respond to both mothers and fathers!

Activity: Sleeping Through a Racket

Invite the parents to experience all of the different sounds that their baby hears regularly in addition to the mother's own sounds. Ask the mom to sit quietly in various rooms of her home and to keep track of all the common sounds she hears there—horns, doors, laughter, television, and other sounds. Ask the parents how they think these sounds might sound to the baby, and what effect the sounds might have on her.

This activity is an opportunity to explain how babies—both in utero and in the first months of life—are able to tune out unwanted noise and interference.

Explain also that babies differ in their ability to handle sound, just as we adults do. Explore whether the mother has ever felt the baby startle in utero in reaction to a loud sound while the mother was asleep.

Tell the parents that after the baby is born you will look at this together and explore how their baby handles sounds. Will their baby be able to sleep through a racket or will she need for those around her to be a little quieter?

Activity: Baby's First Security Blanket

Discuss with the mother what it might be like for her baby to hear her constant heartbeat and her voice. Talk about how, in some ways, the mother's heartbeat may be the baby's first security blanket.

Explain that the mom provides another kind of security for her baby when she lets the baby know what's going to happen. Let her know that telling her baby what is going on around her or what the two of them are doing is a simple and meaningful way to teach her baby about the world. Explain how talking her baby through transitions—even now, in utero—is a wonderful habit. Practicing now to help her baby move from place to place or activity to activity will really pay off later. Ask the mom if she remembers being sung to as a child, and explore how this felt. Encourage the mother to find enjoyable and comfortable ways to talk with her child, both now and after the baby is born.

Parent and Baby Time Activities—Previewing the Newborn

Activity: Story Time

Materials: A book of poems, a Bible, or other book

Introduce the idea that talking with the baby is valuable for both the baby and the parents. Describe how the baby will learn the patterns and rhythms of the mother's own speech—just by hearing it so regularly—and will prefer it right after birth.

Explain that researchers have found that when babies are repeatedly read the same story in utero, they seem to remember it and respond by sucking more when they hear it after birth. Ask the parents if they would like to pick out a very short story to tell or read to their baby before he is born. If they want to, they can tell or read that same story to the baby each day. Some parents may want to read a favorite poem or a Bible verse to their child. Suggest that this is a wonderful tradition to start now and continue after their baby is born. This is a pleasant ritual that is often satisfying for both parents and child, and it can help to calm the child.

A song can take the place of a story in this activity. Ask the parents if there is a song that they would enjoy singing to their baby. Now is a good time to share with the parents that this is a big part of how their baby will learn to talk after she is born—by listening to people speaking directly to her and with each other.

Activity: Symphony of Sound

Explore with the mother what things she thinks her baby likes to listen to most. As appropriate, explain that what the baby hears the most is the mother's voice and that what babies like most is what they know. Are there any sounds that the mother thinks her baby doesn't like? Explore with her how she thinks her baby might have reacted to harsh or angry sounds during her pregnancy.

Talk about the kinds of sounds she thinks she wants her baby to hear after she is born. Discuss everything from kinds of music, to busy households, to the feelings attached to words—both loving and angry words.

Prenatal Home Visit 3
Behavioral States
(30–31 Weeks Gestation)

Remember:

About Your Work

- Preparation
- Parent Time
- Parent and Baby Time
- Family Time
- Reflection and Writing to the Baby

About the Baby

- Before birth, babies have four states: quiet sleep, active sleep, quiet alert, and active alert.
- Toward the end of the second semester, at 24 weeks gestation, the baby begins to develop regular quiet and active states, which later develop into quiet and active sleep states.
- The closer the baby is to delivery, the more she is in quiet sleep and active alert.

Parent and Baby Time Activities—Exploring the Baby's Present Behavior

Activity: Baby's Day

Introduce to the mother the idea that even at this early stage, her baby has definite times during the day when he is asleep and awake. Ask the mom if she can remember times when her baby is in the following states:

- Deeply asleep—pretty quiet with only brief movements, mostly startles and little jumps
- Lightly asleep—frequent movements, no really big kicks
- Quiet and awake—really still, almost no movement
- Awake and active—vigorous, nonstop activity

Wonder with the mom about the baby's day:

- What is the baby usually like in the morning? In the afternoon? After dinner? Before bed? During the night?
- When does she think the baby might be awake and active (vigorous, nonstop movements; feels like baby is rolling around)?
- Does she have any special name for that time of day?
- How does she feel about those times when the baby is so active?
- What does she do then?

- When does she think the baby might be asleep?
- What does she do then?

Let her know that as she gets closer and closer to delivery, more and more often her baby will be either deeply asleep or actively awake—resting up and then revving up to be born!

Activity: Working It Out—You and Me

Ask the mother about her day:

- What time do you usually wake up? Are you full of energy at this time?
- Are you a morning person? Or do you need a fairly long wake-up time?
- Are there times in the day when you feel an energy slump, when—especially in the middle of the afternoon—you would like to take a nap?
- Is there a time when you get your second wind, maybe around 7 o'clock, after dinner?
- Now, here's a really important question: What do you do for yourself, and what do you expect from others, when you're in one of these states?
- When you're full of energy, what kinds of things do you do? Go shopping, do homework, go to class, laugh with friends?
- What happens when you're full of energy and there's nothing to do or no one to be with?
- What about when you have a tired time during the day? What do you do for yourself?
- What happens if someone expects you to do a high-energy activity at this time, like wash a load of clothes or go shopping? What do you feel like then?

Ask the mother what her baby inside her is telling her right now about the state he's in. Then ask her what her own energy and activity state is like right now. Does it match the baby's state? Or is it very different from the baby's state? Has the baby's kicking in the night ever woken her up? How does that feel to her?

Activity: Rock-a-Bye Baby

Ask the mother if she has ever tried to help her baby calm down at a time when the baby is really active. Wonder with her what she thinks might help her baby calm down. If it is appropriate to her situation, introduce her to the idea that sometimes the baby might calm down to the father's deep voice. Invite her to consider encouraging the dad to talk to the baby when the baby is very active and to see what happens. Or, encourage the mom to see how the baby responds when the baby is very active and she puts her arms around the baby while she lays down on her back and rocks side to side.

These are examples of the baby changing states—from active to quiet. The parents will see their baby do this over and over after the baby is born. Let them know that babies in utero begin to get used to sudden sounds that they have heard repeatedly, and they don't respond every time. Ask the mom if she has noticed times when the baby startled to a sudden, loud sound, such as dogs barking, fire engine sirens, or drums, and then was able to tune the sounds out. This is an ability that the baby will develop more and more after he is born so that he will be able to handle unexpected sounds of dogs barking or telephones ringing. Also explain that babies are different—some do this easily, and some find it harder to protect themselves from loud sounds. Tell them that, together, you will look at this when their baby is born.

Parent and Baby Time Activities—Previewing the Newborn

Activity: My Time and Your Time

Materials: Crayons and drawing paper

Ask the parent to select three different colored crayons—one to represent how she feels when she is sound asleep, one for when she is in a light sleep (either falling into or waking up from sleep), and one for when she is wide awake.

Give the parent a piece of paper and turn it horizontally. Ask her to draw a colored circle across the top of the paper, using her crayons, to represent sound sleep, light sleep, and wide awakeness. Then ask her to describe how she likes others to interact with her when she is in each of these three different states. Write her descriptions next to the corresponding colored circle.

A few inches below the color key, draw a line that almost reaches each side of the paper. Just under the line at the far left write "midnight," in the center write "noon," and at the far right write "midnight" again. Then write the number for each hour of a day beginning with 1 a.m. and moving across the page to 12 p.m.

Now ask the parent what time of day she usually wakes up. Ask her to draw a colored circle for waking up along the timeline at the right spot. Next, ask her to draw a wide-awake circle to show the different times of the day that she feels wide awake. Ask her if she usually naps during the day and have her draw circles to represent the general times she might be in a light sleep, either falling into or waking up from naps. Finally, ask her to mark the timeline with the corresponding circles for falling asleep at night and being in a sound sleep for the night. Review the timeline she has drawn and discuss the ebb and flow of her own way of being and what she appreciates from others during the course of all these changes.

Draw another timeline in the middle of the paper; write "midnight" and "noon" in the same places and fill in the hours. Explain that this timeline represents her baby's day during the first weeks of life. Discuss what she has heard or read about how long newborns sleep and stay awake during the course of a typical day. Depending on her knowledge, you can add what you know.

All babies are different and their awake–sleep cycles vary. Newborns can sleep between 12 and 20 hours a day during their first weeks, often taking between 7 and 12 naps every 24 hours.

Ask the parent to draw the colored circles for all of the times she thinks her newborn will be falling into or coming out of sleep, be in a sound sleep, and be wide awake. Talk about how her baby probably will want her to be with him at the various times. Compare the two timelines and explore what the parent thinks about while imagining what life with her new baby will be like for both of them.

Activity: A Baby's Way of Being

Materials: Pictures of newborns; caption clouds

Talk with the parents about what their baby's state can tell them:

"We have been talking about the idea that your baby already—before he is born—has different ways of being. He can be awake and quiet, awake and really active, or asleep. This is important because your baby needs different things from you when he is in different states. Your baby's state gives you a clue about what to do!

"Your baby will be her own unique person. You will be the detective, reading her cues and figuring out as you go what your baby needs. Your baby will always tell you through her behavior if she is on track or if she needs to try a different path."

Collect pictures of newborns and infants in different states. Wonder aloud with the parents about what each pictured baby's state might be saying. For example, an alert and active baby might be saying, "Let's play! I want more!" An exhausted baby might be saying, "This is too much. I need to rest."

You also can prepare blank cartoon caption "clouds" above each pictured baby. Together with the parents, write captions for each picture—what the baby is telling you by her behavior and state. Remind the parents that, together, you will look at and talk about their baby's states after she is born.

Activity: Singing the Blues

Materials: Videotape of a baby going from fussy to upset to calm (you can make one with the help of a new mother and her baby); doll; blanket

Introduce the parents to the idea that for many parents soothing a crying baby is the hardest part of parenting—especially when the baby seems inconsolable. Play the videotape of the baby crying. Explore with the parents what it feels like to hear the baby cry. Share your feelings as well. Talk about the reasons babies might cry and how parents might respond to their baby's cries, and talk about what soothed the baby. Anticipate with them that there will be times when they do not know what to do, and their baby will continue to cry. You can label this "Singing the Blues."

Problems arise when both the baby and the parents are feeling the same way—upset! Explore options that parents have at that point. Identify ahead of time two or three safe people who can help. Consider making a "Singing the Blues" collage with the parents. Include things that they think might help them calm the baby and the people who can help them. Offer to frame or laminate this collage.

If there is a doll available, guide the parents in swaddling the doll, all the while describing how comforting it feels for many babies to be wrapped and held snugly. Let the parents know that you will talk more about soothing upset babies—and adults—as you visit with them during the months ahead and explore with them what will help calm their baby.

Activity: Family Stories

Invite the mother to tell her baby about the following:

- The happiest times they have had together so far
- How she has tried to reduce stress for her baby
- People the baby will meet who will be there to help the mom and love the baby (Jernberg, Thomas, & Wickersham, 1985)

If the mom wants to, she or you can write this down in the family book.

Prenatal Home Visit 4
Touch
(32–33 Weeks Gestation)

Remember:

About Your Work

- Preparation
- Parent Time
- Parent and Baby Time
- Family Time
- Reflection and Writing to the Baby

About the Baby

- Touch is the first sense to develop in the first trimester.
- The mouth and face are sensitive to touch first.
- By 14 weeks, the whole body is sensitive to touch.
- About this time, ultrasound shows the baby self-initiating touch by sucking his fingers and bringing his hands close to his face.

Parent and Baby Time Activities—Exploring the Baby's Present Behavior

Activity: Gentle Touch

Materials: String or dental floss

Explain to the mother that touch is the first sense that her baby develops—before the baby is born and way before the baby can hear or see, he can feel touch. Invite her to see with you just how sensitive her baby's sense of touch is. Show her a fine string or piece of dental floss. Ask her if she would be willing to look the other way while you touch her with the thread and then try to identify when and where you are touching her. Say: "Clearly, the baby cannot feel this from the outside. But your baby's sense of touch is so developed that if his hand lightly touched his face in utero—even as lightly as the string touched you—he can feel it.

Activity: Little Explorers

Materials: 30-week fetal model; picture of a baby in utero at 31–32 weeks

Reflect with the parents on their baby's sense of touch, which is developing in a particular order—a very sensible order, in fact. The first area to become sensitive to touch is the baby's face and mouth. Wonder together about why that might be. Note that our mouths are still very sensitive: "Think about what a small cut on your gum feels like compared to the same small cut on your back."

The next areas to become sensitive are the nose, chin, and eyelids: "By now your baby can feel touch all over—on her legs, feet, hands. She can even find her fingers and suck on them. Some babies are born with blisters on their fingers from so much prenatal sucking!"

Talk with the parents about how important our faces are. Facial expression is one of the major ways that we communicate with others.

Look with the parents at a picture of a baby in utero at 31–32 weeks. Talk about what their baby might be able to touch at that point in her development: "Let's think about all the things your baby can touch right now. She can touch her umbilical cord, feet, hands, and face, and she can suck her thumb." Offer parents an opportunity to hold a 30-week doll as they think about how their baby is developing and how much she can do.

Activity: Brain Care

Explain to the parents how touch builds connections in the baby's brain: "When your baby holds on to his cord, his hands feel a sensation. This sensation is sent to his brain. His brain then has the experience of receiving touch signals. The brain then sends back messages to the hand. The message tells the hand what to do—move this way, hold on that way. The brain also remembers these signals. The next time the baby finds his cord, he is more able to grab on to it. In this way, pathways are built into the brain. Your baby is doing that right now when he feels his body or senses his mother's body move. He is learning all the time!"

Activity: Baby Massage

Ask the mother if she has ever tried massaging her baby. Invite her to take some time now and begin to massage her baby: "Let's take a few moments now for you to hold your baby." Help the mom get comfortable, and encourage her to put her arms around her baby and just hold him for a few minutes. Then encourage her to massage the baby in a way that is comfortable for her and for the baby. Explain that after her baby is born, if she likes, you will help her learn about infant massage.

Activity: When You Were Brand New

While the mother massages her baby, encourage her to tell her a story beginning with the phrase, "When you were brand new..." (Jernberg et al., 1985). She might begin with when her baby was first conceived, or at a later point in the baby's development. Listen attentively, but allow this to be a quiet time between mother and child. Appreciate how much the mother and baby already know about one another and how their relationship is growing.

Parent and Baby Time Activities—Previewing the Newborn

Activity: Snuggling Up

Materials: Baby carrying devices, such as a Snugli and a sling; infant doll

This activity requires that you know or learn about culturally accepted practices for carrying and holding babies in the communities you are serving. Explore with the parents the idea that many babies like to be held close in their parents' arms or in a Snugli or sling, and that some babies are calmed by being carried in this way. Discuss with them that some people think that we do not hold babies enough anymore. They think that the use of baby seats, swings, and walkers can distance parents from their babies. Carrying devices can be very helpful at times, but being close physically may be what their baby needs most to feel safe and secure.

Have several carrying devices available for parents to look at—a Snugli, a sling, or something similar—and offer them an opportunity to try them on. If they seem comfortable, place an infant doll in the one of them so that the parents can try it out.

Play with the idea of holding the baby close. Tell the parents about a study (Aniseld, Casper, Nozyce, & Cunningham, 1990) that showed that young mothers who were given a Snugli developed closer, more secure relationships with their babies than similar mothers who did not have a Snugli. Explore with the parents why this might be: "What could carrying your baby with you more offer the baby and you?"

Prenatal Home Visit 5

Smell and Taste

(34–35 Weeks Gestation

Remember:

About Your Work

- Preparation
- Parent Time
- Parent and Baby Time
- Family Time
- Reflection and Writing to the Baby

About the Baby

- The sucking reflex begins in the first trimester, and babies have a lot of practice sucking and swallowing before they are born.
- At 13 weeks, the baby can be seen sucking her thumb on ultrasound.
- By 16 to 20 weeks, taste buds start to develop.
- Toward the end of the second trimester, the baby swallows up to an ounce of fluid an hour—the equivalent of an 8-ounce baby bottle in an 8-hour day.
- By the third trimester, the baby swallows more than a quart of fluid a day.
- The mother's diet changes the smell of the fluid, which gives the baby varied experience with smell.
- By 32 weeks, swallowing improves, partly because muscle tone for swallowing is improving. Typically, all the oral reflexes are mature and ready to go by 37 weeks.

A Note About This Visit

This promises to be a very exciting visit because the growing baby, if born now, would be able to do nearly everything that a baby born at full-term can do. The mother and baby have done it! Share this exciting fact with her. The rest of baby's growing time—to 40 weeks—allows him to master sucking and swallowing, strengthen his muscles and lungs, and just hang out. If born now, the baby very likely would be ready to suck, swallow, and breathe, all at the same time.

This shows that the baby has a wonderful ability to coordinate these very complex activities. How do babies do it? They are just little miracle workers! It this fascination and wonder at prenatal development that you can pass on to teen parents.

Parent and Baby Time Activities—Exploring the Baby's Present Behavior

Activity: Sweet Connections

Materials: Juice box; pictures of babies; sample pacifiers

Share with the parents that their baby can already taste and smell. She can taste sweet, sour, bitter, and salty tastes. The taste of the amniotic fluid varies depending on how much of the fluid is urine, how much is water, and other liquids, and the smell varies depending on what the mother has eaten—another way that the baby's and mom's experiences are linked!

Offer the mother a juice box. Then imagine with the parents what the baby is tasting inside while the mom drinks the sweet juice. A high intake of sugar often increases a baby's activity. So, ask if the mother if she has noticed her baby's reaction when she eats a candy bar or other intensely sweet food. You can talk with parents about their ideas of what babies like to eat, about what to feed their baby, and about their ideas concerning feeding their baby water, water with sugar, formula, breast milk, and cereal. Take a look at the activity, "Infant Feeding," later in this chapter to get some ideas to guide this discussion on infant feeding.

Activity: Fetal Feast

Materials: Four cups for each participant; sugar; lemon juice; Worcestershire sauce; and salt

Since the 7th month, the baby has been developing his taste buds at a remarkable rate. By the time he is born, he has about 7,000 taste buds. His sense of taste may be more developed at birth than at any other time in his life. By the time he reaches his 70th birthday the number of his taste buds will have decreased to about 4,000.

Enjoy with the parents imagining what their baby is tasting in utero. Mix up some drinks that approximate the four major tastes that the baby can already discern. Pour four cups of water for each person tasting. With the parents, add sugar (sweetness) to one set of cups, lemon juice (sour) to another set, Worcestershire sauce (bitter) to the third set, and salt (salty) to the fourth set. Each of you can taste the different flavors and wonder together what it might be like for the baby in utero.

Use this shared experience to create opportunities for parental wonderment and exploration, as well as a springboard for discussion about topics such as what the parents believe their baby likes or doesn't like in the mother's diet, their ideas about what babies like to eat, and their questions about what to feed their baby. This, too, can be a time to talk about the parents' ideas concerning feeding the baby water, water with sugar, formula, breast milk, cereal, and other foods (see the activity "Infant Feeding" later in this Home Visit for more information).

Finally, as the parents become more aware of the baby's fine sense of smell and taste, you can begin to share information concerning the newborn's ability to know his parents by their smell and even to be able to tell his mother's breast milk from other women's by the smell and taste.

Activity: Soothing

Talk with the teen about what is happening now: "Your baby has been practicing sucking and swallowing since about 3 months in utero. By now, she drinks more than a quart of amniotic fluid a day! She is drinking in nutrients from the amniotic fluid, nutrients that are helping her grow."

Continue: "Some babies are born with blisters on their thumbs from sucking so much. It's a sign of growth for a baby to get her hand in her mouth. After birth, it means that the baby's hands and arms are getting steadier and that she may be able to help herself calm down by finding her fingers and hand to suck."

Talk with the mother about what she observed her baby doing with her hands on the ultrasound. Was the baby putting her hands up by her mouth? Ask the mom about how she feels about babies sucking on their hands or fingers. Explore whether she remembers sucking her own thumb or fingers and how others responded to her doing that.

Explore also what her thoughts are about pacifiers. You can bring a picture of a baby using a pacifier and several different kinds of pacifiers. How does the mom respond to the picture? What does her own mother think about pacifiers? What ways does the teen think that she will use to calm her baby?

Parent and Baby Time Activities—Previewing the Newborn

Activity: That's You, Mom!

Just as you do in the activity "Fetal Feast," share information with the parents about the newborn's ability to know his parents by their smell—even her ability to discern the smell and taste of his mother's milk from that of other women. Describe how—if given the opportunity—a newborn, even before the umbilical cord is cut, may be able to instinctively crawl from his mother's abdomen to her breast and latch on with little or no help.

Encourage the mother to consider the following ideas for after her baby is born:

- Put a small soft toy under her shirt for a while to pick up her scent, then put this toy in the baby's crib or near where the baby sleeps;
- Sleep with the baby's blanket near her skin and use this blanket when she is trying to soothe the baby's crying or when they are separated.

Activity: Infant Feeding

Talk with the mom about her plans for feeding the baby. Has she decided yet whether she will breast-feed or bottle-feed the baby? With whom has she talked this over—her mother, the baby's father, her sisters, her friends? What are their views? What are her own views? If the teen is planning on breast-feeding, talk with her about what she has heard about breast-feeding. What kind of support, if any, does she feel she might need?

New parenthood always comes with a lot of advice from family members, friends, doctors, and even from people on the street. Everyone loves to talk about what the new baby needs to eat. This is a perfect time to explore with the teen mom what she knows, thinks, and feels about what her baby should eat and when and to help her feel comfortable with making her own informed decisions. Share information, but also share yourself as a sounding board while the young mother decides what is best for her baby and herself.

Invite the teen to tell her yet-to-be born baby about how she herself was fed as a baby and about how she plans to feed her. Can she remember what her favorite foods were as a small child? Talk with the mom about how feeding her baby can be a special time for both of them—a time when she can really tune into her baby. No doubt, her baby will also use this time to focus on her. In the beginning, the baby will pay most attention to just feeding, but then as time goes by, she'll pause more to take her mom in. Explore with the mom how she thinks she'll feel about holding her baby while she is being fed.

Activity: Sipping Sisters

Materials: Individually wrapped straws and a glass for each participant

Engaging the parents in a simple activity such as sucking water through a straw is a good demonstration of what you'd like them to know about sucking, swallowing, and breathing. Ask the parents if they're interested in exploring something that their baby will do a lot. Have a straw and glass of water for everyone and ask the parents to drink. Then ask them to think about what they just did and what it might tell them about their baby: "How did you know when you needed to take a break? What could you look for to know when your baby needs to take a break?"

Whether a mother chooses to breast-feed or bottle-feed, this is a good time to talk about the rhythms in a newborn's eating patterns. There are two kinds of rhythms. First, there is the rhythm, unique to the baby, of how long he will suck before taking a breath. Every baby is different. Some babies are so hungry that they have to be reminded to take a breath or they will wind up spitting up or throwing up after their feedings. The second kind of rhythm relates to how often her baby will eat. The baby will teach his mother about both these rhythms very soon after birth.

Prenatal Home Visit 6
Vision
(36–37 Weeks Gestation)

Remember:

About Your Work

- Preparation
- Parent Time
- Parent and Baby Time
- Family Time
- Reflection and Writing to the Baby

About the Baby

- Eye movements can be seen during the 3rd month in utero.
- The baby's eyelids are fused and do not open until the third trimester.
- In the second trimester, eye movements continue, but response to light does not come until the third trimester.
- At 24 to 25 weeks, eye activity in utero increases in response to light.
- By 32 weeks, the baby turns his head to light in utero.
- As the mother's skin stretches over her belly and becomes thinner, letting more light into the uterus, the baby perhaps gets a bit of experience seeing.
- Infants do not see like adults do until they are 4 to 6 months of age.

Parent and Baby Time Activities—Exploring the Baby's Present Behavior

Activity: You Oughta Be in Pictures

Materials: Video camera and videotape

Offer to make a home video of the mother and her unborn baby. If your program has the resources, this can be the first of many videos taken of the parents and their baby together. The tone and comfort level set during the first video will either help or hinder future home videos.

Talk with the parents and plan for what they would like in the video. Depending on their comfort level, there are a variety of opportunities. The mother may want to narrate for the camera what her pregnancy has been like, and what her plans and dreams are for her baby. She may appreciate the opportunity to describe her physical and emotional feelings during the pregnancy. She may want to speak directly to her unborn baby, or to read or sing to her.

Some mothers find it helpful to put their hand on their belly and feel the fullness and activity of their baby while they talk. Some mothers feel good gently massaging their belly as they speak for the camera. The physical connection at times helps to get the mother talking.

After completing this prenatal video, build anticipation toward making a video soon after the baby is born.

Activity: Baby's First Portrait

Ask the mother if she has had daydreams—or dreams while asleep—about how the baby looks. Invite her to describe the baby's features and explore her ideas and feelings. She may enjoy drawing pictures, or simply describing how she imagines the baby will look.

Activity: Baby—What Do You See?

Materials: Flashlight

Discuss with the mother her understanding of how her baby sees already. If the baby is awake, ask the mom where she feels her baby's head and hands, and place a strong light to the side of that position. The mother may feel the baby move toward the light. She and the baby may enjoy playing flashlight tag. She can also try this with a dimmer light, perhaps with paper between the light and the belly, to see if the baby responds differently.

Activity: Seeing You

Materials: Waxed paper; baby doll

Ask the parents what they think babies can see after birth. To help them get an idea of what it will be like for their baby, have the parents either squint their eyes almost shut and look around, or look through a sheet of waxed paper. Explore with them how it is easier to see clearly under these conditions when objects are close. Prepare them by telling them that their newborn baby will see them and objects best when they are about 8–12 inches from his face.

Give the parents a baby doll to hold so that they can begin to imagine what it will be like when they and their baby look at one another. Explain that babies love to look at faces, and explore with them the baby's timeline for being able to see her parents. Remind the parents that after their baby is born, you will look together at all of this.

Activity: Getting to Know You

Discuss with the parents the importance of being good observers of their baby's behavior, mood, likes, and dislikes. Be sure to support the observational abilities that they have already demonstrated over the past weeks of Community-Based FANA home visits. Help the parents develop an appreciation of how they and their baby can become effective communicators. Describe this as being their way of knowing how best to care for their child once the baby arrives.

Activity: Reading Babies Like a Book

Materials: Video of a newborn

Watch a video of a newborn with the parents. Discuss what they see the baby doing. Encourage them to observe and report what they see, to express empathy, and to make some interpretations of the baby's nonverbal expression. Ask the following questions:

- Exactly what do you see this newborn doing?
- From watching her face and the rest of her body, how do you think she feels?
- What might she be telling us with her face and body? If you could speak for her now, what would she be saying?

Parent and Baby Time Activities—Previewing the Newborn

Activity: Brain Power!

Explain to the mother that right after the baby is born, he will enjoy watching her face, especially her eyes and smiles. Remind the mother that looking at, touching, and talking with her baby not only is fun and feels good but also helps the baby learn.

Activity: First Sight

Materials: Video or pictures of a newborn

Ask the parents what they hope to see first about their baby. Watch a video or look at photographs showing some of the different ways babies look immediately after birth. Talk about the various appearances.

Activity: Your Baby's Expressions Are Like a Thousand Words

Discuss with the mother cues and signals that she thinks she will be able to observe after her baby is born that will tell her how her baby feels or what he needs and wants. Guiding questions might include the following:

- What have you learned already—either from our talking or from other babies—about how babies express themselves nonverbally?
- What signals or cues might you see from your baby that will have specific meaning?

Activity: Dreams for the Future

Materials: Stationery

Encourage the mother to discuss her dreams and visions for the future—her own and her baby's. Invite her to write a love letter to her baby in which she talks about the future and how she sees it from this vantage point. She can decide if she wants to keep the letter to read again to herself in the future, or if she would like to read it to her baby at some later time. Fathers can be invited to do this same activity.

References

Aniseld, E., Casper, V., Nozyce, M., & Cunningham, N. (1990). Does infant carrying promote attachment? An experimental study of the effects of increased physical contact on the development of attachment. *Child Development, 61*(5), 1617–1627.

Jernberg, A., Thomas, E., & Wickersham, M. (1985). *Mothers' behaviors and attitudes toward their unborn infants.* Wilmette, IL: Theraplay Institute.

Postnatal Home Visit Activity Guide

Remember:

- Preparation
- Parent Time
- Parent and Baby Time
- Family Time
- Reflection and Writing to the Baby

Parent and Baby Time Activities

- If the baby is fussing or crying, facilitate soothing.
- If the baby is in a quiet alert state, facilitate the visual and auditory orientation activities.
- If the baby is coming out of sleep, has been soothed, or is in an alert state, facilitate the visual and auditory orientation activities.
- If the baby is asleep or coming to alert, facilitate the feel of the baby's muscles and the reflexes.
- If the baby is sound asleep, facilitate the habituation items.

Activity: Soothing the Baby

If the baby comes up into a robust crying state during the home visit, this provides an opportunity for the parents and baby to experience reciprocal interaction. Your first instinct may be to pick up the baby yourself and soothe her in traditional ways that almost always work, such as swaddling, rocking, and engaging the baby in sucking. Remaining calm, observant, and intrigued by the baby's crying, however, enables you to help the parents discover for themselves graduated strategies for soothing their baby, starting with watching to see if the baby is able to do it herself, and moving on to talking, holding the baby's hands across her chest, picking her up, swaddling her, and, finally, pacifying her.

Ask the parents if it is okay to take some time to see what works best. Then, ask them to begin by softly calling the baby's name and gently talking to her. Ask the parents if that seemed to help. If not, try gently holding the baby's hands close to her chest. If the baby quiets, ask the parents about that. If not, invite them to try picking her up. If the baby is soothed, ask the parents if that seemed to help. If not, ask them if it's okay to try swaddling her snugly in her blanket. If the baby continues to cry after she is swaddled, move on and ask the parents if they have ever put a finger in their baby's mouth to let her suck it. Invite them to do that now. If the baby does not quiet, suggest that she be fed: "You know, I think your baby may be just too hungry to go on playing with us. How about some eating time?" If the baby is very hungry, it may be necessary to stop the Community-Based FANA activities at this point and try again at the next visit.

Explain: "When your baby is crying she's either blowing off steam, or she's hungry, or she's wet. In a few weeks, you'll get to know her signals pretty well. Whatever the reason for her crying, she will always love being picked up and held by you when she cries."

If the parents respond that they are afraid of spoiling their baby, explain: "From everything we know, you just can't spoil a baby by holding her and hugging her a lot when she cries. Doing that as soon as she starts to cry lets her know that her cries are important and that she is important!"

"What do you like best from the people around you when you cry or are sad?"

Activity: Staying Asleep—Habituation

Materials: Rattle; flashlight

This activity can be complex for you as the home visitor. Not only do you want to see how the baby responds to having a light shown across his sleeping eyes, but you're also watching the parents' responses to their baby's response!

Ask the parent: "While your baby is asleep, let's see how he'll respond if you shake a rattle near his ear or shine a light in his eyes. Remember, nothing we do today will hurt your baby in any way!"

Turn on the flashlight and model how the parents can observe their baby's response to light in his eyes while he's asleep. Cup one hand loosely into a fist: "Now, if my hand is your baby's eyes, we're going to pass this light across them like this and see how he responds."

Hand the parents the flashlight and ask one of them to pass the light across the baby's closed eyes: "What did you see him do? Yes, he tightened his lids, didn't he?" or "He started to wake up, didn't he?"

Ask the parents: "Let's wait a few seconds while he gets relaxed again (or falls back asleep) and try it again. What did you see him do that time? Yes, he responded less, didn't he?"

Repeat the process again. If the baby stops responding after the third presentation of the light, stop the procedure and say: "Did you see what he did? Yes, he just stopped bothering with that light. He said, 'Mom, go ahead and be pesty if you want, but I'm not going to wake up if I don't have to!'" Repeat the process until the infant stops responding, but not more than 8 or 10 times.

Explain: "This is your baby's way of protecting himself. He's helping you take care of him." If the baby is unable to shut out the light, talk about this as another way that the baby communicates with his parents by saying, "Hey, Mom and Dad! I'm little, and I need your help in staying asleep. Please shut off the lights when I'm trying to sleep."

Draw the parents' own experiences into this event as another strategy for linking the reality of the baby with the parents' realities. You can ask: "What do you do when someone tries to wake you from a deep sleep? Is it pretty easy for you to fall back to sleep?"

Remember that most teens have an enormous need for sleep. What might it mean to a teen mother to be painfully sleep deprived and yet have to protect her infant's sleep state? This may be a good time to say: "How does it feel to you to be so tired and to see your baby sleeping so peacefully?"

Now try the baby's response to sound: "Let's see now how he responds to sound while he's asleep. While I'm holding your baby, you can hold this rattle about this far (about 12 inches) from your baby's ear and then give it one good shake. What did you see? Yes, he startled didn't he? What did you see him do? Yes, his arms just flew out," or "He started to wake up."

Ask the parents: "Let's wait a little bit (about 5 seconds) for him to get relaxed again."

Repeat as above two more times or—if the baby continues to respond—up to eight more times. If he remains asleep, this will be a good time to talk about the baby's ability to shut out noise and discuss what the teen mom's household is like: "Is it pretty noisy in your house? Does this bother you? Well, your baby has just said, 'I'm pretty cool about noise right now. It doesn't have to be completely quiet for me to stay asleep.'"

If, however, the baby never got used to the sound, use this to explain the baby's needs: "Your baby is saying, 'Hey, Mom! I'm so little. Will you do me a favor and have everybody just keep it down for a while when I'm trying to sleep?'" This is also a good time to relate back to the mother's need for or lack of need for quiet.

Activity: Feeling the Baby's Foot and Hand Reflexes and Muscles

With the baby asleep or coming to alert, ask the parents to turn the baby on her back, if she isn't already there. Then ask them to uncover the baby's legs and take off her booties.

"Let's see what your baby wants to show us about her feet and hands."

Hold up the index finger of your preferred hand and say to the parents: "Let me have this finger for a second. Together, we'll look at your baby's foot movements—things she does automatically in response to your touching her in a particular way. We'll take your finger and run it on the outside of her foot. What did you see? Yes, her toes flared out, didn't they? Now, press right here (right under the baby's toes) and what do you see? She curled her toes around your finger, didn't she?"

Ask the parents: "Have you put your finger in your baby's hand? Will you show me what she does when you do that?" or "When you press your finger in the palm of her hand, what did she do? How does that feel to you?"

Very likely the baby will have curved her fingers around the mother's finger and grasped it with her hand. Some parents say that this feels like their baby is hugging them back! This can be a delightful idea to build on with young parents: "This may be the beginning of her hugging you back," or "Your baby is showing that she's responsive to you, right from the start." Help the parents relate this back to what they learned about prenatal development.

If the baby does not show these responses, it is not necessarily a matter for concern. Say: "Well, she's just not in the mood to show us this today. We'll try it again the next time I visit."

After demonstrating the baby's foot and hand reflexes, move to his muscles: "I'd like you to take your baby's legs and slowly bend them and press them gently toward her tummy, then gently pull them out."

Wait for the parents to do this, guiding them along the way if necessary. Ask: "What did you feel? Yes, she was pulling back, wasn't she? You could feel her resisting as you pulled out. She was saying, "Hey, Mom! I may be little but I'm packed."

Or, if the baby felt as though her muscles were loose or floppy, explain: "Yes, it felt as though her muscles were loose. As she grows and you play with her and just regularly change her diaper and let her kick her legs, she will begin to feel stronger. All babies are different."

Next, ask: "Now, let's take her arms and gently pull them across her chest; now, down at her sides. What did you feel? Often, babies' arms move much more freely than their legs. This is part of normal development."

Activity: The Rooting Reflex

Ask the teen to put an index finger to the corner of the baby's mouth and gently stroke until the baby turns in the direction of the stimulation. Ask: "Let's see what happens when you stroke the side of your baby's mouth." Guide the mother's finger. Then, ask: "What did you see happen? I saw that, too. He turned toward your finger. Have you ever seen him do that when you just begin to feed him? What did you think it meant?"

Some mothers will say they thought it meant "No! No! No!"—that the baby just didn't want to eat. This is a good time to give parents information on the rooting reflex as a way for the baby to get his mouth in the best position to ensure that something will get in it! It's his very clever way of being sure he gets fed when there is a chance that he's going to be fed. He is really saying, "Yes! Yes! Yes!"

Activity: Turning to the Parent's Face and Voice—Visual and Auditory Orientation

Materials: Receiving blanket

Most parents describe this activity as the highlight of the Community-Based FANA experience. It shows off their infants as profoundly human and ready for engagement!

Many parents can hardly believe that their baby has a preference for their face, voice, smell, and touch. You can maximize having the baby turn to the parent's face and voice by first snugly swaddling the baby, arms and legs. Remember to ask the parents for permission before picking up their baby and also before swaddling her.

Voice. With the baby well swaddled and in a quiet alert state, hold her with one hand flat behind her head and the other comfortably and firmly supporting her back. Wait until you feel the baby relax in your arms.

Ask: "Let's see what happens when you call your baby's name. Go ahead, keep on calling her."

Speak for the baby: "Oh! Mom! I really like hearing your voice."

Ask: "What did you see her do? Yes, she turned to your voice, didn't she?"

While still holding the baby, ask: "Let's see what she does when you call her name and slowly move your head to the side. Yes, she followed your face, didn't she?" or "No, she wasn't in the mood to do this right now."

This is a good time to discuss the baby's preferences for the parental voice, smell, and touch over anybody else's in the world.

Face. Put the swaddled baby in the parent's hands, facing directly into her line of vision. Invite her to lock her eyes into the baby's eyes, then slowly turn her face and call his name. If the baby does not follow her face, say: "Hey Mom, I'm just getting too much of a good thing. Can we try this later?" If the baby does follow his mother's face ask: "What did you see your baby do just now?"

Activity: Following a Ball—Visual Orientation

Materials: Red ball

When the baby is in a quiet alert state, swaddle her and hold her comfortably. Remember to ask the parents' permission before picking up their baby and before swaddling her.

Hand the mother or father a red ball. Standing close to the parent, hold the baby so that the parents are not in her field of vision. Say: "Mom, show your baby the ball." When you're sure the baby is looking at the ball, move the ball slowly to the side: "Let's see what she wants to do about this."

If the baby does not follow the ball say: "Hey, Mom and Dad, I'm not in the mood to do this just now." If the baby does follow the ball, ask: "What did you see her do just now?"

Activity: Following a Rattle—Auditory Orientation

Materials: Red rattle

Ask: "Do you remember when your baby was asleep and we shook a rattle? Yes, he just stayed asleep, didn't he? Now, let's try it when he's awake. Will you take that little rattle and keep shaking it gently right about here (about 18 inches from the baby's ear)? Let's try the other side, too. What did you see him do? Yes, he turned to it, didn't he? May I try shaking the rattle while I also let him see it?"

Hold the rattle about 6 inches from the baby's face, and be sure he locks his eyes on it. Then, gently shake and move the rattle slowly to the side, slightly up, then around, and then continue to the other side. An alert baby likely will follow it.

Ask: "What did you see him do?"

About the Authors

Ida Cardone, PhD, is a clinical psychologist who has been enthusiastically involved in the area of infant mental health nearly all of her professional life. She is the former director of the Perinatal Family Support Center at Evanston Northwestern Healthcare and in that capacity she founded Connections for Pregnant and Parenting Teens. She also is the founding director of the Perinatal Depression Program of Evanston Northwestern Healthcare and is a ZERO TO THREE senior fellow. Ida is currently in private practice in Winnetka, Illinois.

Linda Gilkerson, PhD, is a professor at Erikson Institute, Chicago, a graduate school in child development, and is director of Erikson's Irving B. Harris Infant Studies Program. She has developed and expanded programs to support parents and infants including Project Welcome, a collaboration of Wheelock College and Boston Children's Hospital, the Infant Care Program at Evanston Hospital, and the Fussy Baby Network at Erikson Institute. She is a board member of ZERO TO THREE.

Nick Wechsler, MA, is an infant specialist who is the assistant director for program development at the Ounce of Prevention Fund in Chicago. Since 1990 his work for the Fund has been devoted to building programs for teenage parents and their very young children. He has also focused on the nature of relationships and supporting efforts to promote secure attachments through previous work as a mental health specialist, family day care provider, director of daycare programs, program developer, and trainer. *Teenagers and Their Babies* enables him to focus on the very start of all relationships, the perinatal period.